W9-CDM-792

DISCARD

ENCYCLOPEDIA OF
FAMILY HEALTH

THIRD EDITION

ENCYCLOPEDIA OF
FAMILY HEALTH

—— THIRD EDITION ——

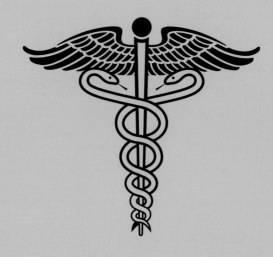

CONSULTANTS

David B. Jacoby, M.D.
Johns Hopkins School of Medicine

Robert M. Youngson, M.D.
Royal Society of Medicine

VOLUME 18

INDEXES

MARSHALL CAVENDISH
New York · London · Singapore

MEDICAL CONSULTANTS

Second Edition
David B. Jacoby, M.D.
Johns Hopkins School of Medicine
Associate Professor of Pulmonary and Critical
    Care Medicine

Third Edition
Robert M. Youngson, M.D.
Fellow of the Royal Society of Medicine
Officer of the Order of St John of Jerusalem
Diploma in Tropical Medicine and Hygiene
Fellow of the Royal College of Ophthalmologists

CONTRIBUTORS TO THIRD EDITION

David Arnot   Tom Jackson
Deborah Evans   Nathan Lepora
Leon Gray   Fiona Plowman
Joanna Griffin   Alison Tarrant
Tim Harris   Aruna Vasudevan
John Jackson

Picture Credits
(b – bottom; t – top; r – right; l – left; c – center)

Cover: Dynamic Graphics: John Foxx & Images 4 Communication b/l, b/r;
PhotoDisc: Don Farrall b/c, Keith Brofsky t/r; Photos.com: c.

Corbis: Warren Morgan 2457; DK Images: 2459, 2465, 2475; Rex Features:
Alix/Phanie 2461; Zefa: 2463b.

Marshall Cavendish
99 White Plains Road
Tarrytown, NY 10591-9001

www.marshallcavendish.com

© 2005, 1998, 1991 Marshall Cavendish Corporation

All rights reserved. No part of this book may be reproduced or utilized in
any form or by any means, electronic or mechanical, including photo-
copying, recording, or by any information storage and retrieval system,
without prior written permission from the publisher and copyright holder.

Library of Congress Cataloging-in-Publication Data

Encyclopedia of family health / David B. Jacoby, Robert M. Youngson.--
3rd ed.
     p. cm.
Includes bibliographical references and index.
  ISBN 0-7614-7486-2 (set)
  ISBN 0-7614-7504-4 (vol 18)
1. Medicine, Popular--Encyclopedias. 2. Health--Encylopedias. 1. Jacoby, David
B. II. Youngson, R. M. III. Marshall Cavendish Corporation. IV. Title
RC81.A2E5 2004
610'.3--dc22   2003065554

Printed in China
08 07 06 05 04 5 4 3 2 1

Marshall Cavendish

Editor: Joyce Tavolacci
Editorial Director: Paul Bernabeo
Production Manager: Alan Tsai

The Brown Reference Group

Project Editor: Anne Hildyard
Editors: Jane Lanigan, Sally McFall
Designers: Jeni Child, Reg Cox, Karen Frazer
Picture Researcher: Clare Newman
Indexer: Kay Ollerenshaw
Illustrations: Samantha J. Elmhurst
Managing Editor: Tim Cooke
Art Director: Dave Goodman

CONTENTS

First Aid Handbook   2453
    Artificial respiration   2454
    Bites and stings   2456
    Bleeding   2458
    Burns   2460
    Car accidents   2462
    Choking   2464
    Convulsions   2466
    CPR (cardiopulmonary resuscitation)   2467
    Electric shock   2468
    Falls   2469
    Fractures   2470
    Heart attack   2472
    Hypothermia   2473
    Poisoning   2474
    Shock   2475
    Sprains and strains   2476
    Unconsciousness   2477
    Wounds   2479

Medical Glossary   2481
Further Reading and Research   2497
Health Organizations   2503

Thematic Indexes
    Human body   2508
    Diseases and other disorders   2521
    Treatments and cures   2534
    Prevention and diagnosis of disease   2539
    Human behavior   2541
    People index   2544

Comprehensive Index   2545

INTRODUCTION

The decision to create this updated and expanded edition of the popular *Encyclopedia of Family Health* reflects the broad scope of new advances in the health care field. This third edition has been extensively rewritten, and many new topics have been added. The new edition is intended to provide students and the general public with up-to-date and accurate information that is also concise and useful, and like previous editions offers an overview of numerous medical topics in such a manner as to allow immediate comprehension of medical conditions and health issues. The encyclopedia's easy and attractive style will help readers understand medical terms and diseases and thereby assist in preventing problems and encouraging well-being. The substantial level of medical knowledge contained here is not readily available in any other single source for general readers and will allow users to dispel misunderstanding and apprehension that often lead to fear concerning health care.

Finding quality information about health care can be challenging in the increasingly complex world of modern medicine, which includes a growing number of alternative therapies. Written for the consumer and organized alphabetically, this work provides a quick way to research health-related subjects. It is easy for the young reader to find reliable information here about a variety of medical conditions from a trusted source. There are extensive, carefully chosen illustrations and tables that make the topics easy to understand and navigate and also give importance to the most relevant science. The immediately accessible question-and-answer feature in every article addresses the most likely concerns. Indexes in every volume help readers find what they want. For more complicated topics and special problems where additional details are needed, volume 18 contains numerous references to books and Websites as well as to medical and counseling organizations that provide more in-depth knowledge.

Although this encyclopedia does not provide a substitute for personal consultation with your doctor, it is my hope that it will be of practical use to all who are seeking general information about their health care. The more you know about human anatomy and physiology, the better prepared you will be to prevent illness and keep your mind and body healthy.

Michael E. Ryan, D.O., Chairman of Pediatrics,
Geisinger Health System, and
Director of the Janet Weis Children's Hospital,
Danville, Pennsylvania
Clinical Professor of Pediatrics,
Jefferson Medical College, Philadelphia

First Aid Handbook

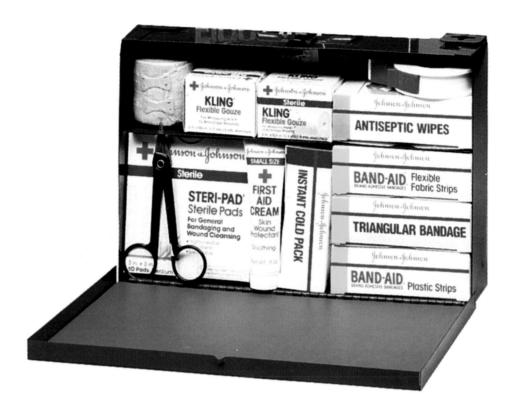

This section will give you all the basic information that you need
to deal with the more common emergencies. It gives a
quick and easy step-by-step guide to emergency first aid.

The aim of all first aid is to keep the patient alive, to protect him or her from
further harm, and to be as reassuring as possible.
In short, the first aid provider's task is to safeguard the victim until
a doctor or nurse arrives to take over.

First you should ensure that the patient is still breathing and try to restore
breathing if necessary. Then you should control any bleeding and treat
for unconsciousness. Next you need to protect the patient
by immobilizing any fractures, treating any burns, dressing
any wounds, and, finally, minimizing shock. Throughout this
process you need to comfort the victim.

Always make sure that you have an accessible record of your doctor's telephone
number, and never hesitate to call the emergency services—it is usually better,
except in extreme emergencies, to telephone an ambulance rather than
drive a patient to the hospital yourself.

Artificial respiration

- Hold patient's head back
- Pinch patient's nose and take a deep breath
- Place your mouth over patient's mouth and breathe into patient
- Check for pulse
- Repeat this procedure, regulating your puffs by the rise and fall of the patient's chest

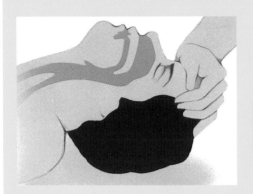

1. To ensure that patient's tongue does not block the throat, place a hand on the forehead and gently tip head back.

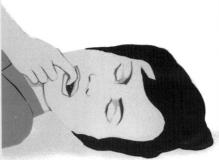

2. If there is an obstruction, turn the head to one side. Use your forefinger to clear out mouth. Tip head back again.

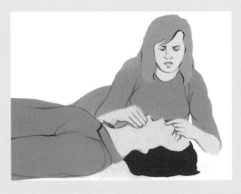

3. If the mouth is closed, grasp chin and pull open gently. Pinch the nose firmly shut and take a deep breath.

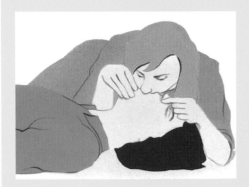

4. Place your mouth over patient's mouth, ensuring a firm seal. Give four breaths in fairly rapid succession.

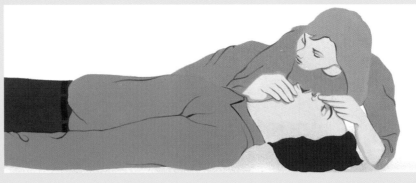

5. Remove mouth. You should feel and hear air leaving the patient's mouth, and the chest will sink. If there is a pulse but no breathing, give two breaths, enough to raise the chest. Continue breaths, about 12 per minute, until breathing resumes.

Take note

- In the case of a young child or baby, cover the mouth and nose. Don't blow too hard—give two slow breaths, just enough to raise the child's chest. If there is a pulse, continue giving breaths, one every three seconds for a baby, one every four seconds for a child.
- If the mouth is injured, hold the mouth shut by applying pressure underneath the chin. Give breaths into the nose and allow mouth to open for exhalation. Repeat.
- If treatment is interrupted (e.g., if the patient vomits), restart by giving four quick breaths, which will supply oxygen immediately.
- An alternative method of opening the patient's mouth is to place a hand under the neck and raise it slightly—the mouth should open on its own.
- To clear an obstruction in the patient's mouth, use a small, hard object if it is available, to keep your finger from being bitten.

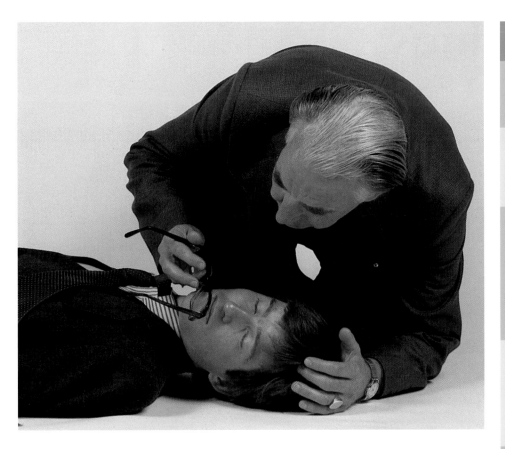

▲ *Before attempting artificial respiration, make sure that the victim has actually stopped breathing. Establish this by holding a pair of eyeglasses in front of his or her mouth: if the glass mists over, then the victim is still breathing.*
Note: If there is any possibility that the patient has suffered trauma or fracture, do not move the neck.

Dos and don'ts

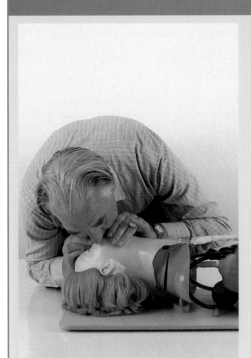

DO keep fingers and hands clear of the patient's lips and neck at all times—they could obstruct breathing.

DON'T blow too hard—just raise the patient's chest visibly; otherwise, you may damage the lung tissue.

DON'T try to drain water or fluid from the lungs of a person who may have drowned. The victim's first need is for oxygen, and air will bubble through liquid in the windpipe.

DON'T practice on a person who is breathing normally. If you enroll in a first aid class, there will be lifelike mannequins provided.

DON'T be worried if the person vomits; this is common. Stop your breathing for long enough to turn his or her head and clear the mouth, then resume by giving the patient four quick breaths.

Checklist

1. Send any onlookers for medical aid. Do not allow people to crowd around or interfere while first aid treatment is being given.

2. Loosen any tight clothing. If possible, the patient should be lightly and loosely covered to prevent heat loss, but the contour of the chest should remain clearly visible.

3. Sometimes it is enough to tilt the patient's head back. He or she may have stopped breathing because of a simple blockage, and holding the head back may free the airway. If this is the case, the patient will probably start to gasp for breath. Placed him or her in the recovery position and take precautions to minimize shock (see Shock).

4. Throughout the first aid treatment, keep checking that the patient's head is tilted back and be sure to keep his or her nose firmly pinched. It is easy to overlook these things if you are concentrating on giving artificial respiration.

5. Check periodically to see if the patient has started to breathe naturally. If breathing has not resumed, begin giving artificial respiration again, starting with four quick breaths and then resuming single puffs. If the patient's breathing has started, keep the head fully back and watch carefully in case the breathing stops again. Once the respiration is steady and natural, treat the patient for unconsciousness (see Unconsciousness).

6. Continue giving artificial respiration until the patient's breathing starts spontaneously or medical help arrives and is able to take over. People have been known to survive for up to eight hours after treatment has begun, so don't give up.

7. If the patient's heartbeat has stopped, heart compression will have to be used (see CPR). The only acceptable indication of a stopped heart is the complete lack of a pulse. Heart compression is a difficult technique to learn and apply, so try to attend a first aid course to supplement the information given here.

8. The risk of contracting HIV through mouth-to-mouth resuscitation is extremely remote, but there are special mouthpieces available that can be used as a safeguard.

Bites and stings

- Various bites and stings need different treatment
- Animal bites need to be washed thoroughly
- Snakebites need special care
- Bee stings have to be removed
- Jellyfish stings need to have tentacles removed

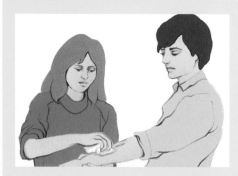

1. Animal bites should be treated like ordinary wounds (see Wounds), except that only the wound itself should be washed thoroughly. Consult a doctor to check for infection.

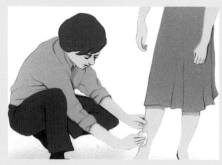

2. If the patient has been bitten by a venomous snake, wipe venom from the wound and bandage a pad tightly onto the wound. Keep patient absolutely still. Seek medical aid.

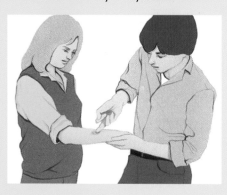

3. Bee and wasp stings are often left in the wound and continue to pump in venom after the insect has gone. Scrape the sting out with a credit card. Wash the wound and cover.

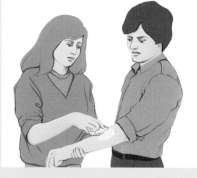

4. If jellyfish tentacles stick, wash with diluted ammonia or alcohol. Remove tentacles with a gloved hand. Soothe wound with calamine lotion. Seek medical aid.

Dos and don'ts

DO clean a bite or sting with warm water and, if possible, unperfumed soap. Then apply a mild antiseptic.

DO reassure the victim of a snakebite. People are often frightened by the idea of snake venom. Remind them that many people have been bitten by far more venomous snakes and have lived to tell the tale. If you have been bitten by a snake in a foreign country, try to remember what it looked like—a good description will save a great deal of medical time.

DO apply calamine lotion or cream to insect bites or stings, including those from gnats and fleas. Antihistamine cream is no longer recommended for home use.

DO get medical help quickly in the following instances:
1. Stings inside the mouth
2. The patient is allergic
3. Signs of shock—pallor, sweating, collapse, and breathing difficulties
4. Stinging by swarms of insects

DON'T apply vinegar to wasp stings or ammonia to bee stings, since these are no longer considered useful remedies.

DON'T use tweezers to remove a bee sting. This will only put pressure on the sting itself and cause it to release more venom. Use a fingernail or credit card.

DON'T treat snakebites by cutting the area, trying to suck out the venom, or applying a tourniquet. These "wild West" treatments can actually aggravate the wound.

Prickly plants

- Plants with prickles and thorns do not sting, but if they break the skin, infections such as tetanus can result. Thorns should be pulled out with fine tweezers. If they are deeply embedded, apply a small dressing and see a doctor or nurse.
- Stings from poison ivy should be washed with hot water and soap. Calamine lotion may help to relieve the discomfort. Cacti can leave fine needles embedded in the skin. Press adhesive bandage or tape onto the affected area, then lift off to remove prickles.

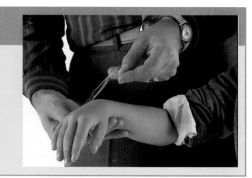

Take note

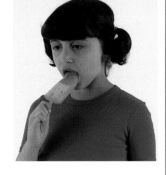

• In the case of a sting inside the mouth, medical aid should be sought immediately. The mouth may swell and breathing can be impaired as a result. While you are waiting for help, swelling can be minimized by using cold mouthwashes, sucking ice cubes, or even eating popsicles.

• The risk of infection is high with any animal bite, so always consult a doctor. This is particularly important if there is even the slightest risk of rabies. If the attacking animal was thought to be rabid, go to the hospital immediately. Report the animal to the local health department so that it can be caught and tested. People helping a victim should take care not to infect themselves.

• If jellyfish tentacles stick to a sting, cover with vinegar and flour, or with wet sand. Using the flat of a knife blade, scrape the sand off the area and wash with rubbing alcohol.

• If you cannot scrape a bee sting out using a fingernail or credit card, you can use a sterilized needle or pin. Hold the pointed end in the blue part of the flame from a lighter or match; this will sterilize the point.

• Ticks are parasites that feed on humans, dogs, and other warm-blooded vertebrates. Some ticks are harmless, but others can transmit disease to humans. A tick must be removed promptly. Cover it with mineral oil or alcohol to immobilize it, and then gently remove with a pair of tweezers, ensuring that the head is completely removed. Wash the area with soap and water, and cover with a bandage. Consult a doctor if fever, rash, or aches and pains occur.

▼ *A picnic in the backyard is one of the delights of childhood. However, it is important for parents to be aware that the undergrowth may contain creatures that bite or sting. Wearing shoes or sandals is a sensible measure.*

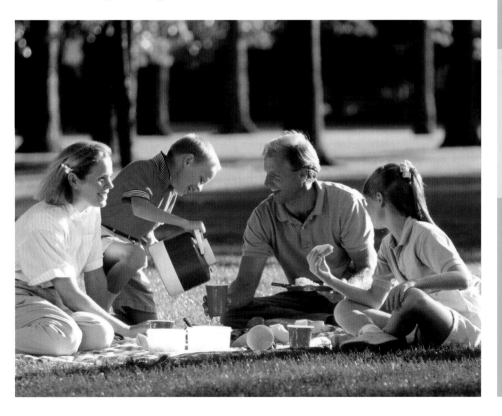

Checklist

1. Make sure that the patient does not scratch the affected area. The irritation and itchiness can be very annoying, but scratching or rubbing often only makes it more intolerable. It also helps to spread the venom, and it certainly increases the chances of developing an infection. A rash may take some time to appear; if a rash does occur, calamine lotion or 1 percent hydrocortisone can help to reduce irritation.

2. Any pain resulting from bites and stings usually resolves itself quickly within the following hour or two. If you do want to take some sort of painkiller, acetaminophen or ibuprofen may speed up the relief of pain. The pain caused by venomous snakebites tends to get progressively worse for some time after the incident, so it is important to give the patient anti-snakebite serum (antivenin) as soon as possible. This should be accompanied by other drugs, such as epinephrine or steroids, to prevent an adverse reaction to the serum. These should always be administered by a doctor.

3. The risk of infection is always high, particularly with bites. If the punctured area becomes red, swollen, harder, or more painful over the next couple of days, it is probably infected, and a doctor should be consulted. It is always sensible to call the emergency service or visit a doctor in the case of animal bites and snakebites, because infections or other complications are likely.

4. Shock can be caused by any form of bite or sting, no matter how minor. It is especially likely if the victim is elderly or very young, but any patient may suffer an allergic reaction to the venom, or just be very frightened. Always treat for shock (see Shock). Send for medical help as quickly as possible, but do not leave the patient alone. Keep the affected area immobilized.

5. Although plant and animal poisons have different constituents, they all contain a substance called histamine, which can produce symptoms that vary from rashes to serious breathing difficulties. In more severe cases, a doctor may administer an antihistamine by either pill or injection. Antihistamine is effective in alleviating the irritation and itching from bites or stings. It blocks the action of the chemical histamine, which the body releases in an allergic response to certain substances.

Bleeding

- Wear protective plastic gloves
- Apply pressure to the wound with your hand to stop the bleeding
- Unless it is known that there is a fracture, raise the injured part to diminish the force of the blood flow at the injury
- Maintain pressure even after a clot has formed
- Move the limb as little as possible, since there may be further injuries

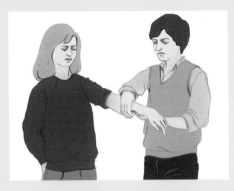

1. Stanch the bleeding by placing your gloved hand immediately over the wound and applying firm pressure; or, if this is easier and equally effective, pinch the edges of the wound firmly together.

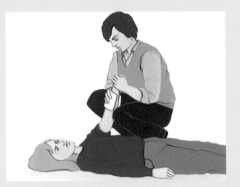

2. Lay the patient down and raise his or her arm. Maintaining pressure all the time, use your free hand to make any available material (such as a handkerchief) into a pad. Hold firmly over the wound.

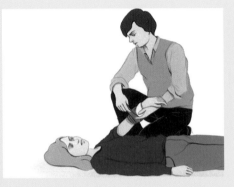

3. Still maintaining pressure, find other material (such as a belt, scarf, or tie) that will act as a bandage. Wrap this tightly around the pad, and secure it with a very firm knot.

What to do in an emergency

Coughing up blood

Place patient in recovery position (see Unconsciousness), but if breathing is difficult, prop up him or her on pillows. If you know from which side the blood is coming, let the patient lie toward that side. Clean away any blood from the mouth. Get medical aid quickly. Any blood coughed up must be reported to a doctor.

Vomiting blood

Place the patient in the recovery position. Clear away any vomit from the mouth. Get medical aid or an ambulance urgently. Keep the vomit for a doctor to examine.

Blood that collects for some time in the stomach before being vomited will be acted on by digestive juices, which will alter its color to brown or black. If red blood is vomited, the bleeding is probably severe and fast.

Slight but sustained bleeding in the stomach will give rise not to vomiting but to black, tarry-looking stools. This situation also requires medical attention.

Internal bleeding

Pain or discomfort can be deceptively slight. If the patient shows signs of shock (faintness, pallor, coldness, sweating, thirst, fast and weak pulse and breathing), place him or her in the recovery position or with the head low and legs raised. Loosen tight clothes and cover him or her with a blanket. Give no additional heat, and nothing by mouth. Send for urgent medical help or an ambulance.

Take note

- Keep checking on a bleeding patient for signs of shock. In an extreme case, he or she will be faint, pale, cold, sweating, and thirsty with a rapid, shallow pulse and breathing rate. At worst, breathing is labored and gasping.
- If any of the above signs appear in a patient without visible injury, suspect internal bleeding.
- Be suspicious of an external blow that has left no significant mark on the skin, but has had the force to imprint a pattern of bruising from overlying objects, such as a buckle or pocket contents. In such a case there may be internal damage with bleeding.
- Stomach bleeding is obvious if the patient vomits blood. The color of the blood depends on how long it has been in the stomach. It may be brown or black and resemble coffee grounds; this indicates that stomach acids have broken it down. Red blood indicates a severe type of internal hemorrhage.

Different types of bleeding

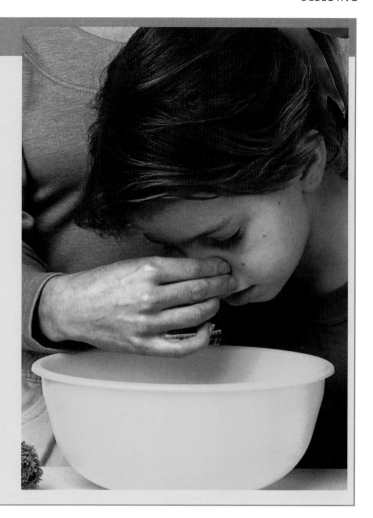

Bleeding from a palm
Keep the patient's arm raised. Make a thick pad from material available and get the patient to clench his or her fist around this. Make an improvised bandage, wrap it firmly around the pad, and knot it securely at the back of the hand.

Nosebleed
Make the patient sit up and bend forward, and pinch the lower half of his or her nose just above the nostrils between finger and thumb for at least 10 minutes without letting go. If necessary, the patient can spit out any blood from the mouth into a bowl. When bleeding has lessened, tip the head backward, maintaining pressure with finger and thumb. Do not let the patient blow his or her nose or sniff. A nosebleed after a blow on the head could be due to a skull injury, so, if appropriate, get immediate medical help.

Bleeding from a tooth socket
This might happen after a tooth extraction. Make the patient bite hard for at least 10 minutes on a thick pad placed over, but not into, the socket. If the patient cups his or her hand under the chin, with the elbow resting on a table, this will help to maintain pressure and be less tiring. Bleeding from the mouth usually looks worse than it is.

Bleeding from the tongue
Sit the patient up, bending forward. Grip the tongue firmly between finger and thumb with a clean handkerchief. Keep up the pressure for 10 minutes, letting the patient take the grip him- or herself.

Dos and don'ts

DO tie the bandage firmly, much more so than you would to secure an ordinary dressing. Once the affected area has been bandaged, check the circulation and ensure that the bandage is not too tight. Check by pressing an area of skin until it looks pale. On release, the color should return at once, if it does not, the bandage is too tight and should be loosened. Circulation should be checked every 10 minutes or so. Watch for signs that the patient's fingers or toes are becoming pale and cold and unable to move. Even with severe bleeding, never apply a tourniquet.

DO get the patient to lie down, or at least sit down, as soon as possible, and then make sure he or she is not moved again.

DON'T waste time washing your hands or looking for orthodox sterile dressings. Speed is the priority; the risk of hemorrhage is far greater than the risk of infection.

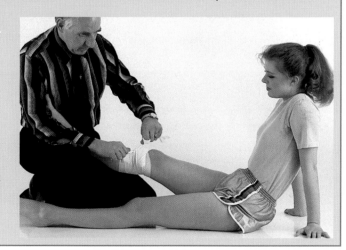

DON'T ask the patient to use his or her hand to exert pressure—he or she may be too weak to do so.

Checklist

1. The risk of shock is high when the patient has lost a lot of blood, so keep him or her warmly but loosely covered; stay with the patient and give reassurance. Keep checking for signs of shock: they are restlessness or irritability; altered consciousness; nausea; pale or ashen, cool, moist skin; rapid breathing; and rapid pulse. Shock can be life-threatening.

2. In severe cases of bleeding, get emergency medical care or call an ambulance immediately and give details of the accident.

3. Let the patient lie quietly and avoid any movement of the injured part; keep the limb elevated and immobilized. Lying down can help minimize pain.

4. Keep a close watch on the bandage. If there are signs of renewed bleeding, do not remove it, but apply more pressure; make another pad and bandage and apply these over the first bandage.

Burns

● If there are flames, smother with cloth or water, and get medical aid

In the event of ordinary household burns:
● To cool the burn, cover it with a thick cloth soaked in cold water or place it in a cold tub
● When the burn is cool, cover it with a clean, dry dressing, and guard against shock
● Lay patient down and call the ambulance or a doctor

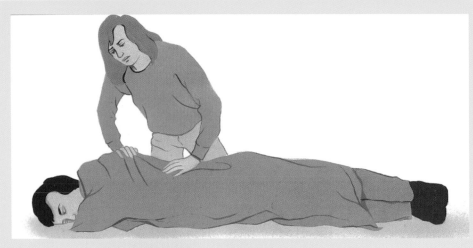

If the patient's clothes are on fire, lay him or her down and smother the flames by pressing down with any thick cloth (towel, curtain, rug, or jacket) that is nearby. Protect the patient's face by bringing the cloth down to fan the fire away from the head and toward the feet. Wrap the cloth firmly around the patient, but don't roll him or her around on the floor. This would expose other parts of the body to the flames. Once the fire is out, pull away charred or smoldering cloth. Leave anything sticking to the skin alone.

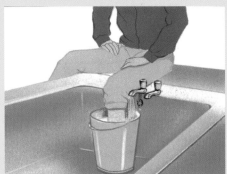

1. Plunge the burned limb into cold water and keep the cold tap running. Immerse it for at least 10 minutes. Or cover the area with a thick cloth soaked in water. Keep it damp.

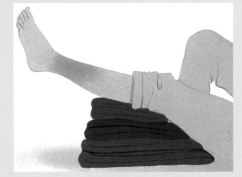

2. In severe cases, keep the patient lying down. If the face is burned, have the patient sit up. Elevate a burned limb to reduce swelling. A leg can be kept high by placing it on pillows.

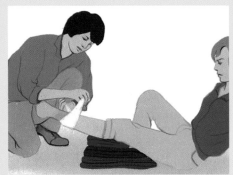

3. Cover the burned area with a clean, dry dressing (see Wounds), which is bandaged or strapped on lightly once the area has been well cooled. Do not apply lotions or ointments.

Dos and don'ts

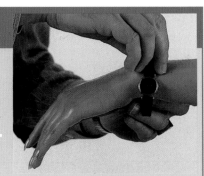

DO remove anything that might constrict if the burned part swells—for example, rings.

DO keep a burned limb elevated to reduce swelling.

DO get someone whose clothes are on fire to cover the face, drop to the floor, and roll around.

DON'T pull away anything that is stuck to the area that has been burned, and never apply any creams or ointments to the burn.

Take note

- Scalds are due to moist heat, such as steam or boiling water. Clothes saturated in steam, boiling water, or hot fat will continue to burn the skin unless they are taken off quickly. For a scalded throat, cool fast with mouthfuls of cold water or by sucking ice.
- Dry heat burns come from flames or from contact with hot objects. Friction can cause burns, as in sliding down a rope using firmly closed hands. Electricity can also cause deep burns.
- Corrosive chemicals such as strong acids can burn severely. For chemical burns, dilute and wash away the substance with lots of water until you are confident that it has all gone. Remove any contaminated clothing. For chemicals in the eye turn the patient, lying down, on the affected side. Gently pull open the eyelids. Pour streams of water into and over the eye to wash out the chemical. Cover with a clean, dry pad. Seek medical help. It is important to act as quickly as possible.
- The significant damage in burns is beneath the skin where the heat is retained. Apart from tissue destruction, the major effect is dilation of the blood vessels, which allows plasma to ooze from them, forming blisters. If the skin surface has been destroyed there will be no cover to hold in the fluid, and the plasma loss can be considerable. The risk of shock is high and must be guarded against. Fluid loss can be offset by frequently giving the patient small amounts of sweetened water.

Checklist

1. Get anyone who has been badly burned or scalded to the hospital as soon as possible. In young children and infants, even small burns should be regarded as very serious. Call an ambulance: it is speedier and allows the patient to remain lying down. If he or she continues to complain of severe pain during transit to the hospital, keep a cold wet cloth on the burned area. Reassure the patient at all times during the journey.

2. With any large burn there is a real risk of shock, and you should follow the advice given in the section on shock in this handbook. In such cases the depth of the burn is not as significant as the surface area affected: the greater the area of skin involved, the greater the volume of plasma oozing from the damaged vessels, and the higher the risk of shock.

3. The burn can be cooled either by immersing it in cold water (never use ice water or put ice directly on the skin), putting it under gently running cold water, or covering it with a cold, clean, wet dressing. If a blister forms, leave it alone. Avoid breathing or coughing on the burn, as this could contaminate it. After the burn has been cooled, pat the area dry and cover it with a dry, clean (preferably sterile) nonadhesive dressing Avoid using fluffy materials; plastic wrap can be used as a temporary dressing.

4. Burns offer an exception to the general first-aid rule of not giving anything by mouth to the injured person. Here you may give the patient about half a glassful of tepid water every 15 or 20 minutes. The water may be sweetened slightly, but remember that fluids can cause vomiting when the patient is suffering from shock. The liquid helps to replace body fluids that have been lost as a result of plasma loss caused by the burn.

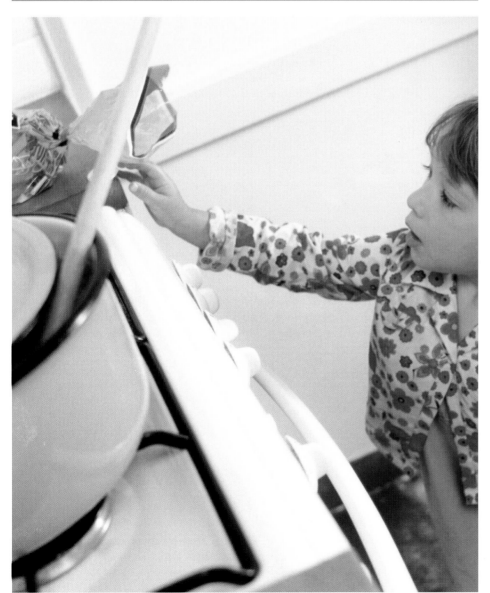

◄ *This child is in danger of suffering a serious but common injury: a bad scald. Make sure that kettles, teapots, saucepans, and the like are kept well out of the reach of inquisitive hands—away from the edge of a table or work surface. Don't place hot containers on placemats, tablecloths, or dish towels, where they can be pulled off easily, and never leave cookies or candies near teapots or kettles. A child will simply be blind to the dangers and, in his or her haste to reach the cookies, may knock the boiling liquid over and sustain an injury.*

Car accidents

- Search the area for any people thrown from the vehicles
- Establish an order of priority for treatment among the victims
- Treat patients for breathing, bleeding, and unconsciousness
- Delegate traffic control to an onlooker
- Send for emergency services, giving thorough details of the accident

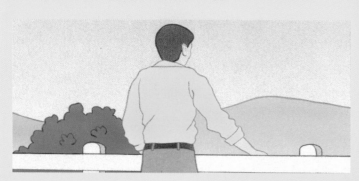

1. Stop your car a short distance away and park well into the side of the road. Turn on hazard lights and headlights to help you see exactly what has happened.

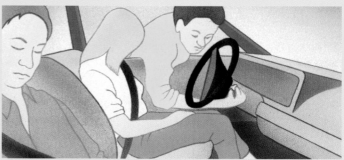

2. Extinguish any smoke coming from vehicles, but leave victims in position unless fire is a risk. Prevent further damage by immobilizing vehicles.

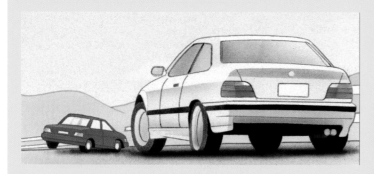

3. Look for victims who might have been thrown from the vehicles—for example, into ditches or over fences. If you have a cellular phone, call the emergency services.

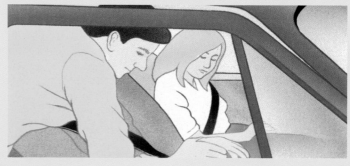

4. Treat victims in order of priority. Deal with breathing, bleeding, and unconsciousness in that order (see Bleeding; Unconsciousness). Move the victims as little as possible.

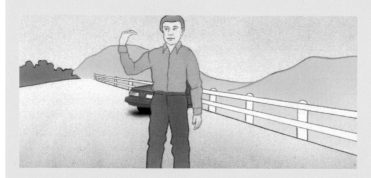

5. Use any onlookers as traffic controllers. Have them stand about 200 yards (65 meters) from the site of the accident and make sure they are clearly visible to oncoming drivers.

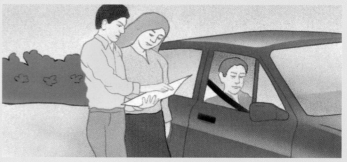

6. Send the first available person for emergency services, giving information about the location, number of vehicles involved, and details of any injured people.

Always be prepared

You should always carry a first aid kit in your car. Many of the accident victims who die before reaching the hospital could have been saved if simple first-aid measures had been taken promptly, so being prepared can be extremely vital. If you carry your own kit, you will be able to give thorough first aid to the victims of an accident that you come across; the kit will also be available should you be involved in an accident yourself.

The first aid kit should be kept in a clearly marked waterproof case, preferably in the glove compartment. The kit should include the following:
- packs of gauze and cotton
- 2- and 3-in. (5- and 7.5-cm) bandages
- medium and large sterile dressings
- a large flashlight (renew batteries every 2 to 3 months)
- a pair of protective rubber gloves
- a large pair of scissors
- pen and paper for messages

If possible, you should also carry a small fire extinguisher.

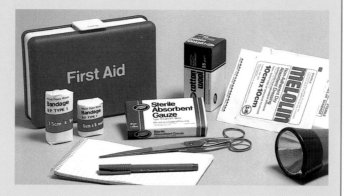

Checklist

1. While you are waiting for the emergency services to arrive, try to discourage other motorists and passersby from hanging around unless they can offer expert or practical help.

2. Keep the area between your car and the crash clear at all times so that the emergency services can stop safely near the accident.

3. Stay with the accident victims until the paramedics arrive. Watch the victims carefully to ensure that breathing does not stop, bleeding does not resume, and no one loses consciousness. Try to be calm and reassuring.

4. Use any spare time to gather information for the emergency services. Collect names and addresses from the least injured victims and take a note of the vehicle licence plates. If victims are unconscious, look for any medical information they may have on them in the way of bracelets, necklaces, or cards. Give the information to the police and paramedics when they arrive, along with any first aid measures that you have taken and any other useful observations.

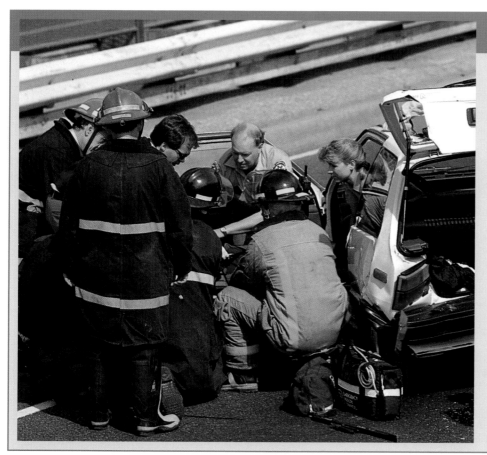

Dos and don'ts

DO ensure that there are no more accident victims in the area. Park your car a short distance away and well off the road. Make sure that the passing traffic is aware that an accident has occurred by asking onlookers to control the traffic.

DO check that all the vehicles are safe—switch off the ignition, apply the brakes, and, if possible, put the car in gear.

DO use any available material, such as car mats or coats, to keep the victims warm. If they are suffering from shock, however, you must avoid overheating them.

DON'T move accident victims from vehicles unless there is a danger of fire. It is a natural human tendency, but you may waste valuable time and even exacerbate existing injuries. The rescue services have special tools to cut people out of damaged vehicles, and this difficult task is best left for them to deal with.

DON'T ever smoke anywhere near the location of the car crash—leaking gasoline may catch fire.

Choking

- As long as the patient can cough vigorously, do not interfere
- If the patient cannot cough, alternate blows to the back with abdominal thrusts
- Should the patient collapse, give artificial respiration
- When airways are completely blocked, try to remove the obstruction
- Have a doctor examine the patient if blows or thrusts have been used

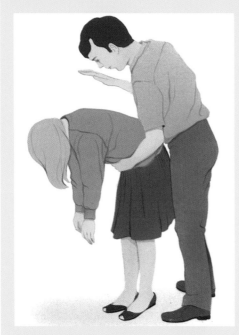

1. If the patient is not able to dislodge the object by coughing, bend him or her over and slap with the heel of your hand between the shoulder blades.

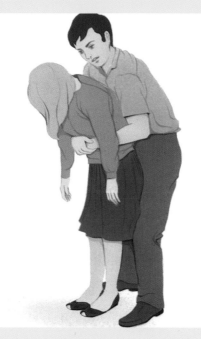

2. If four backslaps fail to loosen the object, give abdominal thrusts. Should the obstruction remain, try alternating back slaps with thrusts.

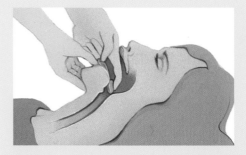

3. If the patient's airways are obstructed and you cannot get air into the lungs by artificial respiration, you must find and remove the object (see Artificial Respiration). Place a curved finger into the mouth, ensuring that the patient does not bite you, and probe the area gently. Do not ram the finger straight in, since this might push the object deeper into the throat. Start at the side of the cheek, moving the finger to the back of the mouth, then hook the finger forward to dislodge the object. Pull the object out quickly, so that the patient cannot suck it back into the throat.

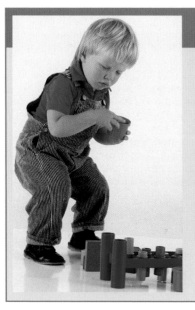

Dos and don'ts

DO stay with the patient, even if he or she is able to speak and cough.

DO try to keep the patient as calm as possible. If the irritating object is in the throat, the trachea (windpipe), which is encircled by muscles, will react by going into spasm. Any anxiety on the part of the patient could increase the tension of the muscles, and the problem will worsen, since the object causing the obstruction is held more tightly.

DO give very hard blows high on the back if this is necessary. Most people do not appreciate how hard these should be to dislodge the object. If you have had to give back blows or abdominal thrusts, ensure that the patient is checked by a doctor. Both processes can cause internal damage.

DO make sure that small children are provided with safe toys. Avoid those with any small parts that can be easily removed and inhaled. Keep all small objects well out of a baby's or toddler's reach. At these ages, most children are particularly likely to put anything into their mouths.

DON'T resort to backslaps and abdominal thrusts before allowing the patient to try to dislodge the object by coughing vigorously. The object may be dislodged easily.

Take note

- If the patient can still speak to you, despite coughing, stand by. Encourage but do not interfere. Advise him or her to try separate heavy coughs with slow inhalation.
- Should this technique fail, bend the patient forward and give him or her a hard blow between the shoulder blades with the heel of your hand. If one blow fails, try up to four blows. This can be done when the patient is standing or sitting. If the patient is on the ground, turn him or her on one side.
- Bend a child over your lap or lay him or her along a thigh. Lay a baby along your arm, head down, and supporting the head and chest.
- If the object is still in place and the older child or adult is weakening, give abdominal thrusts. Encircle patient's waist from behind. Place one fist, thumb side first, halfway between the navel and lower end of the breastbone. Cup your hand over the fist and give a hard thrust (inward and a little upward). This may shoot the obstruction into or out of the mouth. If one thrust fails, try up to four.
- If the patient is on the ground, turn him or her onto his or her back and kneel astride his or her thighs. Place the heel of one hand halfway between the navel and the lower end of the breastbone. Place the heel of the other hand over the first, and continue as above.
- In the case of a baby, hold him or her faceup and head down. Support the head. Place your other hand along the end of his or her sternum and press with your fingers up to four times.
- If necessary, alternate five back blows with five abdominal thrusts.
- If the patient stops breathing, start artificial respiration.

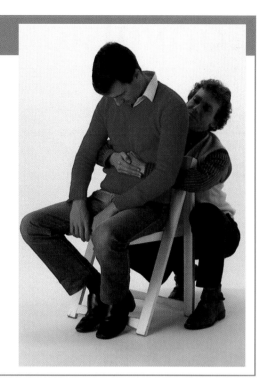

Checklist

1. When something "goes down the wrong way," it can obstruct the back of the throat or it could have moved a little farther down and be blocking the windpipe.

2. If the obstructing object comes free and moves into the patient's mouth, seize it and pull it out quickly so that the patient's next sudden breath will not suck it back in again.

3. If the patient feels faint or vomits, put him or her in the recovery position (see Unconsciousness).

4. If you have used the abdominal thrust, you must watch your patient carefully, even if he or she seems fit again.

5. Even if the patient seems fine, he or she should be seen by a doctor or sent to the hospital for observation as soon as possible, particularly if he or she is still coughing intermittently. In rare cases, the thrust damages an internal organ and medical treatment will then be necessary. This is a calculated risk you must take—the alternative might be suffocation and death.

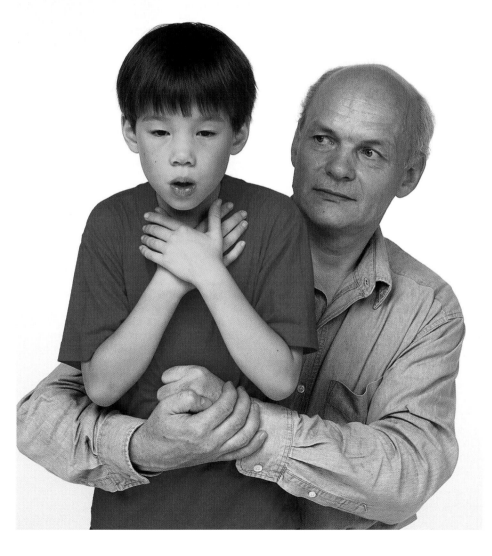

◄ *If a child is choking and four backslaps have failed to dislodge the object, encircle the child's waist from behind, cup your hand over your fist, and give a hard thrust.*

2465

Convulsions

- Call an ambulance immediately
- Don't try to control thrashing limbs; surround patient with cushions
- When the jerking stops, keep the head tipped well back
- If the patient is uninjured and safe to move, place him or her in the recovery position

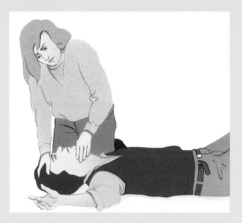

1. The patient lies rigid. To ensure a clear airway, the head should be tipped well back. Any tight clothes should already have been eased. Remember that the patient may have sustained an injury in falling.

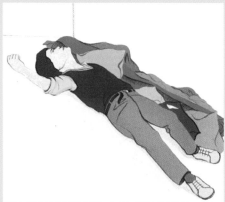

2. When convulsions start, do not attempt to control thrashing limbs. Instead, surround the patient with soft buffers to protect him or her from self-inflicted injuries and move dangerous objects out of reach.

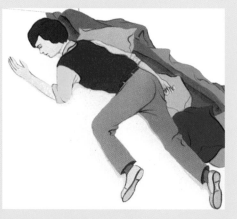

3. The patient stops jerking and relaxes, but remains unconscious. Keep the head tilted back, and look for injuries. If it is safe to do so, put the patient on one side in the recovery position.

Fever convulsions

- A child aged six months to five years with a high fever may have a brief convulsion.
- Tip the head back, and put him or her in the recovery position. Take off his or her clothes and cool him or her with a cold, wet sponge. Check his or her temperature with a thermometer in the armpit and try to reduce it by 1 or 2 degrees.
- Get medical attention as soon as possible. After recovery, keep the child lightly covered.

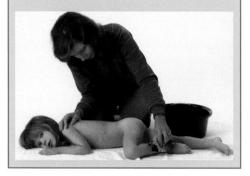

Dos and don'ts

DO check if the person has a medical tag stating that he or she is epileptic.

DO stay by the person's side until his or her recovery or until expert medical attention has arrived.

DO ease any tight clothing at the start of the convulsion. Tip the person's head well back to ensure that he or she does not choke during the attack.

DO mop away any froth that has come from the patient's mouth during the course of the convulsion.

DON'T try to control jerking or thrashing limbs. Just try to prevent self-inflicted injuries by moving furniture and other hard objects out of the way.

DON'T attempt to push anything between the teeth.

Take note

- An epileptic attack or a child's feverish convulsion may be alarming, but generally such seizures are short-lived.
- Most attacks of convulsion come without warning and the patient will usually fall unconscious. He or she may cry out and not be aware of doing so.
- The patient begins jerking limbs and face or thrashing about—this can last 30 seconds. There may be frothing at the mouth and breath holding, and the patient may bite his or her tongue, or may be incontinent.
- When the patient stops jerking, he or she will remain unconscious for some minutes. When the patient comes to, perhaps drowsily, he or she may wave any helping hands away. Many epileptics prefer to take care of themselves after an attack.
- Unless there are familiar people to look after the patient, you should get him or her to the hospital—by ambulance, if this is at all possible.

CPR (cardiopulmonary resuscitation)

- CPR, or heart compression, should be learned through formal instruction
- If the patient is not breathing, begin CPR, which alone may be sufficient to start circulation and promote sufficient air flow; this is more effective with two people
- Continue to alternate heart compression and respiration until the patient shows signs of recovery or until medical help arrives

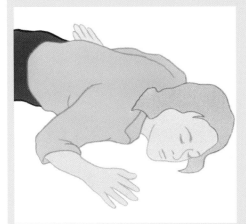

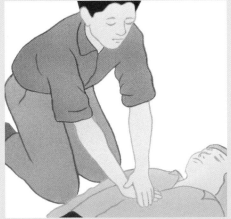

1. Start by sending someone for help. If the patient is breathing, place him or her in the recovery position (above). If there is no movement, no breathing, and no response to any stimulus, start heart compression at once. Do not waste time trying to find a pulse in the neck or doing artificial respiration.

2. Kneel beside the patient, placing the heel of one hand on top of the other. Using the full weight of your body, apply pressure to the lower part of the breastbone, clear of the victim's ribs. If you are alone, the rate of compression should be 80 per minute, giving two breaths after every 15 compressions.

Take note

- Cardiopulmonary resuscitation is a life-support technique that is difficult to carry out effectively without proper training. Thus, although CPR can be performed following the instructions described here, the procedure is best learned by following a formal first-aid course.
- When attempting resuscitation, always follow the basic ABC of priorities: airway, breathing, and circulation.
- When performing CPR, position your shoulders directly over your hands and keep your arms straight and elbows locked, so that the whole of your body weight goes into each compression. Make sure that compressions are carried out smoothly and evenly.
- If you are performing heart compression on children, you will need much less force. With very small children, during resuscitation you may find it more effective to blow into both nose and mouth simultaneously.

Checklist

1. Make sure that the patient is lying down on a firm, level surface. CPR is much less effective if the patient is in a sitting position or if he or she is lying on a soft surface such as mattress.

2. To find the correct position for your hands to enable you to perform heart compressions, search for the notch at the lower end of the patient's breastbone, where it meets the ribs. Put your middle finger on the notch and your index finger next to your middle finger. Place the heel of one hand above your middle finger and your other hand directly on top of the first hand.

3. Use only the heel of your hand when making heart compressions, not the fingers. To keep your fingers out of the way, interlock them together or stick them up and away from the hand.

4. Recheck for signs of circulation and breathing only after you have done three cycles of 15 compressions and two rescue breaths. The check should last no more than 10 seconds.

With two rescuers

If CPR is prolonged, two people will be needed to sustain the treatment. Effective heart compression needs a lot of energy, so get help. If two people are available, one should perform artificial resuscitation while the other carries out heart compression (see Artificial Respiration). The rate of compressions should be 60 per minute, with two seconds' pause after five compressions. One breath should be administered for every five compressions.

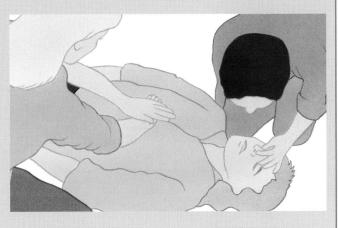

Electric shock

- Turn the electricity off at the fuse box
- Do not touch the victim until you have done this
- Check that the victim is breathing
- Use artificial respiration if necessary
- Check for bleeding and bone fractures
- Treat any burns by cooling
- Send for medical help urgently

GENERAL POINTS

- The vast majority of electrical injuries occur in the home, so make sure that your electrical appliances and home wiring are in good working order.
- Do not touch a shock victim until he or she has been separated from the current, or the electricity supply has been turned off. Otherwise, you too may receive a shock.
- If you cannot turn the current off, use a dry implement made of nonconductive material, such as a broom or chair, to separate the victim from the live apparatus. Act quickly.
- When the victim is free, check that he or she is breathing. He or she may need artificial respiration at once (see Artificial Respiration).
- Try to ascertain the extent of the injury. A severe shock will cause burns and even cuts and fractures if the victim has fallen or been thrown. Use a dry dressing to protect cuts and burns (see Wounds). If burns are minor, cool them (see Burns).
- Immediately call for an ambulance. Stay with the victim. Watch for signs of collapse (pallor and sweating) until the ambulance arrives. Place the victim in the recovery position.

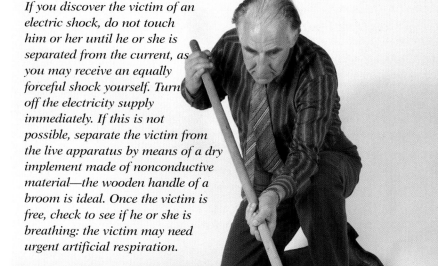

If you discover the victim of an electric shock, do not touch him or her until he or she is separated from the current, as you may receive an equally forceful shock yourself. Turn off the electricity supply immediately. If this is not possible, separate the victim from the live apparatus by means of a dry implement made of nonconductive material—the wooden handle of a broom is ideal. Once the victim is free, check to see if he or she is breathing: the victim may need urgent artificial respiration.

Falls

- Don't try to pick the patient up immediately, but check for injuries
- If a fracture is suspected, don't move the patient
- If the patient is uninjured, help him or her onto all fours, placing a stool in front of the patient. Get him or her to bend one knee and lean forward. Move to one side, and help the patient to push him- or herself up

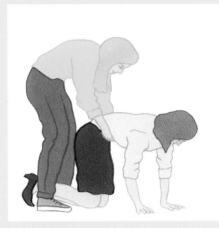

1. Clear the area of any extraneous objects. If the patient has use of arms and legs, turn him or her facedown. Stand over the patient's legs and help him or her onto all fours.

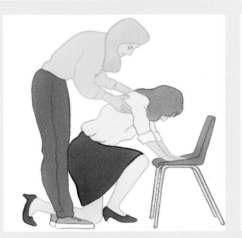

2. Place a stool or chair in front of the patient. Help the patient to put his or her hands on the seat. Still straddling the patient's legs, get him or her to bend one knee and lean forward.

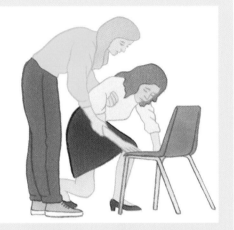

3. Move to one side of the patient. Put one hand in the armpit on that side and the other on the elbow. Gently help the patient to push him- or herself up, using the chair for additional support.

Take note

- Before trying to pick the patient up, it is essential to ascertain whether he or she is conscious—and if so, to ask him or her if there is any pain—and to establish whether he or she has sustained any injuries. Check for bleeding, wounds, or fractures (see Fractures).
- Consider whether it is safe to move the patient. This will not be advisable if there is any chance of a fracture—a fall from a height, a blow to the back, or pain in the back or neck may indicate a fractured spine. If you suspect this, don't move the victim. Make him or her comfortable and call for medical help.
- If you have decided that the patient can be moved but you need help, spread out a blanket and with someone's aid, roll him or her onto the center. Rolling each edge toward the patient, grasp the blanket firmly, one person at each end, and carry him or her to a couch or bed.

Dos and don'ts

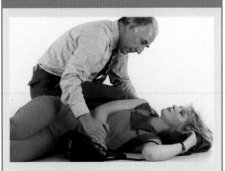

DO examine the patient carefully for injuries; give treatment when appropriate. When lifting him or her, have regard for your own back: lift correctly and as gently as possible.

DON'T attempt to move the patient if there is the slightest chance that he or she may have sustained a fracture. Leave the patient where he or she is until expert help arrives.

Checklist

1. If the patient's condition is uncertain, get a doctor, especially if the patient is unconscious, has difficulty moving a part of the body, or seems to have developed a psychological change—owing to a blow to the head, for example.

2. If the patient's legs are weak, get the patient to sit on the floor and place a low stool behind him or her. Have the patient place his or her hands on the seat and bend forward; the patient can then use his or her arms to push up and sit on the stool. Put a higher stool or chair behind the first one; repeat the maneuver to get him or her sitting on this one. The elderly and the weak, in particular, may need more help in getting up after a fall.

3. Ask yourself why the patient fell. If general weakness was the cause, discuss medication or the need for a walker with the doctor.

Fractures

- Keep the patient still and cover him or her with a blanket
- Attend to such injuries as an open wound or bleeding before dealing with the fracture
- If necessary, protect the broken bone
- Stay with the patient, and make him or her comfortable until professional help arrives

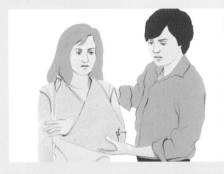

1. Simple arm sling: support elbow, keeping hand raised. Pass bandage between chest and arm.

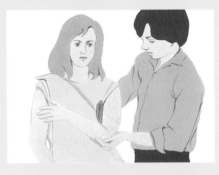

2. Bring bandage over forearm and around back of neck; tie together over hollow above clavicle. Pin at the elbow.

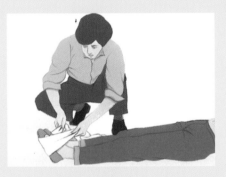

3. Figure-eight bandage: place patient's feet together. Lay middle of bandage across the soles of the feet.

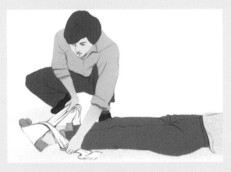

4. Bring ends of bandage to front of feet and cross over insteps. Wrap again by carrying ends to back of ankles.

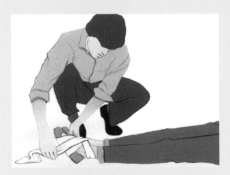

5. Cross ends and bring them back to front of ankle. Cross again. Take ends back under soles; tie ends in place.

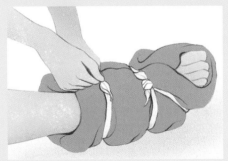

6. Foot-and-ankle bandage: use folded cloth or flat cushion around ankle and foot, then tie with narrow bandages.

Dos and don'ts

DO ensure that the patient cannot move. Place cushions or other soft articles between his or her body and any pieces of furniture.

DO use a sound part of the patient's body as a splint (for example, leg to leg, arm to chest) if you have to immobilize a fracture. Whenever possible, move the uninjured part to the injured part.

DO place thick padding (absorbent cotton, towels, scarves, socks, and so on) to fill spaces between two parts of the body.

DO tie the parts of the body together with firm bandages (if these are not available use scarves, neckties, handkerchiefs, and so on).

DO avoid placing a bandage directly over a fracture of the limb and tie any bandage knots over the uninjured part.

DO check that any bandages or slings are not so tight that they cut off the patient's circulation.

DON'T ever give any food, liquid, or medication to the patient before professional help arrives.

Immobilizing fractures

Jaw:
Gently clear mouth of any blood or dentures. Put thick pad under and around jaw. (Patient's cupped hand can support it temporarily.) Secure by placing bandage over pad; bring ends up over ears and tie on top of patient's head.

Clavicle:
Keep point of elbow supported until sling can hold it; support arm on side of fracture with a sling (see opposite page, figures 1 and 2). Place soft pad under armpit. Secure upper arm against chest: place wide bandage over arm and across back and chest, and tie under armpit on unaffected side.

Leg:
Keep patient lying down. Place padding between legs from groin to just above ankles. Put bandage around knees and tie on side. Make figure-eight bandage around feet and ankles (see opposite page, figures 3, 4, and 5) .

Arm:
If elbow can be bent without pain, place pad in armpit and support forearm with sling (see opposite page, figures 1 and 2). Ensure that forearm slopes slightly upward. If elbow is straight and painful to bend, keep patient lying down. Place padding between arm and body. Secure arm to body with three wide bandages (as for clavicle, figures 1 and 2).

Foot and ankle:
Wrap folded cloth around foot. Secure with narrow bandages (see opposite page, figure 6).

Checklist

1. In the case of a broken backbone, the fracture of a vertebra might create loose pieces of bone that could enter the spinal cord, causing permanent paralysis and loss of feeling. If there is any possibility of such a fracture, leave the patient as you found him or her and wait for professional assistance.

2. Deciding whether someone has broken a bone can be difficult—many of the classical features of a fracture can also indicate other injuries, such as a sprain. For example, an initial symptom that is common in a fracture is pain. Yet a severe contusion, without a break, can be extremely painful, and sometimes a major fracture hurts only a little. Restricted movement of the injured part and swelling of tissues in the area can be symptomatic of both sprains and fractures. Also, many fractures retain the broken bone ends in good anatomic position so that another classical feature, deformity, is not always present.

3. In diagnosing a fracture, the history of the injury should be taken into account. The likelihood of bone damage is high if there was a considerable force, such as a hard blow or a fall. Yet this can be deceptive, too, since diseased bones—or, in the elderly, brittle ones—can break relatively easily. However, anyone who administers first aid can do no harm by suspecting a fracture when circumstances suggest it, and thus acting accordingly.

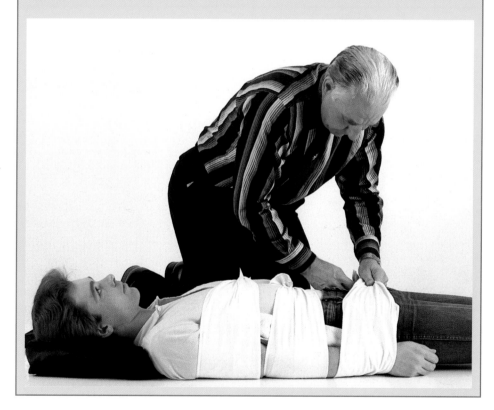

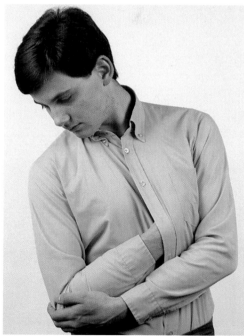

▶ *If a triangular bandage is not available, an adequate emergency sling can be rapidly improvised from clothing. The patient's arm can be placed inside the shirt, supported by the fastened buttons. A necktie can be used, or the hem of the patient's jacket can be taken up over the fractured arm and then pinned to a lapel.*

Heart attack

- Call or send for an ambulance immediately
- Place the patient in a resting position
- Keep the upper part of the body raised
- Loosen any tight clothing at neck and waist
- If breathing stops, give artificial respiration
- Keep patient warm by covering with a blanket

When a person suffers a heart attack, prompt action is of crucial importance. Make sure you perform the following in the correct order:

1. Call or send someone for an ambulance immediately. Specify the nature of the problem.

2. Place the patient in a resting position at once—in bed, on a sofa, or in an armchair.

3. Loosen clothes at the neck and at the waist.

4. If the patient appears very breathless, let him or her sit up against a headboard banked with pillows. The headboard can be improvised with a light chair set upside down against the wall.

5. If there is nothing suitable against which the patient can rest, use your body as a prop.

6. Keep him or her loosely covered. Open the window so that the room is well ventilated.

7. Alleviate the patient's fears by keeping a calm and sympathetic attitude, and express confidence about recovery.

8. Reassure the patient that medical help has been sent for and that it will arrive shortly.

9. Remain with the patient to comfort him or her, but avoid fussing and prevent others from crowding around.

10. If the patient loses consciousness and stops breathing, begin performing artificial respiration at once (see Artificial Respiration).

11. If the heart stops beating, the patient will also need heart compression (see CPR).

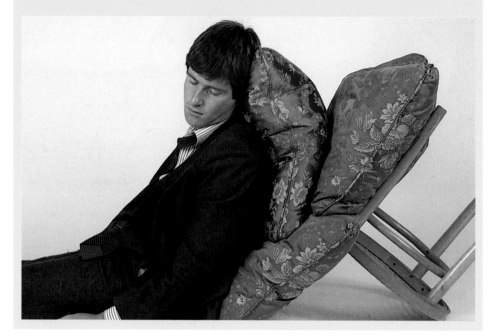

Hypothermia

- Exposure to cold can cause lasting damage to the body's tissues
- Complications associated with exposure include frostbite and hypothermia
- The extremities—nose, fingers, and toes—are most affected
- Any attempt at rapid rewarming can cause further tissue damage

Exposure

Symptoms of exposure include physical and mental slowing down, a decrease in reasoning power, mood changes, slurred speech, shivering, and cramps, followed by possible collapse. Once any symptoms are detected, stop the patient from moving and get him or her to take shelter. Remove any wet clothing and replace with blankets, a sleeping bag, or fresh clothing. Cover the patient's head and face, but leave the mouth, nose, and eyes free. If the patient is conscious, give him or her warm, sweet drinks, but never administer alcohol.

Frostbite

If subjected to intense cold, the tissues under the skin may freeze. Freezing is caused by the formation of tiny ice particles and disruption of the blood supply brought on by clumps of red blood cells that then block the vessels. When frostbite (numb, white tissue) is suspected, remove wet clothing and constricting objects (such as a ring) from the affected area. Apply a dry, protective cover after dabbing away any moisture. If possible, immerse the part in warm, not hot, water. Or, use a warm blanket. Do not rub area.

Hypothermia

A patient with hypothermia is extremely cold all over, with puffy skin that is white or blue—except for a child, who looks pink. The heartbeat will be slow and weak. When this occurs, keep the patient in bed in the recovery position. Cover the patient with blankets, but keep them loose. Do not use hot water bottles or an electric blanket, since excessive heat may damage the patient. Make sure that all open windows are shut and then warm the room with any available heater. If the patient is conscious, give him or her warm, sweet drinks.

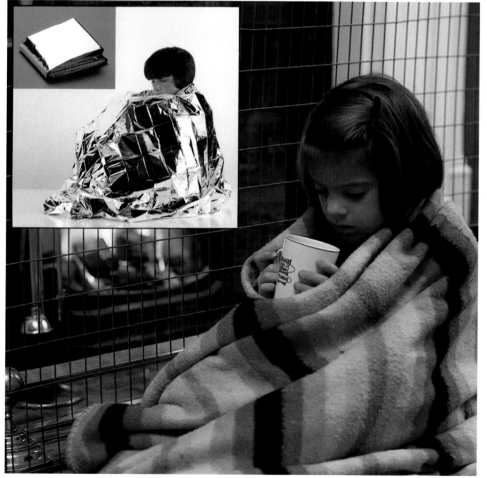

Dos and don'ts

DO cover the head in extreme cold to protect against excessive loss of body heat.

DO ensure that the young and elderly sleep in warm conditions, since they are particularly vulnerable to low temperatures.

DO use suitable protective clothing in extremely cold conditions. On long trips, take high-energy foods (such as chocolate and glucose) and flasks of hot, sweet drinks.

DON'T give a patient alcohol; it encourages the body to lose rather than retain heat.

◄ *Children who go on camping or hiking expeditions in which they risk exposure to cold or damp weather should be supplied with thermal blankets; they are excellent at retaining the body's heat, take up very little space, and are light to carry. Warming a cold child in front of a fire is effective in cases of chill and slight exposure—for example, after a soaking—but victims of severe exposure and frostbite should never be put near a roaring fire: rapid reheating may cause further tissue damage.*

Poisoning

- Call an ambulance and a Poison Control Center
- A conscious patient should be given fluids
- If patient is unconscious, put in the recovery position
- If he or she is not breathing, give artificial respiration

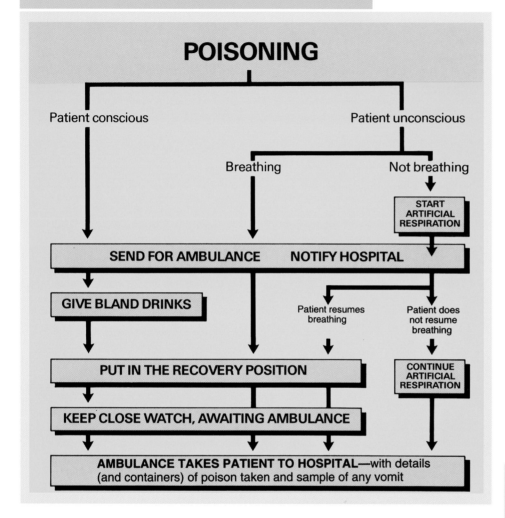

POISONING

Patient conscious → Patient unconscious

Breathing / Not breathing

Not breathing → START ARTIFICIAL RESPIRATION

SEND FOR AMBULANCE — NOTIFY HOSPITAL

GIVE BLAND DRINKS

Patient resumes breathing / Patient does not resume breathing

PUT IN THE RECOVERY POSITION

Patient does not resume breathing → CONTINUE ARTIFICIAL RESPIRATION

KEEP CLOSE WATCH, AWAITING AMBULANCE

AMBULANCE TAKES PATIENT TO HOSPITAL—with details (and containers) of poison taken and sample of any vomit

Take note

- Quickly determine the nature of the poison swallowed and inform your local Poison Control Center immediately.
- If the patient is alert enough to swallow, give him or her at least two glasses of milk or water to sip slowly—but no salty drinks.
- Don't try to make the patient vomit unless directed to do so by a doctor. If he or she vomits spontaneously, clear the throat and mouth to protect breathing. Send a small sample of the vomit to the hospital, with an estimate of the amount vomited, along with a container of the substance swallowed.
- Watch the patient closely in case he or she vomits, loses consciousness, or stops breathing. A person who attempted suicide must be kept from another attempt.

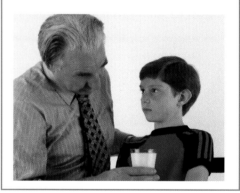

Pesticides

- Pesticides are variable in their action. The more dangerous ones, if used as sprays, can cause harm if swallowed, breathed in, or absorbed through the skin.
- The effects of pesticide poisoning can be cumulative, causing headaches, muscle ache, weakness, sweating, lassitude, vomiting, and difficulty in, or even cessation of, breathing.
- Get the patient out of the spray area and put him or her to rest. Wearing gloves, remove any contaminated clothing and thoroughly wash his or her skin. Check the pesticide container label for advice (always keep pesticides in the original containers—apart from being a safety measure, it usually gives instructions on what to do in an emergency).
- Summon medical help immediately and, if necessary, give artificial respiration (see Artificial Respiration).

Fumes and smoke

- Make sure that you do not rush into the danger area unprepared. Have a safety line tied around you, with its end in the hands of someone outside.
- If possible, put a moist handkerchief or towel over your mouth and nose. Take a couple of deep breaths before you go in. Hold your breath.
- If the smoke is from a fire, travel along the floor.
- Support the patient as you lead him or her out. If the patient cannot walk, drag him or her out with your hands under his or her armpits.

Shock

- Shock is caused by many types of severe injury—it is due to failure of the circulation
- Always tend to major injuries first
- Minimize shock by laying the patient down at the site of the accident, keeping his or her head low and legs raised
- Loosen tight clothing and keep the patient lightly covered

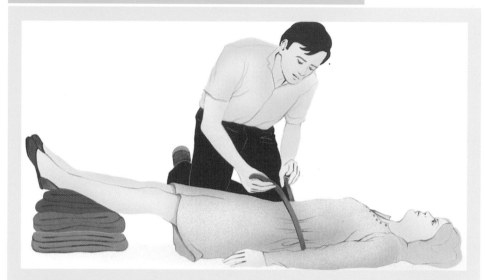

1. Stop bleeding (see Bleeding). If possible, treat patient on the spot. Lay him or her down with head low and legs raised about 12 in. (46 cm). Keep movement to a minimum.

2. Loosen tight clothing. Dress wounds with clean, dry material (see Wounds). If injuries allow, place the patient in the recovery position (see Unconsciousness).

Checklist

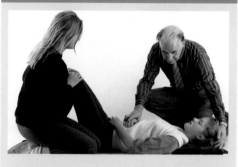

1. Keep a careful watch on the patient to make sure that he or she is breathing properly, does not start—or resume—bleeding, and does not vomit. Lightly cover with blankets so that the patient remains cool, but is not cold. Do not heat with hot water bottles or electric blankets—these will draw blood away from the vital organs where it is needed.

2. Do not give the victim any food, drink, or medication. Stimulants, such as alcohol and cigarettes, should be avoided completely.

3. Even if the patient seems to be unconscious, do not talk to bystanders about his or her condition. He or she may well hear you and understand what is being said. The patient needs to be reassured, not made more anxious.

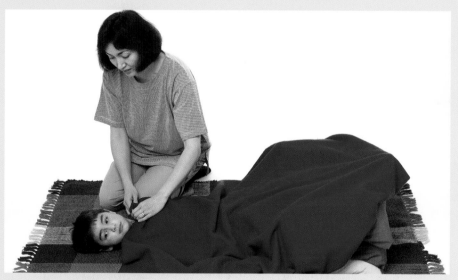

3. In cold conditions in which the person might shiver, cover loosely, but do not allow the skin to warm up. Do not cover routinely. As you give first aid, explain what you are doing so that the patient is reassured. Stay with the patient until medical aid arrives.

Sprains and strains

- Let the patient rest the injured part in the most comfortable position, slightly raised if possible
- Cover the affected area with a cold compress, keeping it in position for approximately 30 minutes
- Protect the area with a pad of wool or cotton cloth
- Bandage from well below hurt area to well above

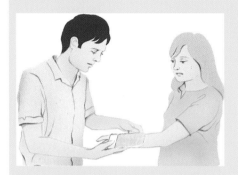

1. Spraining means damaging the ligaments around a joint. Apply a cold compress, then remove it and cover the area with a pad.

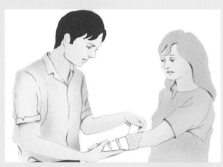

2. Starting well below the damaged joint, firmly wrap a bandage up and around the joint, leaving a few strips of padding visible.

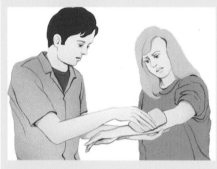

3. A strain involves a muscle in any part of the body. Apply a cold compress, then remove it and cover the area with a thick pad.

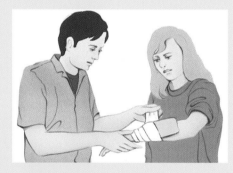

4. Wrap an elasticized bandage around the injured area. Do this firmly but not tightly, and cover the padding completely.

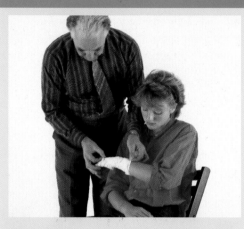
Take note

- In both strains and sprains the muscle or ligament has been overstretched by a powerful movement. Sometimes small blood vessels will also be torn and a bruise forms. The area will be painful, discolored, and swollen.
- Swelling can be minimized by cooling the area with a cold compress for up to 72 hours after the accident. After this, no amount of cooling will help to reduce the swelling.
- To make a cold compress: use thick cloth, such as a folded towel; soak it in cold water; wring it out so it is just moist; place on the sore area; keep in place for about half an hour; moisten if it begins to dry out too much.
- If you think there is the slightest chance that the patient has fractured a bone, treat as for fractures (see Fractures). Many doctors do exactly this until they have the results of an X ray.

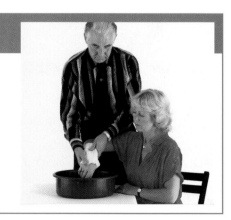

Unconsciousness

- If the patient is not breathing, begin artificial respiration immediately
- Clear the patient's mouth of any vomit, blood, or displaced dentures
- Control any bleeding; check for other wounds and for possible fractures
- If it is safe to move the patient, move him or her gently into the recovery position
- If possible, stay with the patient and send someone for medical help

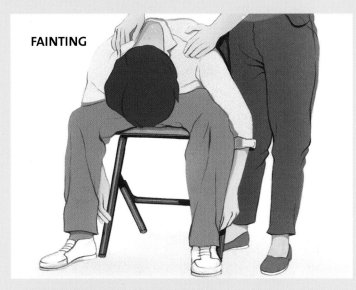

FAINTING

1. When a seated person feels faint and it is impossible to lay him or her down (for example, in a concert hall), tell him or her to bend all the way forward, with the head between the legs, and to try to relax completely. Do not leave the patient in case he or she loses consciousness.

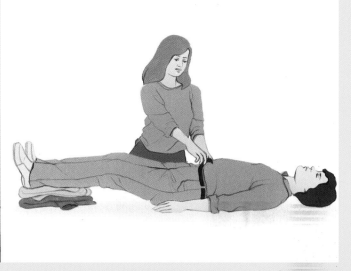

2. If possible, lay the patient down, with legs raised at least 12 in. (30 cm). Loosen tight clothing at neck. If the patient is conscious, tell him or her to take deep, slow breaths. As the patient recovers, give him or her cold water to drink. Ask him or her to stay still for 5 minutes before trying to sit up slowly.

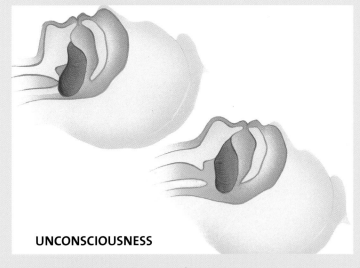

UNCONSCIOUSNESS

1. In an unconscious person, the tongue may sometimes flop backward and obstruct the opening of the windpipe. Bend the head back, without twisting the neck: the tongue will be carried up with the jaw and the airway will open. Give artificial respiration if necessary.

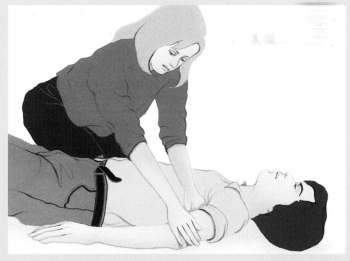

2. Stop bleeding (see Bleeding), dress wounds (see Wounds), and check for fractures (see Fractures) by feeling firmly but gently with hands flat, from one end of the body to the other for any swellings. If you suspect a fracture, avoid moving the patient; otherwise put him or her in recovery position.

Dos and don'ts

DO remember to check the patient's breathing before you do anything else. If he or she is lying on the back, the tongue may be obstructing the airways, and this must be treated as an emergency.

DO remove anything, such as a pillow, from under the patient's head if he or she is having any difficulty breathing.

DO follow the routine to safeguard breathing, stop bleeding, and protect against further harm before you move the patient into the recovery position.

DON'T twist or turn the neck when moving the head, in case there has been some injury to the upper part of the spinal column.

DON'T try to make an unconscious person drink. The fluid would run into the windpipe. Even if the patient responds vaguely to touch, his or her ability to swallow may be impaired.

If you find someone lying unconscious, you should search the person for clues about his or her medical history: he or she may suffer from epilepsy or diabetes.

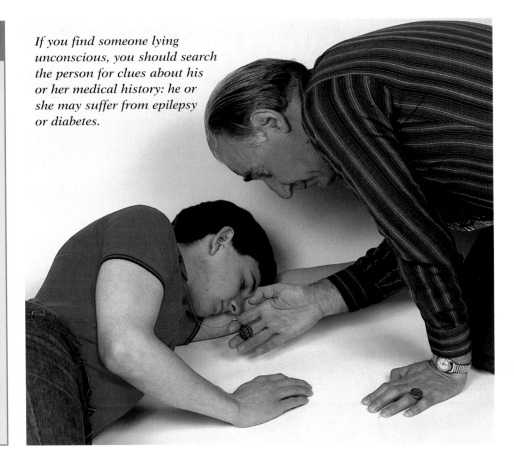

Take note

● Examine the patient to see if he or she is breathing. If not, then begin artificial respiration immediately (see Artificial Respiration).
● If the patient is breathing noisily and with some difficulty, use a curved finger to scoop the mouth clear of any obstruction in the airway, such as vomit or blood. Bend the head back and keep it in this position.
● Look for any severe bleeding. Control it at once (see Bleeding).
● Check for any other wounds. Cover them at once with a dressing (you may have to improvise one; see Wounds).
● Search for any possible fractures (see Fractures). If you suspect a fracture (which would be made worse by moving the patient), leave him or her as is. Note that a fractured spine is almost impossible to discern in an unconscious patient, but the circumstances (for example, a fall from a height or a blow to the back) may suggest it. If so, **do not move the patient under any circumstances.**
● If it is safe to move the patient, turn him or her gently into the recovery position (see below).
● Send for medical help.

RECOVERY POSITION

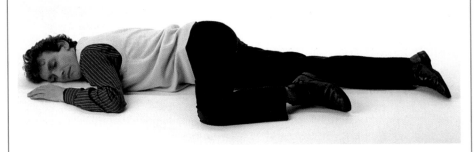

Checklist

1. The cause of the patient's unconsciousness may be unknown. This is for the doctor to diagnose and to treat. Your first responsibility is to call for medical aid and to administer first aid, if necessary.

2. Even if there is no sign of emergency at first, keep watching the patient carefully in case his or her breathing stops and needs artificial respiration, or the patient vomits. If he or she does vomit, clear his or her mouth using a curved finger.

3. If the patient is unknown to you and you will not harm him or her with your movements, search for any cards, bracelets, or other medical tags that may tell you if the patient suffers from a condition such as diabetes. Also search the person for any drugs that may indicate what could have led to a drug overdose. These items should be handed to the doctor or paramedics.

4. If you suspect that the patient has a fracture, and medical help will be delayed, or you have to transport the patient to the hospital, immobilize the part that has been fractured.

Wounds

- Elevate the injured part of the body; make sure the patient keeps still
- If bleeding is heavy, apply pressure on the wound with your hand until bleeding subsides
- Wash the wound, then put gauze over it, then a thick pad, and finally a firm bandage
- Protect the patient against shock and seek medical attention

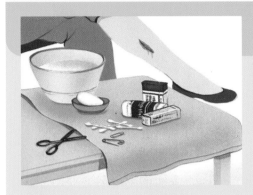

1. For dressing a wound you need several articles from a first aid box: cotton, gauze, bandages. You will also need soap and warm water.

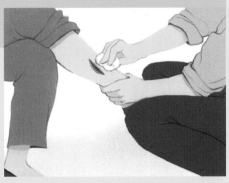

2. Elevate the wound. Wash it and skin around it. Use cotton moistened with water and soap; flush with clear water. Work outward from the wound.

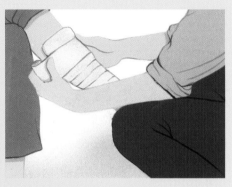

3. Put gauze over the wound, covering beyond the wound area. Place thick pad over the gauze. Bandage dressing firmly, preferably with a pressure bandage.

MAKING A RING PAD

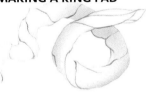

1. Use a long, thin, twisted fold of cloth such as a large handkerchief. Form one end into a circle.

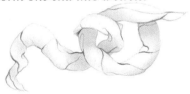

2. Hold the circle and slip the end through the loop. Keep looping the long, free end around the circle.

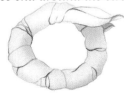

3. When all the cloth is used up, it forms a firm, thick ring that protects the wound when it is bandaged.

OBJECTS IN WOUNDS

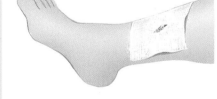

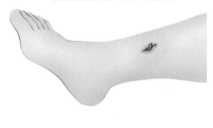

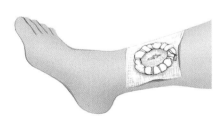

1. If an object is lying on the surface of a wound, brush it away with a clean piece of gauze. However, if an object has become embedded, you must leave it undisturbed. It will be removed properly when medical assistance becomes available.

2. Carefully cover the wound with a piece of sterile gauze; it should be sufficiently large so that it extends well beyond the area of the wound itself. If the piece of gauze is too small, it may slip and a part of the wound may become exposed.

3. Make a ring pad (see box, left) from a large handkerchief or a small towel and place this around the object in the wound. This will prevent the object from being pressed on by the thick pad and bandage that you will place over it. Once the wound has been bandaged, expert medical advice should be sought.

Take note

- Get the patient to sit or lie down and elevate the injured part of the body.
- Temporarily protect the wound with the cleanest cover that you can find. Wash your hands and collect the material needed: soap, water, cotton balls, gauze, bandages (or improvised substitutes). Place them on a clean surface nearby.
- Wash the wound and the skin around it. Use cotton moistened with water and soap; follow with clear water. Use a clean piece of cotton for each separate stroke, moving the cotton outward from the wound.
- Put nonstick gauze over the wound; make sure it is large enough to extend well beyond the wounded area and cover the cleaned skin.
- On top of the gauze, gently set a thick pad of cotton.
- Bandage firmly (but not too tightly). Each successive bandage turn should overlap the previous one by two-thirds of its width.
- Keep the wounded part at rest.
- Protect the patient against shock (see Shock).

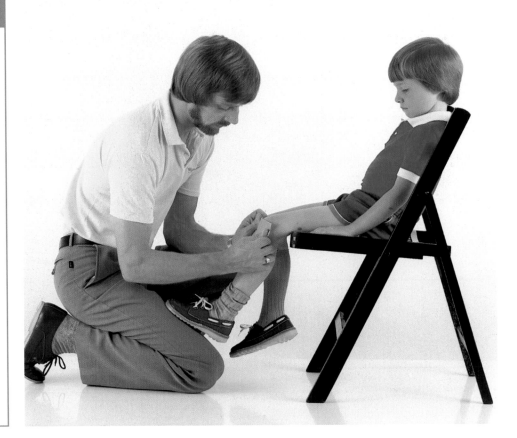

Dressings

- Convenient, ready-made, all-in-one dressings come with the gauze and the pad attached to the bandage.
- Adhesive dressings are either in continuous strips to be cut to size or in different sizes of single dressings. They are useful for dressing small, superficial wounds. After partly peeling off the protective cover, apply the gauze pad that is now exposed onto the wound, then pull away the cover.
- Tubular gauze is fitted over toes and fingers by means of a metal or plastic applicator.
- An improvised gauze dressing can be made from most smooth, clean materials such as a handkerchief, pillowcase, or towel (but not fluffy cotton). One or two folded handkerchiefs can serve as a pad. Cloths folded lengthwise (a handkerchief, scarf, sock, stocking, and so on) can serve as bandages. Make sure that the material is large enough to extend at least 1 in. (2.5 cm) beyond the edges of the wound.

Dressing an eye wound

- For an eye wound, bandage or tape a large, soft, clean pad over the whole eye, without putting any pressure on it. Never use fluffy material as a bandage.
- If it hurts the patient to move his or her eye, cover both eyes, because the two automatically move together.
- Seek medical help immediately—trying to remove foreign bodies may do more damage.

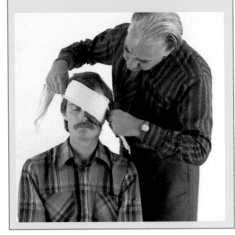

Checklist

1. The slight bleeding of most wounds is soon brought under control by the pressure of ordinary dressings and bandaging. However, if the patient's bleeding is severe, it will have to be controlled by applying pressure on the wound with your hand (see Bleeding).

2. In the case of wounds, the aim of first aid is to protect the wound from becoming infected and damaged. The person administering first aid should limit his or her help to cleaning around the wound (if circumstances permit) and to covering it.

3. In giving first aid, do not use antiseptic or antibiotic lotions and creams. These may interfere with the healing process.

4. With any wound there is the risk of tetanus, and the deeper the cut, the higher the risk. Tetanus vaccinations are given routinely in childhood, but immunity lasts only five to 10 years. Even if the patient has been immunized in the last 10 years, he or should consult a doctor to determine whether a tetanus booster is needed.

Medical glossary

A

ABDOMEN The abdominal cavity that lies between the diaphragm and the pelvis, containing the stomach and intestines, as well as the kidneys, liver, and pancreas. The front wall is a muscular sheet, and the internal surface is lined by the peritoneum.

ABLATION The deliberate removal of tissue, such as a growth, for treatment purposes.

ABORTION "Spontaneous abortion" is the medical term for a miscarriage—the loss of an embryo, or fetus, before 28 weeks. The term "therapeutic abortion" refers to the surgical termination of pregnancy.

ABSCESS A cavity containing pus.

ACHONDROPLASIA Genetic disorder causing severe limitation of skeletal growth.

ACIDOSIS Abnormally high level of acidity in the blood, often as a result of kidney failure, diabetes, or poisoning.

ACNE Skin condition affecting face, neck, chest, and back, resulting in blackheads.

ACQUIRED IMMUNODEFICIENCY SYNDROME *See* AIDS.

ACROMEGALY Abnormal enlargement of face, hands, and feet as a result of a tumor of the pituitary gland.

ACUPUNCTURE Traditional Chinese medical technique in which fine needles are inserted into specific sites on the body along a series of energy lines, or meridians, in order to treat a disorder or relieve pain.

ACUTE Term used to characterize a medical condition that develops over a short time.

ADDISON'S DISEASE Failure of the adrenal glands, leading to low blood pressure, increased pigmentation of the skin, and possible collapse.

ADENOIDS Small masses of lymphatic tissue, found in the pharynx at the back of the nose, which are prone to swell up during childhood.

ADIPOSE Term meaning "fatty," used to describe tissue composed of fat cells.

ADRENAL GLANDS Two glands situated on top of the kidneys, of which the outer layer (the cortex) is responsible for the production of cortisone, and the inner core (the medulla) for the production of epinephrine.

AFTERBIRTH The placenta and other fetal tissues expelled from the uterus after childbirth.

AIDS (acquired immunodeficiency syndrome) A disease that causes fatal depression of the immune system owing to infection with HIV.

ALBINISM Condition characterized by a lack of pigment in hair, eyes, or skin.

ALBUMINURIA Presence of albumen (a form of protein) in the urine, usually the result of kidney disease, or of renal complications of another disease such as heart failure. Also called proteinuria.

ALCOHOLISM Addiction to alcohol, which can lead to deterioration in psychological and physical health, family life, and social position.

ALLERGEN A substance that causes an allergy.

ALLERGY Hypersensitive reaction, such as wheezing or rashes, to a foreign substance that stimulates the immune system.

ALOPECIA Hair loss. Alopecia areata is a disease with no known cure. It leads to patchy hair loss on the scalp.

ALTITUDE SICKNESS Headache, breathlessness, and weakness found in people who have not acclimatized to the reduced barometric pressure found at high altitudes.

ALVEOLUS The word "alveolus" means a small hollow, cavity, or socket. It can apply to a tooth socket, but in the lungs, alveoli are tiny air sacs through which gases diffuse in and out of the bloodstream.

AMEBIC DYSENTERY Inflammation of the intestines, caused by infestation with the amoeba *Entamoeba histolytica*, and characterized by blood-flecked diarrhea.

AMENORRHEA The absence of menstruation during pregnancy, or as a result of emotional disturbance or hormonal imbalance.

AMNIOCENTESIS An obstetric procedure in which a sample of the amniotic fluid surrounding a fetus is taken for testing.

AMNIOTIC FLUID The clear fluid surrounding a fetus in the uterus.

AMYOTROPHIC LATERAL SCLEROSIS (ALS) A progressive disease characterized by weakness in the muscles, and caused by degeneration of cells in the spinal cord. It is one form of motor neuron disease.

ANALGESIC Any drug that relieves pain.

ANAPHYLACTIC SHOCK Severe allergic reaction leading to collapse.

ANEMIA A lack of hemoglobin in the blood, often caused by a decrease in red cell production, by destruction of red cells, or by blood loss.

ANESTHESIA Pain relief given for the purpose of treatment or surgery. It can be administered as gas or injection that leads to unconsciousness (general anesthesia), or by injection in or around the affected part (local anesthesia).

ANEURYSM A dilation (widening) of a blood vessel as a result of a weakening in its wall.

ANGINA A cramplike pain often felt in the chest, arms, and legs that results from narrowing of the arteries. This narrowing starves the heart muscle of oxygen.

ANGIOGRAM An X-ray picture of blood vessels made after the injection of a contrast medium.

ANOREXIA NERVOSA An emotional disorder in which an abnormal drive to be thin leads to self-starvation, emaciation, and even death. The disorder is most often found in adolescents, predominantly in girls. Compare with bulimia.

ANTACID A medicine that neutralizes the effects of stomach acid.

ANTIBIOTIC Drug that acts against bacteria and other infecting organisms. Antibiotics are derived from naturally occurring substances made by other organisms. Examples include penicillin and tetracycline.

ANTIBODY A protein produced in the blood that attaches itself to invading organisms (or other foreign substances), making the foreign substances susceptible to destruction by immune system cells, especially phagocytes.

ANTICOAGULANT Any drug that delays or prevents coagulation (clotting) of the blood.

ANTICONVULSANT A drug that is used to prevent seizures.

ANTIGEN A substance that triggers the immune system into producing antibodies. *See* antibody.

ANTIHISTAMINE A drug that counteracts the effects of histamine in the body.

AORTA The main vessel in the arterial network.

AORTIC VALVE The heart valve between the left ventricle and the aorta.

APHASIA Loss of ability to speak or understand speech or the meaning of words.

APPENDECTOMY Surgical removal of an appendix.

ARTERIOGRAM An X-ray picture of arteries taken with the help of a radiopaque medium.

ARTERIOLE The smallest vessel of the arterial system.

ARTERY Blood vessels carrying oxygen-rich blood from the heart to the tissues.

ARTHRITIS Inflammation leading to pain and swelling of joints.

ARTIFICIAL INSEMINATION The insertion of sperm into the vagina or uterus by mechanical means rather than by sexual intercourse.

ASBESTOSIS Lung disease resulting from the effects of inhaled asbestos.

ASPHYXIA Lack of oxygen in the blood due to restricted respiration. Strangulation, inhalation of toxic fumes, and drowning are possible causes.

ASPIRIN A valuable mild painkiller and anti-inflammatory drug that works by blocking the production of prostaglandins. Aspirin reduces the risk or severity of thrombosis.

ASTHMA Respiratory disorder caused by narrowing of the bronchial tubes, leading to breathlessness and wheezing.

ASTIGMATISM Nonspherical curvature of the cornea causing visual blurring that is most severe in a particular meridian (orientation).

ATHEROMA Soft fatty substance laid down in the walls of the arteries, leading to narrowing, reduced blood flow, and sometimes heart attacks, strokes, or gangrene.

ATHEROSCLEROSIS The most common disease of arteries, featuring hardening of the walls and the deposition of atheroma in the lining. Atherosclerosis is the cause of heart attacks and strokes and is the major cause of death in the western world.

ATHLETE'S FOOT Common chronic fungal infection of the foot, usually found between the toes. Also called tinea pedis.

ATRIUM One of the two (left and right) low-pressure pumping chambers of the heart.

ATROPHY Wasting of an organ or tissue.

ATTENTION DEFICIT DISORDER *See* hyperactivity.

AUTISM A condition in which the sufferer is abnormally self-absorbed, and unable to relate to people or deal with everyday events.

AUTONOMIC NERVOUS SYSTEM The part of the nervous system that controls automatic functions, such as heartbeat and sweating.

AZT The trademark drug used to inhibit HIV.

B

BACTERIA Small, single-celled organisms that cause infection. Bacteria vary in shape, being spheric (cocci), rod-shaped (bacilli), spiral (spirochetes), or comma-shaped (vibrios).

BASAL METABOLIC RATE A measure of the basic level of the body's metabolic processes. The rate is raised by thyroid overactivity and lowered by thyroid underactivity.

BCG (bacille Calmette-Guérin) A form of tuberculosis (TB) bacterium that is able to stimulate immunity without causing disease, and is used as a vaccination against TB.

BEDSORES Painful ulcers that develop on the skin of bedridden patients, such as stroke victims. Also called decubitus ulcers or pressure sores.

BEHAVIOR THERAPY Psychological technique that aims to alter abnormal behavior patterns.

BENIGN Term used to describe tumors that do not spread to other parts of the body. Compare with malignant.

BENZODIAZEPINES A class of drugs used as sedatives and mild tranquilizers and for the short-term treatment of insomnia. They have largely replaced barbiturates for these purposes.

BETA-BLOCKERS A family of drugs that block the effects of epinephrine, principally used to treat heart disorders and high blood pressure.

BILE Greenish-brown fluid produced by the liver that carries away the liver's waste products and helps to break down fats in the small intestine, which it enters via the bile duct.

BILHARZIA *See* schistosomiasis.

BIOPSY A sample of tissue taken from the body for microscopic examination.

BIORHYTHMS Physiological functions that vary over time in a rhythmic way, of which the menstrual cycle is a good example.

BIPOLAR DISORDER A mental disorder that fluctuates between deep depression and excessive elation. Also called manic depression.

BLADDER The hollow, muscular organ in the pelvis that acts as a reservoir for urine.

BLOOD CLOTTING The vital mechanism whereby components of the blood solidify after any damage, thereby stopping bleeding.

BLOOD GROUPS A system of classifying blood according to the identifying chemical markers on the red blood cells. Classification is vital in order to ensure compatibility for blood transfusion, thereby avoiding adverse reaction.

BLOOD PRESSURE The pressure of blood in the larger arteries. The peak pressure with each heartbeat is called the systolic pressure, and the running pressure between beats is called the diastolic pressure. It is written as, for instance 120/80. These figures are of pressure in terms of the height in millimeters of a column of mercury. Blood pressure is a function of the force of the heart muscle contraction as affected by the resistance offered by the arteries.

BLUE BABY A baby born with a heart defect that results in a lack of oxygen in the blood and a characteristic bluish complexion.

BM STRIP A simple test for blood sugar levels used by many diabetics.

BOIL An abscess in the skin, usually arising from a hair follicle infected with the bacterium *Staphyloccocus aureus*.

BOTULISM A rare but highly dangerous form of food poisoning caused by the toxin produced by the bacterium *Clostridium botulinum*, which thrives in improperly canned or improperly preserved foods.

BRADYCARDIA An abnormally slow heartbeat, which in an adult is anything below 60 beats per minute.

BREAST PUMP An electric or hand pump used to express milk from a nursing mother.

BREATHLESSNESS Shortness of breath leading to rapid conscious breathing.

BREECH BIRTH Birth where the baby is born feet, knees, or buttocks first.

BRONCHIAL TUBES The airways that connect the trachea to the lungs.

BRONCHIECTASIS Persistent infection in the lungs due to destruction of lung tissue.

BRONCHITIS Inflammation of the bronchial tubes, characterized by coughing and difficulty in breathing.

BRONCHOGRAM X ray using contrast medium to outline the bronchial tubes.

BRONCHOSCOPE Instrument for looking into the lungs via the trachea and bronchial tubes.

BUBONIC PLAGUE The most common form of plague, characterized by painful buboes (large inflammatory swellings) and fever.

BUERGER'S DISEASE A disease causing blockages in arteries of the legs and arms that may lead to gangrene and loss of limbs. It occurs mainly in young men who smoke.

BULIMIA Disorder characterized by gross overeating, and often followed by self-induced vomiting. Associated with anorexia nervosa.

BUNION Inflammation and painful swelling over the joint at the base of the big toe.

BURN Any area of tissue that is destroyed or damaged by heat, electricity, chemicals, gases, or radiation.

BURSA (pl. bursae) Fibrous, fluid-filled sac acting as a cushion between some tendons, or the skin and bones beneath them.

BYSSINOSIS A respiratory disease primarily affecting workers in the cotton industry. Caused by inhalation of cotton-fiber dust.

C

CALCIFICATION The accumulation of calcium in tissue; a normal process in bone.

CALORIE A unit used by dieticians to express the amount of energy taken into the body from digested food. A calorie is defined as the amount of heat that will raise 1,000 ml (1 liter) of water by 1 degree Celsius. In physics, a calorie is the amount of heat that will raise 1 ml of water by 1 degree Celsius.

CANCER Any sort of malignant tumor that spreads by setting up new foci of tumor (metastases) in different parts of the body instead of being confined to where it grew.

CAPILLARIES The tiny blood vessels that connect the arterioles to the venules, and the sites at which the contents of the blood pass through to the tissues.

CARBOHYDRATE One of the three basic food types. Carbohydrates are the sugars and starches (chemical combinations of sugars) found in cereals and potatoes.

CARBUNCLE A large boil with numerous pockets of pus.

CARCINOGEN Any cancer-causing substance.

CARCINOID SYNDROME A rare condition characterized by facial flushes and diarrhea, caused by an intestinal or lung tumor called a carcinoid.

CARCINOMA The most common form of tumor, occurring in the lining membrane of such organs as the lungs, breasts, and stomach. Compare with sarcoma.

CARDIAC ARREST A cessation of the heart's pumping action. The most common cause is heart attack, but other causes are anaphylactic shock, hypothermia, and electric shock.

CARDIOVASCULAR Of or pertaining to the heart and blood vessels.

CARRIER A person who has an infectious disease without having any of its symptoms, and who is able to transmit the disease to other people.

CARTILAGE Gristly connective tissue that forms an important part of the skeletal system, such as the joints.

CAT SCAN (computerized tomography; or computerized assisted tomography) An X-ray technique that creates detailed pictures of the body's internal structures by producing detailed images of tissue composition in cross section.

CATARACT An area of opaque tissue that develops in the internal lens of the eye and impairs sight.

CATARRH An increase in mucus, usually due to inflammation of the mucous membrane.

CATATONIA Extreme muscular immobility suffered by some patients with schizophrenia.

CATHETER Any tube passed into the body for diagnostic or treatment purposes.

CELIAC DISEASE A condition leading to malabsorption of food from the intestines, caused by sensitivity of the intestinal lining to gluten. Also called sprue.

CEREBELLUM The part of the brain that coordinates movement and maintains balance.

CEREBRAL HEMORRHAGE Bleeding into the brain, causing stroke.

CEREBRAL PALSY Disturbance in the function of the brain and nervous system as a result of injury often caused through lack of oxygen during birth.

CEREBROSPINAL FLUID Fluid that bathes and cushions the brain and spinal cord.

CEREBRUM The largest, uppermost, and most complex part of the brain, dealing with the sensory, motor, and intellectual functions, including speech and memory.

CERVICAL SMEAR A specimen taken from the secretions and superficial cells of the cervix for laboratory investigation.

CERVIX Any neck, but usually the neck of the uterus, which is the central channel which opens during labor to allow childbirth.

CESAREAN SECTION Surgery to remove a baby from the uterus through an incision in the abdominal wall.

CHEMOTHERAPY The use of chemical compounds to destroy cancer cells.

CHICKEN POX An extremely infectious disease common during childhood, of which the symptoms include a rash of fluid-filled spots.

CHILBLAINS Hot, red, itchy patches of skin on toes or fingers caused by exposure to cold.

CHIROPODY Care of the feet, with particular emphasis on the care of nails and the removal of hard skin, corns, warts, and calluses.

CHIROPRACTIC A therapy based on the belief that an individual's health is directly related to the condition of his or her spinal column. Treatment does not include drugs or surgery, but centers on the manipulation of the patient's spine. A practitioner is termed a chiropractor.

CHOLANGITIS Inflammation of the bile ducts.

CHOLECYSTECTOMY Surgery to remove the gallbladder.

CHOLECYSTITIS Inflammation of the gallbladder.

CHOLECYSTOGRAM An X-ray picture of the gallbladder.

CHOLERA An acute bacterial infection of the small intestine, characterized by diarrhea and vomiting, and caused by ingestion of foods and drinks that have been contaminated with the feces of those infected with the bacterium.

CHOLESTEROL A fatty substance that is essential to the structure of cell walls. However, when present in the blood in excessive quantities (usually owing to a diet too rich in animal fats), it is laid down in the walls of arteries, causing atheroma. Cholesterol can also crystallize as gallstones in the bladder.

CHROMOSOMES Threadlike structures within the cell nucleus that carry genetic information. Humans have 23 pairs of chromosomes, plus one pair of sex chromosomes.

CHRONIC Term used to describe an illness that persists over a long period of time.

CIRCUMCISION Removal of the foreskin from the penis, for religious or health reasons, or both.

CIRRHOSIS Liver disease resulting from a continuing process of liver cell destruction.

CLEFT PALATE Congenital abnormality of the palate in which the two sides of the palate fail to fuse, leaving a gap between them.

CLINICAL PATHOLOGY The laboratory-based study of disease.

CLITORIS A small erectile organ on the exterior of the vulva, analogous to the penis.

CLUBFOOT Deformity of the foot present from birth in which the sole is turned inward. Medical name is talipes.

COAGULATION The process in which blood solidifies to form a clot.

COLD SORE A painful sore on the lips that usually arises when the immune system is under stress, for example, during a cold. Caused by the herpes simplex virus.

COLIC An attack of pain in the abdomen that comes in waves.

COLITIS Painful inflammation of the large intestine (colon) leading to diarrhea and occasional bleeding.

COLON The tube stretching from the end of the small intestine through to the rectum. Also called large intestine.

COLOR BLINDNESS Inability to distinguish between some colors, most commonly between red and green.

COLOSTOMY The temporary or permanent surgical rerouting of the colon through the abdominal wall in order to create an artificial anus—used to relieve a blockage in the intestine, such as a cancerous growth.

COMA A state of profound unconsciousness, commonly brought on by head injuries, blood clots, poisoning, or strokes.

COMPOUND FRACTURE A fracture that breaks through the skin.

CONCEPTION The fertilization of the ovum by the sperm, leading to embryo formation.

CONCUSSION A brief loss of consciousness owing to a head injury; often followed by temporarily disturbed vision and loss of memory.

CONDOM A sheath slipped over the erect penis to prevent conception and transmission of STDs such as HIV.

CONGENITAL Term used to describe disease or abnormality which is present from birth, but which is not necessarily hereditary.

CONGESTIVE CARDIAC FAILURE Inefficient heart action that leads to a buildup of pressure in the veins and lungs, resulting in breathlessness and edema.

CONJUNCTIVA The mucous membrane lining the inner surface of the eyelids and the white part of the eyeball.

CONJUNCTIVITIS Inflammation of the conjunctiva due to infection or allergy, causing red eyes and a thick discharge.

CONNECTIVE TISSUE The basic cement and packaging of the body that holds the organs in place and fills spaces. Fibers of the protein collagen provide strength; the protein elastin provides elasticity.

CONSTIPATION Difficulty in passing feces, usually because they are too hard and dry.

CONTAGIOUS Term used to describe a disease that can be contracted from other people by physical contact.

CONTRACEPTION Any method of preventing pregnancy.

CONTRAST MEDIUM A radiopaque substance injected into the body in order to enhance detail on X rays.

CONVULSION A seizure. Sudden involuntary spasms, with or without loss of consciousness, due to abnormal cerebral stimulation.

CORNEA The transparent outer lens of the eye.

CORONARY THROMBOSIS The blockage of a coronary (heart) artery with a clot, leading to a heart attack.

CORPUS LUTEUM The yellowish mass of tissue that forms at the point of rupture after the ovary releases an egg. It produces the sex hormone progesterone.

CORTISONE A hormone produced by the adrenal glands.

CPR (cardiopulmonary resuscitation) A resuscitation technique used both to support the circulation after the heart has stopped beating, and to stimulate the heart back into action. Also called heart massage.

CREUTZFELDT-JAKOB DISEASE (CJD) An uncommon but inevitably fatal spongy degeneration of the brain caused by a protein molecule called a prion that can be acquired by eating beef from animals suffering from bovine spongiform encephalopathy (BSE).

CRIB DEATH The sudden, unexplained death of an apparently healthy baby. Also called sudden infant death syndrome.

CROUP Acute viral infection of the respiratory tract in children, causing fever and a characteristic harsh cough.

CRYOSURGERY Surgery carried out by destroying tissue with cold temperatures, or otherwise using low-temperature objects as surgical instruments.

CURETTAGE Scraping out of any hollow space, such as an abscess cavity.

CYST Any abnormal fluid-filled cavity.

CYSTIC FIBROSIS Hereditary disease, appearing in infancy and characterized by excessive mucus, breathing difficulties, and abnormal secretion and function of many of the other secretory glands of the body.

CYSTITIS A painful inflammatory infection of the bladder.

CYSTOGRAM An X-ray picture of the bladder.

CYSTOSCOPY Looking into the bladder using a special narrow optical viewing tube passed through the urethra.

CYTOLOGY The study of cells, particularly the microscopic examination of cells in such substances as sputum, cervical smears, and urine, to see if cancer cells are present.

CYTOTOXIC Term used to describe drugs that destroy cancerous cells.

D

D & C (dilatation and curettage) Surgery to scrape away the lining of the uterus.

DANDRUFF Scaling of the scalp. Acute dandruff is called seborrheic dermatitis.

DECONGESTANT A drug used to reduce congestion of the air passages.

DEEP VEIN THROMBOSIS A clot in the deep veins of the legs, causing swelling and discoloration of the skin. It may cause a life-threatening pulmonary embolism.

DEFIBRILLATOR A machine that delivers an electric shock to the chest in an attempt to reestablish proper rhythm of the heartbeat.

DEHYDRATION Excessive loss of fluid from the body, normally accompanied by an imbalance in the levels of sodium, potassium, and chloride.

DELIRIUM A state of altered consciousness in which a patient is unaware of his or her surroundings, or finds them strange or frightening—usually brought about by fever, shock, or drug abuse.

DELIRIUM TREMENS (DTs) Acute reaction caused by cessation of excessive intake of alcohol over a long period of time.

DEMENTIA A state of disordered brain function due to generalized loss of brain cells, often in old age. Memory is lost early, and in the final stages of dementia patients may be completely disoriented, unable to care for themselves, and incontinent.

DENTAL CARIES Tooth decay caused by bacterial action, and prevented by effective dental hygiene.

DERMATITIS Inflammation of the skin.

DERMATOLOGY The branch of medicine concerned with diseases of the skin.

DIABETES One of two conditions that cause excessive urination, but "diabetes" usually refers to diabetes mellitus.

DIABETES INSIPIDUS A metabolic disorder caused by deficient production of the antidiuretic hormone (called ADH), or by the failure of the kidney to respond to ADH.

DIABETES MELLITUS Complex metabolic disorder primarily caused by deficient production of insulin in the pancreas.

DIAGNOSIS The identification of disease based on observation of the patient's signs and symptoms. Compare with prognosis.

DIALYSIS Artificial method of taking over the function of the kidneys in order to keep the blood free from waste products, or to purify it of poisons and drugs.

DIAPHRAGM The sheet of muscle that forms a barrier between the contents of the chest and those of the abdomen.

DIARRHEA Increased frequency of defecation with liquid or unformed stools.

DIASTOLE The period during which the heart is relaxing between heartbeats. Compare with systole.

DIASTOLIC PRESSURE See blood pressure.

DIPHTHERIA An acute infectious disease characterized by the formation of a membrane in the throat that can obstruct breathing.

DIPLOPIA Double vision.

DIURETIC A drug prompting increased urine production.

DIVERTICULUM (pl. diverticula) Any pouchlike outward protrusion from a tubular or saccular organ such as the bladder, stomach, or intestine.

DNA (deoxyribonucleic acid) The genetic material that is passed from generation to generation in the chromosomes.

DOWN SYNDROME The most common chromosome abnormality, in which there are three number 21 chromosomes instead of just two. The condition is characterized by mental retardation and multiple defects. Formerly called mongolism.

DUCTUS ARTERIOSUS The vascular channel in the fetus that bypasses the lungs by joining the left pulmonary artery to the aorta. It generally closes after birth when the oxygen supply is provided by the lungs.

DUODENAL ULCER A breakdown in the lining of the duodenum due to the effects of stomach acid.

DUODENUM The first segment of the small intestine as it leaves the stomach.

DWARFISM Abnormal shortness of stature.

DYSENTERY Severe diarrhea due to an infection, often with blood present in the matter evacuated.

DYSLEXIA A pathological impairment of the ability to read.

DYSMENORRHEA Severe menstrual pains.

DYSPAREUNIA Pain during sexual intercourse.

DYSPEPSIA Indigestion; usually resulting from the effects of stomach acid.

DYSPNEA Breathlessness; often a symptom of heart and lung disease.

DYSURIA Pain during the passing of urine; often a symptom of an infection of the urethra.

E

ECG (Electrocardiogram) A graph showing the sequence of electrical changes occurring in the heart during a succession of heartbeats. Characteristic changes in the graph are helpful in diagnosing heart disorders.

ECHOCARDIOGRAM An ultrasound technique used to build up a moving picture of the heart.

ECLAMPSIA A rare complication of pregnancy characterized by high blood pressure and seizures.

ECT (electroconvulsive therapy) An electric shock to the brain given under anesthesia in order to produce a convulsion. Used to relieve symptoms of clinical depression.

ECTOPIC PREGNANCY A pregnancy developing outside the uterus, usually in one of the fallopian tubes.

ECZEMA Any superficial dermatitis, characterized by a red, scaly, itchy, and sometimes weeping skin rash.

EDEMA Any swelling of tissues due to an increase in fluid content.

EEG (electroencephalogram) A multi-channel recording of the electrical activity of the brain.

ELECTROLYTES Soluble mineral compounds that conduct electric currents, of which the body has a large number. These include sodium, potassium, calcium, magnesium, and chloride, and they must be kept within narrow limits for the normal function of cells, especially nerve cells.

ELECTROLYTES AND UREA The name of a common blood test whereby the levels of important minerals (electrolytes) in the body are measured, also the level of urea.

ELEPHANTIASIS Massive swelling of the legs or areas of the trunk or head due to blockage of the lymph vessels by a tiny worm called *Wuchereria bancrofti*.

EMBOLISM The result of a blood vessel's becoming blocked by an embolus.

EMBOLUS A foreign object, usually part of a thrombus, a tumor, or other tissue, or a mass of air, that drifts in the bloodstream until it becomes lodged in a blood vessel. *See also* embolism.

EMBRYO The early stages of a baby's development in the uterus, from the second week or so after conception until the seventh or eighth week of pregnancy. Compare with fetus.

EMPHYSEMA A chronic lung disease, resulting from overenlargement of the lung's air spaces, that causes the destruction of the lung tissue.

ENCEPHALITIS (pl. encephalides) Inflammation of the brain.

ENDEMIC Term used to describe a disease that is native to a particular area or population. Compare with epidemic, epizootic, and pandemic.

ENDOCARDITIS Infection on the inner surface of the heart, usually occurring only when there is already some minor abnormality of structure.

ENDOCRINE SYSTEM The system of endocrine glands (pituitary, thyroid, parathyroid, and adrenal) that produces the body's hormones.

ENDOSCOPY Examination of any part of the interior of the body by a narrow rigid, or flexible optical viewing device which is introduced via a natural anatomical opening or through a short incision.

ENDOTRACHEAL TUBE A tube that is passed into the windpipe to enable artificial ventilation by means of a respirator.

ENEMA Fluid passed into the rectum by syringe in order to help treat constipation.

ENTERITIS Infection of the intestines, leading to diarrhea and abdominal colic.

ENURESIS Passing urine without control, usually during sleep—a condition that occurs commonly in childhood.

ENZYMES Protein catalysts necessary for the innumerable biochemical reactions that occur in living cells and elsewhere in the body. Almost all the genes are codes for the production of enzymes.

EPIDEMIC A widespread outbreak of an infectious disease. Compare with endemic, epizootic, and pandemic.

EPILEPSY A disease of the nervous system that causes recurrent convulsions due to an overwhelming electrical discharge in the brain.

EPINEPHRINE A hormone produced by the adrenal glands that has many effects that together produce a bodily state appropriate for coping with sudden physical emergency. The hormone is produced synthetically as a treatment for cardiac arrest, anaphylactic shock, and acute asthma. It is also known as adrenaline.

EPISIOTOMY A cut made to widen the external opening of the vagina in order to ease childbirth.

EPIZOOTIC An outbreak of infectious disease that spreads through an entire species of animal in the same geographic area.

ESOPHAGUS The muscular canal that leads from the back of the throat down to the stomach.

ESTROGEN One of the two important female hormones. Variations in estrogen levels occur during the menstrual cycle and are responsible for many of the changes that occur in the uterus.

EUSTACHIAN TUBE The tube that connects the middle ear (the part of the ear inside the eardrum) to the back of the throat.

EXFOLIATION The process whereby cells are lost from the surface of any lining or surface layer, such as the lining of the gut or the skin.

EXPECTORANT A drug (e.g., acetylcysteine) designed to promote expectoration.

EXPECTORATION The ejection of mucus, sputum, and other fluids from the lungs by coughing or spitting.

F

FALLOPIAN TUBES The two tubes arising out of the uterus and ending near the ovaries through which eggs produced in the ovaries normally pass on their way to the womb. Also called oviducts.

FAMILY PLANNING Strategic contraception.

FAT One of the three basic food types. It is the most concentrated provider of energy, and is stored in the body as adipose tissue.

FECES The residue after the nutrient value of food has been absorbed by the small intestine—ejected from the body through the anus.

FERTILIZATION The process whereby a sperm enters an egg and fuses with it to start the process of cell division that may end in the production of an embryo.

FETUS Human conceptus growing in the uterus—usually so called from the seventh or eighth week of pregnancy. Compare with embryo.

FEVER A high body temperature, above the normal 98.6°F (37°C). Most infectious illnesses cause fever, which is a sign that the body's temperature-regulating mechanism has been reset by the infection.

FIBROIDS Benign fibromuscular tumors which grow in the uterus, and which may cause heavy menstruation and disturbances in urination.

FIBROSING ALVEOLITIS A disease whereby the alveoli of the lungs become closed by scar tissue so that they no longer allow oxygen to pass into the blood.

FIBROSIS A proliferation of fibrous connective tissue, as part of the formation of scar tissue after injury or infection, or other tissue disease.

FISSURE A split in the skin or other surface.

FISTULA An abnormal channel leading from one body cavity to another, or from an internal organ to the skin.

FLATULENCE The presence of excessive gas in the stomach or intestines.

FOLLICLE A small sac or tubular gland.

FONTANELLES The gaps between the developing bones of a baby's skull—covered and protected by soft membranous tissue and skin.

FORAMEN An opening, usually referring to the opening in a bone through which blood vessels or nerves pass.

FORCEPS Instrument used during surgery that picks up tissue in a pincerlike fashion. Obstetric forceps are used to assist in difficult births.

FORENSIC MEDICINE The branch of pathology that deals with unnatural or criminal injury or deaths.

FORMALIN Solution of formaldehyde in water used for preserving tissue after removal for examination.

FRACTURE Term used to describe an injury to a bone in which the continuity of the tissue is broken.

FROSTBITE Traumatic tissue injury due to cold.

FROZEN SECTION Tissue taken during surgery on which a very rapid microscopic examination is carried out in order to determine the course of the operation.

FUNGAL INFECTION An inflammatory infection caused by a fungus.

G

GALLBLADDER A saclike organ attached to the liver that collects bile and then discharges it into the intestine in response to a fatty meal.

GANGLION A small fibrous swelling on the wrist or the back of the hand. Also the knots of nervous tissue that act as relay stations in the nervous system.

GANGRENE Death of tissue following a breakdown in the blood supply.

GASTRECTOMY The surgical removal of the stomach.

GASTRIC ULCER A break in the inner lining of the stomach, usually resulting from the effects of stomach acid.

GASTRITIS Inflammation of the mucosa of the stomach, causing indigestion and vomiting.

GASTROENTEROLOGY The branch of medicine concerning the stomach, intestines, liver, and pancreas.

GASTROSCOPY Inspection of the inside of the stomach and duodenum using a flexible endoscope passed through the mouth.

GENES The biological units that determine inherited characteristics such as eye color. Each characteristic is controlled by one or more genes passed on from one's parents.

GENETICS The study of genes and inherited characteristics and diseases.

GERIATRICS Branch of medical and social science dealing with the health of the elderly.

GERMAN MEASLES *See* rubella.

GINGIVITIS Inflammation of the gums.

GLAND Any organ that produces a secretion.

GLANDULAR FEVER *See* infectious mononucleosis.

GLAUCOMA An eye disease caused by excessive pressure of fluid in the eye, which may lead to loss of sight.

GLUCOSE A simple sugar that is the main source of energy for the body's cells.

GLUTEN A protein constituent of wheat and wheat products, and the constituent responsible for producing celiac disease.

GLYCOGEN A form of glucose stored in the liver and muscles and released as needed for energy.

GOITER A visible swelling of the thyroid gland.

GONORRHEA A sexually transmitted

disease that produces a greenish-yellow urethral or vaginal discharge.

GOUT Swollen painful joints. Gout especially affects the joint at the base of the big toe, and is caused by excessive accumulation of uric acid.

GRAFT Transfer of a piece of tissue to another site, or replacement of diseased tissue with tissue from another individual. Artificial tissue may also be used.

GRAND MAL SEIZURE Epileptic convulsion characterized by jerking movements and loss of consciousness. Compare with petit mal seizure.

GRANULOMA Term used by pathologists to describe some forms of localized inflammation or infection.

GREENSTICK FRACTURE A partial fracture of a child's bone, which, because the bone is so pliable, splits rather than breaks.

GROUP THERAPY Treatment of psychological problems by discussion within a group of people and under the direction of a trained therapist.

GROWTHS Popularly used to refer to tumors both benign and malignant.

GYNECOLOGIST A specialist in the diseases of the female reproductive system.

H

HALITOSIS Bad- or foul-smelling breath.

HALLUCINATION An imaginary sensation perceived through any of the five senses—the result of drug use, alcohol withdrawal, severe illness, or schizophrenia.

HALLUCINOGENIC Term describing a drug that produces hallucinations.

HAMMERTOE A common deformity usually affecting the second toe (the one next to the big toe) in which the toe is permanently flexed in a clawlike position.

HAMSTRING MUSCLE The group of three muscles at the back of the thigh.

HAY FEVER Runny nose and coldlike symptoms owing to pollen allergy.

HEART ATTACK A sudden, acutely painful, distressing, and often fatal event in which part of the heart muscle is deprived of its blood supply and dies, because of blockage of a branch of one of the coronary arteries. In those who survive, the dead tissue is replaced by scar tissue but the heart is usually weakened in its pumping power.

HEARTBURN A burning sensation behind the sternum, caused by stomach acid in the esophagus.

HEART FAILURE A condition in which the heart can no longer pump enough blood to meet the metabolic requirements of the body.

HEART MASSAGE *See* CPR.

HEART MURMUR Any of several sounds heard in addition to the regular heartbeat.

HEAT EXHAUSTION Condition caused by loss of body fluids due to prolonged exposure to high temperature, causing cramps, nausea, and finally loss of consciousness. Compare with heatstroke.

HEATSTROKE The medical term for sunstroke. A severe and sometimes fatal condition resulting from the collapse of the body's ability to regulate its temperature, due to prolonged exposure to hot sunshine or high temperatures. Also called heat hyperprexia.

HEMATOMA A trapped mass of blood in the tissues of an organ or in the skin.

HEMATURIA Blood in the urine.

HEMIPLEGIA Paralysis of one half of the body.

HEMODIALYSIS The use of a kidney machine to remove waste products from the blood after a patient's kidneys have ceased functioning.

HEMOGLOBIN The oxygen-carrying substance in red blood cells.

HEMOPHILIA An inherited disorder of blood clotting due to absence of one of the factors needed for clotting (factor VIII). Generally only males are affected, though females may be carriers.

HEMORRHAGE Medical term for bleeding.

HEMORRHOIDS Varicosity in the blood vessels of the anus that can give rise to bleeding and discomfort. Also called piles.

HEPATITIS Inflammation of the liver, usually caused by one of the hepatitis viruses.

HERNIA A weakness in the muscular wall of the abdomen that allows tissue (often the small intestine) to push through.

HERPES A group of viruses responsible for cold sores, chicken pox, shingles, and genital sores.

HIATUS HERNIA Condition in which the stomach pushes up through the diaphragm through the hole occupied by the gullet.

HIV (human immunodeficiency virus) The retrovirus that causes AIDS.

HODGKIN'S DISEASE Cancerlike disease of the lymph nodes.

HOMEOPATHY Treatment of disease involving minute doses of a substance that produces symptoms similar to those of the disease itself.

HORMONE One of the complex chemicals produced in the body that regulate the body's metabolism and functions.

HORMONE REPLACEMENT THERAPY (HRT) Synthetic or natural hormones that were used to counteract hormonal deficiency during menopause. HRT carries a slightly higher risk of heart disease, strokes, and breast cancer.

HYDATID DISEASE A disease caused by larval forms of tapeworms, and characterized by cysts in the liver and other organs.

HYDROCEPHALUS Increase in volume of the cerebrospinal fluid within the brain's ventricles. In children it may lead to enlargement of the head, and it is often associated with spina bifida.

HYMEN The thin membrane which partly covers the entrance to the vagina, and which may be torn or stretched during first sexual intercourse or by the use of tampons.

HYPERACTIVITY A term used to describe excessive activity in children, associated with brain damage, epilepsy, and psychiatric trouble, but only very rarely with food allergy. Also known as attention deficit hyperactivity disorder.

HYPERSENSITIVITY Tendency to experience allergic reactions, especially to drugs.

HYPERTENSION Raised blood pressure, which puts extra strain on the heart and arteries, thereby increasing the risk of heart attacks, strokes, and kidney damage.

HYPERTHYROIDISM Overactivity of the thyroid gland that can lead to weight loss, tremor, protrusion of the eyes, hyperactivity, moist skin, and jumpiness.

HYPERTROPHY Abnormal enlargement of an organ or tissue in order to meet extra demands made on it by the body.

HYPERVENTILATION Abnormally rapid breathing, leading to dizziness, tingling in the hands, or even loss of consciousness.

HYPOCHONDRIA Neurotic preoccupation with one's own health and with disease.

HYPODERMIC Term meaning literally "under the skin," as in hypodermic injections.

HYPOGLYCEMIA An abnormally low level of sugar in the blood, causing such symptoms as confusion, coma, trembling, and sweating, and even death.

HYPOTENSION Low blood pressure.

HYPOTHALAMUS The area at the base of the brain that controls many of the body's automatic and hormone-related activities.

HYPOTHERMIA Abnormally low body

temperature—below 95°F (35°C)—usually caused by prolonged exposure to cold, and leading to a faint heart rate, pallor, and eventual collapse.

HYPOTHYROIDISM Underactivity of the thyroid gland, leading to weight gain and thick, dry skin.

HYPOXIA A low level of oxygen in the tissues as a result of lung or heart disease.

HYSTERECTOMY Removal of the uterus.

I

IATROGENIC Term used to describe a condition caused by medical treatment.

ICHTHYOSIS A skin condition in which the skin is abnormally thick and scaly.

IDIOPATHIC Denoting a disease or symptom of which the cause is unknown.

ILEOSTOMY Surgery performed to bring the end of the ileum onto the surface of the abdomen, creating a stoma through which intestinal contents can be discharged.

ILEUM Medical term for the small intestine. Absorbs nutrients.

ILEUS Obstruction of the ileum.

IMMUNE SYSTEM The complex system by which the body defends itself against infection.

IMMUNIZATION Preparing the body to fight and prevent an infection through the injection of material from the infecting organism, or by using an attenuated (non-disease-causing) strain of the organism itself.

IMMUNOGLOBULIN See antibody.

IMMUNOSUPPRESSIVE DRUGS Drugs that suppress the immune system.

IMPACTED TEETH Teeth that are jammed in position beneath the gum and thereby fail to grow from the jaw into the mouth properly.

IMPETIGO An acute staphylococcal skin infection characterized by pustules and yellowish crusts.

IMPOTENCE Failure to achieve or sustain an erection of the penis.

IN VITRO FERTILIZATION (IVF) A method of enabling women who are unable to conceive to bear children by fertilizing egg cells with sperm outside the body ("in vitro" literally means "in glass," i.e., in an artificial environment), and then inserting some of the fertilized eggs in the uterus. Popularly called test-tube babies.

INCONTINENCE Failure to control the bladder or bowel movements, or both.

INCUBATION PERIOD The period between exposure to a contagious or similar infection and the first appearance of any symptoms of the disease.

INDIGESTION A nonmedical term used to describe pain, discomfort, and other symptoms arising from the stomach or intestines after the intake of food.

INDUCTION (OF LABOR) Procedure in which labor is started artificially.

INFARCTION Tissue damage due to a blockage in blood supply.

INFECTIOUS MONONUCLEOSIS Viral infection causing swollen lymph nodes and a sore throat. Also called glandular fever.

INFERTILITY Inability of a couple to conceive and reproduce after a reasonable period of time (about a year to 18 months).

INFLAMMATION A reaction of the body's tissues to injury or illness, characterized by redness, heat, swelling, and pain—a mechanism of defense and repair.

INGROWN TOENAIL Inflammation of the soft tissues at the edge of the nail with swelling, so that the tissue extends over the edges of the nail, causing an appearance of ingrowing. Nail edges never grow sideways.

INHALERS Aerosol or powder-dispersing containers that release doses of drugs for inhalation—used in the treatment of asthma and other respiratory disorders.

INOCULATION Administration of a vaccine in order to produce immunization.

INSULIN A hormone secreted in the pancreas that regulates blood sugar levels.

INTENSIVE CARE UNIT (ICU) A hospital unit that provides specialized treatment for severe medical and surgical disorders.

INTERFERON A protein produced by the body cells when triggered by a virus infection—used as a drug to treat certain diseases.

INTERTRIGO Irritated skin in body folds, such as under the breasts.

INTESTINES The long continuous tube connecting stomach to anus. The first part (small intestine or ileum) absorbs nutrients; the second (large intestine or colon) processes the waste.

INTRAUTERINE DEVICE (IUD) A small device inserted into the uterus in order to prevent pregnancy.

INTRAVENOUS (IV) Within or into a vein.

IRRADIATION Exposure to any form of radiant energy, such as light, heat, and X rays, for therapeutic or diagnostic purposes.

IRRIGATION The process of washing out a wound or body cavity—for example, the colon—with fluid.

IRRITABLE BOWEL SYNDROME A common condition that is characterized by episodes of abdominal pain and disturbance of the intestines (constipation or diarrhea). Also called irritable or spastic colon.

ISCHEMIA Condition in which tissue receives an inadequate blood supply.

ISOTOPE SCANNING A diagnostic technique based on the detection of radiation emitted by radioactive isotopes introduced into the body. Also called radionuclide scanning.

J

JAUNDICE Yellowness of the skin most commonly due to liver conditions, such as hepatitis, in which bile does not pass through the liver properly, resulting in its accumulation in the blood.

JUGULAR LINE A fine tube placed in the jugular vein for the purpose of measuring pressure in the heart (jugular venous pressure, or JVP) and giving drugs.

JUGULAR VEINS The veins that drain blood from the head.

K

KELOID An excessive thickening of skin around a scar.

KERATIN The protein that makes up the outer layers of the skin, nails, and hair.

KERATITIS Inflammation of the cornea.

KETONES Acid waste products from the burning of fats by the body's cells.

KIDNEY FAILURE Malfunction of the kidneys, causing waste products such as urea to accumulate in the blood.

KIDNEY MACHINE A machine that artificially cleans the blood of waste products using a process called dialysis.

KNOCK-KNEE A deformity in which the legs bend inward at the knees so that they knock each other on walking. Medical name is genu valgum.

KWASHIORKOR A disease in children caused by a protein-deficient diet, resulting in retarded growth, edema, lassitude, and diarrhea. It is common in most parts of Africa.

KYPHOSIS Outward curvature of the dorsal part of the spine.

L

LABOR The process of childbirth, which starts with the first contractions of the uterus proceeding to full opening of

the neck of the uterus (first stage), then the birth of the baby (second stage), and ends with the passage of the placenta from the uterus.

LACTATION Milk production by the breasts.

LAMINECTOMY Surgical removal of the arch of a vertebra to gain access to the spinal cord. It is usually performed to treat injury, or remove a tumor or slipped disk.

LANOLIN A naturally occurring substance that softens and lubricates skin.

LAPAROSCOPY The use of a special endoscope that is passed through the abdominal wall in order to view the abdominal organs.

LAPAROTOMY Surgical incision to open the abdominal cavity. In practice, the term means an exploratory operation for diagnostic purposes.

LARYNGITIS Inflammation of the mucous membrane lining the larynx, caused by an infection or irritation, and accompanied by hoarseness or complete loss of voice.

LARYNX The organ of the voice, sited in the air passage between the pharynx and the trachea.

LASSA FEVER A frequently fatal viral disease occurring in sub-Saharan Africa.

LAVAGE The process of washing out hollow organs such as the stomach.

LAXATIVE Medicine that stimulates the intestines to open, relieving constipation.

LAZY EYE Dimmed vision in an eye that otherwise appears structurally normal. Also called amblyopia.

LEAD POISONING The effect of toxic levels of lead present in the body either by ingestion or by inhalation, producing convulsions, weight loss, poor coordination, and mental impairment.

LEGIONNAIRES' DISEASE A bacterial pneumonia caused by infection with the bacterium *Legionella pneumophila*.

LEPROSY A chronic but not especially contagious disease of the skin and nerves produced by the bacterium *Mycobacterium leprae*.

LEPTOSPIROSIS Acute infectious disease caused by the organism *Leptospira interrogans*, and transmitted to humans via the urine of rats and dogs. Symptoms include jaundice and fever. The most serious form is called Weil's disease.

LESION An area of tissue in which the structure and function are altered or impaired owing to injury or disease.

LEUKEMIA A blood disease in which cancerous change in the bone marrow produces abnormal numbers and forms of immature white blood cells.

LEUKOCYTOSIS An excess of white cells in the blood, often due to infection.

LEUKOPENIA A lack of white blood cells, often the result of blood disease or as a side effect of anticancer or other drugs, and causing a reduced resistance to infection.

LEUKOPLAKIA A condition featuring white patches of thickened mucous membrane, especially in the mouth. Can proceed to cancer.

LEUKORRHEA Whitish vaginal discharge.

LEUKOTOMY Surgical removal of some of the connections to the brain's frontal lobes in order to relieve psychiatric symptoms. Also called lobotomy.

LICHEN PLANUS A nonmalignant, chronic skin disease characterized by thick, hardened red patches.

LIGAMENT One of the many strong fibrous bands, usually forming parallel bundles, which hold the bones together at a joint, and which also support the organs.

LIGHT THERAPY Exposure of the skin to infrared and ultraviolet rays for therapeutic purposes, as in the treatment of SAD.

LINCTUS A medicine for the relief of coughs.

LINIMENT An oily preparation rubbed into the skin to relieve pain in the underlying muscle.

LIPOMA A benign fatty tumor.

LIVER The largest gland of the body, situated in the upper right-hand corner of the abdomen just beneath the diaphragm. It is a highly complex gland, with more than 500 functions. These include the production of bile, the conversion and storage of many substances vital for the body's well-being (such as glycogen and urea), and the detoxification of ingested substances, such as alcohol and various drugs.

LIVER FAILURE Inability of the liver to fulfill its function, causing fatigue, anorexia, jaundice, coma, and death.

LIVER FUNCTION TEST A common blood test in which the level of various substances helps to indicate how well the liver is working.

LOBOTOMY *See* leukotomy.

LOCHIA The discharge that flows from the vagina after childbirth.

LORDOSIS An abnormal degree of forward curvature of the lower part of the spine, which results in excessive curvatures elsewhere in the spine.

LOWER-BACK PAIN Ache or pain in the lower back caused by muscular strain or disk trouble.

LUMBAGO *See* lower-back pain.

LUMBAR DISK A condition in which the central part of the disks that lie between the vertebrae bursts or becomes displaced and presses against the nerves of the spinal cord. Also called slipped disk.

LUMBAR PUNCTURE The introduction of a hollow needle into the spinal canal in order to remove cerebrospinal fluid for examination. Also called spinal tap.

LUNG FUNCTION TESTS Diagnostic tests performed to determine the volume of air that can be inhaled into and exhaled from the lungs.

LUPUS ERYTHEMATOSUS A chronic inflammatory disease of the connective tissue, affecting the skin and various internal organs. It is an autoimmune disease. *See* systemic lupus erythematosus.

LYMPH Pale watery fluid which carries, among other things, leukocytes around the body's tissues, and which is filtered by the lymph nodes.

LYMPH NODE A small structure that filters infection; part of the lymphatic system.

LYMPHATIC SYSTEM A network of vessels transferring lymph from the tissue fluids to the bloodstream. Lymph nodes occur at intervals along the lymphatic vessels.

LYMPHOCYTE A type of white blood cell produced in the bone marrow and present mainly in the lymph and blood. Lymphocytes are involved in immunity.

M

MALABSORPTION Failure of the small intestine to absorb nutrients properly.

MALARIA Serious infectious illness common in the tropics, caused by four species of the organism *Plasmodium*, which is passed to humans via an infected anopheles mosquito. Typical symptoms are fever and an enlarged spleen.

MALIGNANT Term used to describe tumors that spread into surrounding tissues and elsewhere in the body. The term is also used to describe other dangerous diseases or states.

MALNUTRITION A nutritional deficiency due to the lack of the basic elements of a balanced diet. Usually brought on by a severe shortage of food, it can also sometimes be caused by inadequate absorption of food or an intake of inappropriate food. The term "malnutrition"

also increasingly refers to the kind of excessive eating that causes obesity.

MALOCCLUSION Improper alignment of the upper and lower teeth on biting.

MAMMOGRAPHY X-ray pictures of the breast, used to help detect tumors.

MANIA A state of excessive and sometimes dangerous excitement, in which patients lack insight into their behavior.

MANIC DEPRESSION *See* bipolar disorder.

MANTOUX TEST A skin test used to determine exposure to infection with tuberculosis.

MARFAN'S SYNDROME An inherited condition causing elongation of the bones, and often accompanied by cardiovascular abnormalities.

MARROW The soft matter found in the middle of bones that plays a vital function in the formation of blood. Also called bone marrow.

MASTECTOMY Surgical removal of a breast, usually in cases of breast cancer.

MASTITIS Inflammation of breast tissue, which may occur soon after the birth of a child (acute mastitis) or which may describe chronic fibrous changes in the breast (chronic mastitis).

MASTOIDITIS Inflammation of the air-containing sinuses in the bone behind the ear.

MEASLES An acute, highly contagious viral disease which occurs principally in childhood, and which is characterized by red eyes, fever, and a rash. Also called morbilli and rubeola.

MECKEL'S DIVERTICULUM A pouch found in the wall of the small intestine in 1 or 2 percent of the population, and usually asymptomatic.

MECONIUM The first feces of a baby, usually dark green or black in color, and consisting of epithelial cells, mucus, and bile.

MEGACOLON Abnormal enlargement of the large intestine, usually as a result of constipation.

MELANIN The black or dark brown pigment that is present in the skin, hair, and eyes.

MEMBRANE Any thin layer of tissue.

MÉNIÈRE'S DISEASE A chronic disease of the inner ear, found in older people and characterized by recurrent deafness, buzzing in the ears, and vertigo.

MENINGES (sing. meninx) The three membranes that surround the brain and spinal cord.

MENINGITIS (pl. meningitides) Any infection of the meninges.

MENOPAUSE The cessation of menses.

MENORRHAGIA Excess menses.

MENSES The flow of blood that occurs during menstruation. Also called period.

MENSTRUATION The period of bleeding as the uterus sheds its lining each month during a woman's reproductive years.

MENTAL RETARDATION A low or very low level of mental ability, which is usually congenital.

METABOLISM The chemical processes that enable the body to work.

METASTASIS (pl. metastases) The process by which tumor cells spread from the site of the original tumor to remote parts of the body. Also the name given to such a secondary tumor.

MICROSURGERY The minute surgical dissection and manipulation of human tissue.

MICTURATING CYSTOGRAM An X-ray picture of the bladder taken while the patient is passing urine.

MIDWIFERY Qualified supervision of pregnancy and childbirth. Compare with obstetrics.

MIGRAINE Recurrent severe headaches, associated with nausea and visual disturbance.

MINERALS Metallic elements, such as sodium, that are vital to many of the body's functions.

MISCARRIAGE Loss of an embryo or fetus from the uterus before 28 weeks of pregnancy, but usually occurring during the first 16 weeks. Medical term is spontaneous abortion.

MITRAL STENOSIS An obstructive lesion in the valve between the left atrium and ventricle, usually due to rheumatic fever.

MOLE A pigmented spot on the skin.

MONGOLISM *See* Down syndrome.

MORBILLI *See* measles.

MORNING SICKNESS Nausea and vomiting widely experienced in early pregnancy (from the sixth to the 12th week), but not necessarily only in the mornings.

MORPHINE A narcotic painkiller derived from a type of poppy.

MOTION SICKNESS Condition arising from erratic movement that upsets the organs of balance, leading to nausea, vomiting, and vertigo.

MOTOR Pertaining to action or movement.

MOTOR NEURON DISEASE One of various

progressive diseases that cause degeneration of the spinal cord.

MUCOSA (pl. mucosae) Various types of moist membrane that line the tubular structures, cavities, and organs of the body. Also called mucous membrane.

MUCOUS MEMBRANE *See* mucosa.

MUCUS Viscous substance secreted by the mucous membranes as a lubricant and barrier against damage and infection.

MULTIPLE SCLEROSIS (MS) Chronic disease of the nervous system. Characterized by loss of the myelin sheath surrounding the nerves, it produces many symptoms, including weakness and loss of coordination. Its course is episodic, with frequent remissions.

MUMPS An acute viral disease primarily affecting the parotid glands in the cheeks.

MUSCLE Powerful tissue that is responsible for all movement.

MUSCULAR DYSTROPHY (MD) A group of inherited diseases causing progressive atrophy of groups of muscles.

MYASTHENIA GRAVIS Rare autoimmune disease featuring weakness of isolated muscle groups, especially in the face and neck.

MYCOSIS Infection by fungi.

MYELOMA Malignant disease of the bone marrow.

MYOCARDITIS Severe inflammation of the heart muscle.

MYOPATHY Any disease of muscle.

N

NARCOTIC A drug that dulls the senses; used to induce sleep or as a painkiller.

NATUROPATHY A system of health care that relies on natural substances, exercise in water, and a natural environment in order to maintain health and effect cures.

NAUSEA The sensation of wanting to vomit.

NECROSIS Death of tissue.

NEOPLASM Term used to refer to tumors, both benign and malignant.

NEPHRECTOMY Surgical removal of a kidney.

NEPHRITIS (adj. nephritic) Any inflammation of the kidneys.

NERVES Bundles of nerve cells enclosed in conducting tissue that carry messages between the brain and the other organs.

NERVOUS BREAKDOWN An informal term to describe a sudden emotional disorder that disrupts normal functioning.

NEURAL Of or pertaining to the nerves.

NEURALGIA Pain felt along a nerve.

NEUROFIBROMA A fibrous tumor of the nervous tissue.

NEUROFIBROMATOSIS Congenital condition characterized by multiple neurofibromas, and accompanied by areas of abnormal pigmentation of the skin.

NEUROLOGY Branch of medicine concerned with the treatment of diseases of the nervous system.

NEUROSIS An emotional disorder such as mild depression, anxiety, or any of the phobias.

NEUROSURGEON A surgeon who operates on the brain, the spinal cord, and other parts of the nervous system.

NOCTURIA Passing urine during the night.

NONSPECIFIC URETHRITIS (NSU) Inflammation of the lining of the urethra caused by germs or agencies other than those commonly known to cause urethritis. The condition formerly described as nonspecific urethritis is now known to be a chlamydial infection.

NUCLEAR MEDICINE The use of radioactive substances to assist in the investigation and treatment of disease.

NUCLEUS The central part of any cell (except red blood cells), which contains the genetic material.

NYSTAGMUS Neurological disorder in which the eyes jerk rapidly and uncontrollably, usually from side to side.

O

OBESITY An excessive amount of body fat.

OBSESSION An unhealthy preoccupation.

OBSTETRICIAN A doctor specializing in the care of women during pregnancy and childbirth.

OBSTETRICS The branch of medicine concerned with pregnancy and childbirth.

OCCLUSION Blockage of a tube in the body.

OCCUPATIONAL THERAPY (OT) The rehabilitation of patients after illness, accidents, or psychiatric breakdown.

ONCOLOGY The branch of medicine concerned with the diagnosis and treatment of cancer.

OOPHORECTOMY Surgical removal of the ovaries, sometimes performed in conjunction with a hysterectomy.

OPHTHALMOLOGY The branch of medicine concerned with the diagnosis and treatment of eye disease.

OPHTHALMOSCOPE Instrument used to inspect the inner eye and retina.

OPTIC NERVE Either of the pair of nerves that carry visual stimuli from the retina to the brain.

OPTOMETRY The practice of testing sight and prescribing corrective lenses.

ORCHITIS Inflammation of the testis.

ORTHODONTICS The branch of dentistry concerned with straightening irregular teeth and making sure that the teeth of the upper and lower jaws align correctly.

ORTHOPEDICS Branch of surgery concerned with the diseases and injuries of bones and the muscles, tendons, and ligaments attached to them.

OSTEOARTHRITIS A long-term inflammatory disease that leads to the destruction of one or more joints.

OSTEOLOGY The branch of anatomy concerned with the bones.

OSTEOMALACIA Softening of the bones, usually caused by a deficiency of calcium and vitamin D.

OSTEOMYELITIS Local or generalized infection of the bone or bone marrow, causing muscle spasms, pain, and fever.

OSTEOPATHY A therapeutic system that, although reliant on orthodox methods of medical treatment (such as drugs, surgery, and irradiation), is based on a much closer interaction between skeletal structure and body function than is found in conventional medicine.

OSTEOPOROSIS A condition in which the bones become thin and brittle.

OTITIS Inflammation or infection of the ear; otitis media is inflammation of the middle ear and is common in children.

OTOSCOPE Instrument used to examine the outer and middle ear.

OTOSCOPY The use of an otoscope to look into the ear and inspect the patient's eardrum.

OVARY The female organ in which eggs are made and stored. Sited inside the abdomen at the ends of the fallopian tubes.

OVULATION Release of one or more ova from an ovary. Unless the egg is fertilized, this usually occurs about 14 days prior to the onset of the next menstrual period.

P

PACEMAKER An electrical device used to regulate a very slow heartbeat (heart block).

PAGET'S DISEASE A disease characterized by bone deformation, usually found in the elderly.

PALLIATIVE Treatment that relieves symptoms rather than providing a cure.

PALPATE To feel for abnormalities with the hands during a physical examination.

PALPITATION Pounding or racing of the heart rate under conditions of stress, or as a result of coronary disease.

PANCREAS The organ at the back of the abdomen, which is responsible for producing the digestive juices. It also produces the hormone insulin.

PANCREATITIS Inflammation of the pancreas, which may produce severe abdominal pain and eventual collapse.

PANDEMIC Any disease that spreads over a very wide area, and sometimes worldwide. Compare epidemic.

PAP SMEAR A simple method of detecting cervical cancer that involves the staining of a sample of exfoliated cells taken from the cervix. Also called Papanicolaou smear.

PAPILLEDEMA A condition in which raised pressure in the fluid around the brain leads to visible swelling of the optic nerve within the eye.

PARALYSIS Inability to move a part or all of the body, caused by disease or injury of the nervous system.

PARAPLEGIA A condition in which the legs are paralyzed owing to disease or injury in the spinal cord.

PARASITE An organism that lives on another living organism. Viruses, bacteria, and fungi are all parasites, as are larger organisms such as worms, lice, and fleas.

PARATHYROID One of four glands found behind the thyroid that control the level of calcium in the body.

PARATYPHOID FEVER A disease caused by food contaminated with a salmonella bacterium. Symptoms resemble those of typhoid fever.

PARKINSON'S DISEASE A disease of the nervous system, characterized by tremor and slowness of movement.

PARONYCHIA See whitlow.

PAROTITIS Inflammation or infection of the parotid glands in the cheek, most commonly due to mumps.

PATENT DUCTUS ARTERIOSUS (PDA) Failure of the ductus arteriosus to close after birth, which places an additional workload on the left side of the heart.

PATHOGEN Any organism that causes disease.

PATHOLOGY The study of the causes, characteristics, and effects of disease.

PEDIATRICS The branch of medicine

concerned with the treatment of children and childhood diseases.

PENICILLIN An effective antibiotic derived from the fungus *Penicillium*.

PEPTIC ULCER An ulcer in the stomach or duodenum resulting from the effects of stomach acid. *Helicobacter pylori* infection is often associated with peptic ulcers; the bacterium interferes with the mucus layer in the stomach so that acidic juices can erode the lining.

PERCUSSION A diagnostic method involving tapping part of the body to determine the condition of internal organs.

PERICARDITIS Inflammation of the fibrous sac holding the heart.

PERICARDIUM The fibrous sac that surrounds the heart.

PERISTALSIS The rhythmic waves of muscular contraction that move food along the digestive tract.

PERITONEUM The membrane lining the abdominal cavity and covering the organs.

PERITONITIS Inflammation of the peritoneum.

PERNICIOUS ANEMIA Anemia resulting from a failure to absorb vitamin B12 from the intestine.

PESSARY A medicated vaginal suppository. Also a plastic ring inserted to treat prolapse of the uterus when surgery is inappropriate.

PETIT MAL SEIZURE Epileptic seizure that takes the form of a sudden, momentary loss of consciousness (or absences). Also called absence seizure.

pH (potential hydrogen) The scale of measurement for acidity.

PHALANGES The small bones that make up the fingers and toes.

PHARMACOLOGY The branch of medicine concerning the effects and properties of drugs.

PHARYNGITIS Inflammation of the pharynx.

PHARYNX The upper part of the throat at the back of the mouth and the nose.

PHEOCHROMOCYTOMA A rare tumor of the adrenal gland.

PHLEBITIS Inflammation of the veins, often associated with thrombosis.

PHLEGM Mucus produced by the nose and sinuses, or by the airways in the chest.

PHYSICAL THERAPY The physical rehabilitation of people recovering after an illness, accident, or surgery.

PHYSICIAN A person who is licenced to practice medicine, but who uses drugs and other treatments rather than surgery.

POSTMORTEM EXAMINATION An examination of a body after death, whereby direct inspection of the organs and microscopic examination of tissue specimens help to explain the cause of death.

POSTPARTUM HEMORRHAGE Bleeding after the birth of a baby.

PREECLAMPSIA Development of high blood pressure during pregnancy. The symptoms of the full condition are high blood pressure, edema, and protein in the urine.

PREMEDICATION Drugs given to patients in order to relax them before surgery.

PREMENSTRUAL SYNDROME (PMS) Irritability occurring before the onset of the monthly period; PMS is due to hormonal changes.

PRESSURE SORES *See* bedsores.

PROCTALGIA A pain in and around the anus.

PROCTITIS Inflammation of the rectal lining.

PROCTOSCOPE An instrument for inspecting the anal canal and rectum.

PROGNOSIS Assessment of the likely outcome of a disease. Compare diagnosis.

PROLAPSE The falling or sliding of an organ from its normal position.

PROPHYLACTIC A form of treatment designed to prevent disease.

PROSTAGLANDINS Chemical compounds that perform a range of hormonelike functions.

PROSTATE GLAND The gland at the base of the bladder in males which is involved in semen production, and which may enlarge later in life and obstruct urine flow.

PROSTHESIS Any artificial replacement for a part of the body.

PROSTRATION Profound collapse, often accompanied by low blood pressure.

PROTEIN The substance made from strings of amino acid molecules that forms the basic building blocks of the body.

PROTEINURIA *See* albuminuria.

PRURITUS Medical term for itching.

PSORIASIS A skin rash with red, scaly patches, found most commonly on the knees and elbows.

PSYCHIATRY The branch of medicine concerned with disorders of the mind.

PSYCHOANALYSIS A form of therapy in which the analyst helps the patient to explore his or her own unconscious mind in order to relieve psychiatric difficulties.

PSYCHOLOGY The study of the mechanisms by which the mind works.

PSYCHOSIS A severe psychiatric illness.

PSYCHOTHERAPY Treatment of emotional problems or psychiatric illness by discussion with a therapist, either on an individual basis or as part of a group.

PUBERTY The sequence of events that changes a child to an adult.

PULMONARY Of or pertaining to the lungs.

PURPURA Tiny spots of bleeding into the skin.

PUS Yellowish-white substance consisting of the debris of bacteria and white blood cells.

PYLORIC STENOSIS Obstruction at the outlet of the stomach, occurring in adults as the result of an ulcer, or as a congenital problem in babies.

PYREXIA Medical term for a fever.

Q

Q FEVER A feverish illness of cattle, goats, and sheep caused by the organism *Coxiella burnetii*.

QUARANTINE Keeping animals or people isolated from the community at large because of the risk of spreading an infectious disease.

R

RABIES A potentially fatal viral disease affecting the nervous system—passed to humans by bites from infected (rabid) animals, and characterized by hydrophobia (fear of water).

RADIATION SICKNESS Sickness arising from exposure to ionizing radiation, characterized by symptoms ranging from nausea and vomiting to fetal damage and cancer, depending on the length of exposure.

RADIOLOGY The use of X rays in order to produce pictures of internal structures and thus diagnose disease.

RADIOTHERAPY The use of X rays to treat disease.

REFERRED PAIN Pain felt at a site remote from the source of the pain.

REFRACTORY A word commonly used by doctors to describe the failure of a condition to respond to treatment.

RELAPSE The return of an illness after apparent recovery.

REMISSION A period free from the symptoms of a chronic illness.

RESUSCITATION The technique used to bring critically ill patients back from the brink of death; in particular the use of artificial respiration and chest compression after cardiac arrest.

RETINA The delicate, multilayered membrane of the eye that receives visual stimuli from the outside world.

RETINAL DETACHMENT The separation of the retina from the back of the eye.

RETROVIRUS A family of viruses, including HIV, which contain RNA, and which are able to produce DNA, using their RNA as a template, and incorporate this into the genome of infected cells.

RH (RHESUS) FACTOR An inherited substance present on the red blood cells that characterizes membership of the Rh blood group system. The importance of the Rh group is that a fetus with a different group from its mother may have its red blood cells destroyed by her antibodies.

RHEUMATIC FEVER A feverish illness following an infection by a streptococcus, which may lead to heart damage.

RHEUMATISM A nonmedical term referring to aches and pains of the joints and related tissues.

RHEUMATOID ARTHRITIS Inflammation of the joints, which may also effect internal organs.

RHINITIS Inflammation of the lining of the nose, usually due to a cold or hay fever.

RICKETS Deficiency disease that affects children during skeletal growth, causing soft and deformed bones and caused by an inability to process calcium due to a deficiency in vitamin D.

RNA (ribonucleic acid) Together with DNA, one of the two substances that carry the inherited genetic instructions in cells. In humans, DNA supplies the genetic codes, and RNA helps to decode them.

RODENT ULCER An ulcer found on the face that is, in fact, a mild form of skin cancer capable of eating away tissue unless removed.

ROSEOLA A common minor viral infection in children and babies that causes a rash.

RUBELLA A virus infection which usually produces only rash and fever, but which can severely damage the fetus in early pregnancy. Also called German measles.

S

SAD (seasonal affective disorder) A mood disorder associated with the decrease in hours of sunlight during the autumn and winter.

SAFER SEX Sexual intercourse in which the risk of transmitting viruses such as HIV is reduced by using protective measures such as condoms. There is no such thing as safe sex.

SALINE A simple salt solution, commonly administered intravenously.

SALIVA Fluid present in the mouth and secreted by the salivary glands as an aid to digestion.

SALIVARY GLANDS One of the three pairs of glands that secrete fluids (including saliva) into the mouth to aid digestion.

SALMONELLA A genus of bacteria that causes typhoid, paratyphoid, and certain kinds of food poisoning.

SALPINGECTOMY Surgical removal of the fallopian tubes.

SALPINGITIS An inflammation of the fallopian tubes, which is usually a symptom of pelvic inflammatory disease.

SALVE Healing or soothing medicated ointment.

SARCOMA A malignant tumor arising in muscle, bone, or other connective tissue.

SCABIES Skin infection caused by mites.

SCARLET FEVER An acute, but now rare, infectious childhood illness characterized by sore throat, fever, swollen lymph nodes, and a pronounced red rash. Also called scarlatina.

SCHISTOSOMIASIS A common tropical parasitic infestation, afflicting over 200 million people worldwide. Also called bilharzia.

SCHIZOPHRENIA A psychotic illness featuring delusions, hallucinations, and a variety of thought disorders that usually start in the late teens or early adult life.

SCIATICA Pain running down the leg, arising from irritation of the sciatic nerve, usually due to disk trouble.

SCLEROSIS Hardening of any body tissue.

SCOLIOSIS A lateral curvature of the spine.

SEASONAL AFFECTIVE DISORDER *See* SAD.

SEBACEOUS GLANDS Glands that lubricate and protect the skin.

SEBORRHEA Abnormally high production of sebum leading to dandruff and acne.

SEBUM The oily substance produced by the sebaceous glands.

SEDATIVE A drug that decreases functional activity and has a generally calming effect.

SEMEN The fluid which is discharged by the male when he ejaculates, and which contains spermatozoa and secretions from other glands such as the prostate.

SENILE DEMENTIA The loss of mental capacity in the elderly due to the death of brain cells.

SENILITY Old age. Often used incorrectly to refer to the presence of various mental and physical disorders common in old age.

SEPSIS Infection with bacteria.

SEPTICEMIA Invasion of the blood by infectious microorganisms, causing fever and chills. Also called blood poisoning.

SEROTONIN Naturally occurring substance found in the brain, blood, and intestines that elevates mood and has many other actions.

SEX HORMONES Hormones that control sexual functions and their development, such as the menstrual cycle and the production of eggs or sperm. There are three main types: androgen hormones (male sex hormones, of which testosterone is the most important); estrogen (female sex hormones); and progesterone (important in the female reproductive cycle).

SÉZARY SYNDROME An intensely irritating form of dermatitis with severe skin shedding, caused by skin infiltration with T cells.

SEXUAL INTERCOURSE The reproductive act, in which the male penis penetrates the female vagina, culminating in the ejaculation of semen. Medical name is coitus.

SHINGLES A skin rash that follows the underlying distribution of nerves. Due to infection with the varicella zoster virus, which also causes chicken pox.

SHOCK A critical drop in blood pressure that, if untreated, may lead to coma and death.

SIAMESE TWINS Identical twins in which the embryo has not split in half, resulting in the twins' being joined. Also called conjoined twins.

SICKLE CELL A crescent-shaped red blood cell containing the abnormal hemoglobin that causes sickle-cell anemia.

SICKLE-CELL ANEMIA An incurable inherited disease in which abnormal hemoglobin causes the red blood cells to become distorted, resulting in joint pain, thrombosis, fever, and chronic anemia.

SIDE EFFECT An undesirable effect accompanying the desired effect of a drug.

SIDS *See* crib death.

SILICOSIS Lung disease due to exposure to the silicon dioxide present in stone dust.

SINUS An air-filled cavity within the facial bones, connected to the nostrils.

SINUSITIS Infection of the sinuses.

SKIN GRAFT Skin transplanted from one part of the body to another in order to repair damage or to correct a deformity.

SLEEPING SICKNESS A disease of tropical Africa caused by the presence in the blood of minute protozoans called trypanosomes, which are transmitted by the tsetse fly. It runs a slow course, and is fatal if left untreated. Also called African trypanosomiasis.

SLIPPED DISK Backward protrusion of pulpy material from the center of an intervertebral disk with painful pressure on emerging spinal nerves.

SMALLPOX An acute and often fatal disease which produced a rash and a fever, but which is now eradicated.

SMEGMA The secretions of glands under the foreskin of the penis.

SPASTIC COLON *See* irritable bowel syndrome.

SPASTICITY A neurological term used to describe resistance of a limb to passive movement. Usually accompanied by weakness, it is caused by damage to nerves in the brain or spinal cord.

SPECULUM An instrument that can be inserted into a body opening (such as the vagina) for the purposes of examination.

SPEECH THERAPY Treatment and counseling to correct speech difficulties.

SPERM *See* spermatozoon.

SPERMACIDES Contraceptive preparations that kill sperm.

SPERMATOZOON (pl. spermatozoa) Male germ cell that is produced in the testes and carried in the semen. Also called sperm.

SPHINCTER Any muscular ring around any body orifice, which closes it off, as in the anus.

SPHYGMOMANOMETER Instrument used to measure blood pressure.

SPINA BIFIDA Congenital defect in which part of the backbone fails to close, exposing the spinal cord. Often associated with hydrocephalus, it may cause paralysis of the legs.

SPINAL CORD The cord of nervous tissue which runs down from the brain inside the central bony canal of the backbone, and from which all the nerves to the body below the brain branch off.

SPINE The column of bone and cartilage that extends from the base of the skull to the pelvis, contains the spinal cord, and supports the trunk and head.

SPLEEN An organ in the upper left-hand corner of the abdomen, responsible for filtering worn-out blood cells.

SPLINT A device for holding a joint in a suitable position to prevent deformity, or to support a limb after a fracture.

SPONDYLITIS Painful inflammation of the spine, often leading to disabling fusion of adjacent vertebrae.

SPRAIN A common injury to joints in which the ligaments that hold them together become overstretched or torn.

SPRUE A malabsorption disease of the small intestine.

SPUTUM The secretions of the bronchial tubes.

SQUINT Condition in which one eye is not properly aligned. Also called strabismus.

STEATORRHEA Excessive fat in the feces.

STENOSIS A narrowed or blocked tube or passage in the body. The term is often used to describe blockages in the arteries or across the valves of the heart.

STERILIZATION Surgery to prevent eggs from reaching the woman's uterus, or sperm from being emitted in a man. Also means the killing of all infective microorganisms on surgical equipment.

STERNUM The breastbone.

STEROIDS Complex chemical molecules, such as the sex hormones; sometimes used to describe cortisone and those drugs that have a cortisonelike effect.

STETHOSCOPE Instrument used for listening to the sounds of the heart, the lungs, and other internal organs.

STIMULANT A drug that stimulates the brain.

STOMA An artificial opening in a body organ or channel (e.g., the intestine).

STOMACH PUMP Equipment used for washing out the stomach, for example, after a drug overdose or poisoning.

STOMATITIS Inflammation of the lining of the mouth.

STRABISMUS *See* squint.

STRANGULATED HERNIA A hernia in which the contents of the small intestine have become stuck, constricting the blood supply and posing the risk of gangrene.

STREPTOCOCCUS A type of bacterium.

STREPTOMYCIN An antibiotic, used mainly against tuberculosis.

STRICTURE A local narrowing in any tubular structure.

STROKE Sudden loss of an area of brain function, causing a defect in movement, sensation, vision, speech, comprehension, or personality. Strokes commonly affect one side of the body only.

STY An infection around the root of an eyelash.

SUBLINGUAL Term meaning "under the tongue"—a route by which drugs may be given.

SUDDEN INFANT DEATH SYNDROME (SIDS) *See* crib death.

SULFONAMIDES A group of drugs that are effective against bacteria.

SUNSTROKE *See* heatstroke.

SUPPOSITORIES Drugs that are inserted into the rectum or vagina.

SUPPURATION Formation of pus as a result of infection.

SURGEON A doctor specially trained in treating diseases by operation.

SUTURE The medical name for a wound stitch.

SYMPTOMS The characteristics of an illness.

SYNCOPE Sudden loss of consciousness. Also called fainting.

SYNDROME A number of specific features that together characterize a disorder.

SYNOVIAL MEMBRANES The membranes that line and lubricate the joints.

SYNOVITIS Inflammation of the synovial membranes.

SYPHILIS A sexually transmitted and inheritable disease caused by the organism *Treponema pallidum*.

SYSTEMIC LUPUS ERYTHEMATOSUS (SLE) A disease involving many of the body's organs, including the skin, joints, and kidneys.

SYSTOLE The time during which the heart is contracting. Each heartbeat is a systole. Compare with diastole.

SYSTOLIC PRESSURE *See* blood pressure.

T

T CELL A type of white blood cell that is involved in immunity.

TACHYCARDIA An abnormally fast heart rate.

TEARS The watery, salty secretion of the lacrimal glands that keeps the cornea and conjuctiva of the eye moist.

TELANGIECTASIA Conspicuously widened small blood vessels often seen in the skin; also known as broken veins.

TEMPORAL ARTERITIS Inflammation of the forehead arteries causing acute pain, tenderness, redness, and the risk of incipient blindness unless urgently treated with steroid drugs.

TENDON Fibrous cord that binds muscles onto bones and transmits the force of their contraction.

TENDONITIS Inflammation of a tendon, usually caused by injury.

TENNIS ELBOW Inflammation of the tendons on the outer side of the elbow as a result of overuse of the arm.

TENOSYNOVITIS Inflammation of the sheath surrounding a tendon.

TERATOGENESIS Malformation of a fetus due to genetic or environmental causes.

TEST-TUBE BABY *See* in vitro fertilization.

TESTES (sing. testis) The male sexual organs responsible for the production of both sperm and male sex hormone.

TESTOSTERONE The male sex hormone produced by the testes.

TETANUS A disease of the nervous system caused by a toxin produced by the bacterium *Clostridium tetani*, which contaminates wounds.

TETANY A condition in which the muscles of the hands and feet go into uncontrollable spasm.

THALASSEMIA An inherited abnormality of the hemoglobin that produces severe anemia in affected children.

THALIDOMIDE A type of tranquilizer and sleeping drug that produced deformity in babies when taken by pregnant women; now used strictly as a treatment for leprosy.

THORAX Medical term for the chest.

THROAT Nonmedical term for the pharynx.

THROMBOCYTE Blood platelet, necessary for blood clotting.

THROMBOSIS The formation of a blood clot within an artery or a vein. While such clotting is a normal reaction in a damaged blood vessel, it occurs in an intact vessel only if it is diseased. Thrombosis in arteries leading to the heart muscle can cause a heart attack, and a thrombus in one of the arteries supplying the brain is a common cause of stroke.

THROMBUS (pl. thrombi) A blood clot.

THRUSH *See* yeast.

THYMUS A flat organ in the neck that processes immune system T cells early in life but later shrinks.

THYROID The gland in the neck that produces the hormone thyroxine, which is important in controlling the body's metabolism.

TIC Involuntary twitching or spasm.

TINEA Fungal skin infection of which athlete's foot is a common example.

TINNITUS Ringing or buzzing in the ears.

TISSUE Collection of similar cells and connecting substance to make material from which organs and other structures are formed.

TISSUE TYPING A series of tests to evaluate compatibility of tissues, necessary when transplanting organs.

TONSILLECTOMY Surgical removal of the tonsils.

TONSILS Two patches of lymphoid tissue that lie at the back of the throat on either side.

TOPICAL APPLICATION The application of a drug directly onto a surface, for example, the eyes, gums, tongue, vagina, or anal canal; or an internal surface during surgery.

TOURNIQUET A device that stops the blood flow to a limb by constricting it.

TOXEMIA Blood poisoning caused by bacterial toxins circulating in the bloodstream. *See* preeclampsia.

TOXICOLOGY The study of toxins.

TOXINS Poisons produced by germs.

TRACHEOSTOMY The opening in the windpipe produced by a tracheotomy.

TRACHEOTOMY Surgical procedure whereby an opening is made in the windpipe to ease breathing in diseases of the larynx, or to enable people to remain on respirators for prolonged periods.

TRACTION Use of a system of weights to pull broken bones into place.

TRANQUILIZER A nonmedical term used to describe drugs that act on the nervous system to produce a calming effect.

TRANSFUSION Intravenous administration of fluids, especially blood or plasma.

TRANSPLANT The transfer of any piece of living tissue from one location in the body to another, or from one body to another.

TRAUMA (literally "damage") Any physical injury or severe emotional shock.

TREMOR A regular, involuntary rhythmic shaking of some part of the body.

TRICHINOSIS Infestation with the larvae of *Trichinella spiralis*, usually acquired by eating infected pork products.

TRICHOMONIASIS VAGINALIS A vaginal infection caused by *Trichomonas vaginalis*, characterized by a greenish, odorous discharge.

TRISOMY The presence of an additional chromosome in an individual's cells, so that there are three rather than two of a particular number. The most common disorder associated with a trisomy is Down syndrome, which is also known as trisomy 21 syndrome.

TROPICAL DISEASES Diseases endemic in undeveloped areas where standards of hygiene, sanitation, and public health administration are low. These areas are found mainly in the tropics, but environmental temperatures are not the fundamental factor.

TUBERCULOSIS (TB) A bacterial infection which most often produces disease in the lungs, but which may affect other organs.

TUMOR A benign or malignant growth.

TWINS Two offspring resulting from one pregnancy. Identical (or monovular) twins develop from a single ovum that divides early in its development. Binovular twins develop separately from two ova.

TYPHOID FEVER A bacterial fever that is caused by ingestion of food, water, and milk contaminated with *Salmonella typhi*, with symptoms resembling those of typhus (typhoid means "typhus-like"): fever, diarrhea, and a rash.

TYPHUS A disease spread by tics, lice, or fleas, producing fever, rash, and, in severe cases, death.

U

ULCER A break in a smooth lining membrane or surface—for example, in the skin or stomach—that fails to heal and may become inflamed.

ULCERATIVE COLITIS A disease causing chronic diarrhea as a result of inflammation and ulceration of the lining of the colon.

ULTRASOUND Sound waves of very high frequency used to produce images of the body's internal structures.

UMBILICAL CORD The cord that carries blood, nutrients, and oxygen from a mother to her unborn child.

UMBILICUS The point on the abdomen where the umbilical cord once joined the fetal abdomen. Also called navel.

UREA A white, soluble waste product of protein formed in the liver and excreted in the urine.

UREMIA A high level of urea in the blood.

URETER One of the two tubes carrying urine from the kidney to the bladder.

URETHRA The tube that carries urine from the bladder out of the body.

URETHRITIS Infection of the urethra.

URIC ACID A breakdown product of DNA found in urine.

URINE The product of the kidneys, containing many of the waste products accumulated in the body.

UROLOGY The branch of medicine concerned with the diseases and treatment of the urinary system of both men and women, and the male genital organs.

UTERUS The organ found in all female mammals that contains and nourishes unborn offspring. Also called womb.

UVEITIS Inflammation affecting the middle part of the eye (the iris and related structures).

V

VACCINATION The administration of a vaccine to prevent one of the infectious diseases.

VAGINA The female genital passage that leads to the uterus.

VAGINISMUS Spasm of the muscles that surround the vagina, causing rejection of sexual intercourse.

VAGOTOMY Surgical cutting of the vagus nerve, usually in order to reduce acid secretion. Formerly used in the treatment of ulcers.

VAGUS NERVE One of a pair of cranial nerves that exert control on the throat, esophagus, larynx, bronchi, lungs, heart, stomach, and intestines.

VALVE A mechanism that allows fluid (such as blood) to flow only one way down a tube.

VARICOSE VEIN A distended and twisted vein.

VAS DEFERENS The tube that carries sperm from the testes to the ejaculatory duct.

VASECTOMY The surgical severing of the vasa deferentia in order to produce sterility.

VASOCONSTRICTION Narrowing of the blood vessels, due to either external factors such as cold, fear, and stress, or to the action of internal secretions such as epinephrine and serotonin.

VEIN A vessel carrying blood from the body tissues to the heart.

VENTRICLE One of the two lower chambers of the heart that receive blood from the atria; also one of the four fluid-filled cavities in the brain.

VENTRICULAR FIBRILLATION Rapid, chaotic beating of the heart, which, if uncorrected, causes death.

VERRUCA (pl. verrucae) A wart.

VERTIGO Dizziness and spinning sensation.

VIREMIA The presence of a virus in the blood.

VIRILISM A condition in which a female starts to acquire male sexual characteristics as a result of a hormonal imbalance.

VIRULENCE The relative capacity of a microorganism to cause disease, assessed according to such factors as incidence of infection among a population, and the rate of mortality.

VIRUS A small infective agent that consists of a protein shell containing a core of DNA or RNA. Viruses require animal cells to reproduce within living cells. They do not respond to antibiotic treatment.

VISCERA Collective term used to describe the internal organs.

VITAL CAPACITY The largest volume of air that can be expelled after a maximal inspiration.

VITAMINS A group of substances that cannot be synthesized by the body but are essential, in tiny amounts, for its healthy growth and development. Vitamins are usually present in a balanced diet, but can also be taken in pill form.

VITILIGO A skin disorder characterized by loss of pigment and patches of pale skin.

VOLVULUS A condition in which part of the digestive tract twists around on itself, cutting off its own blood supply.

VULVA The female external genitalia, including the area of the labia, the clitoris, and the urethral opening.

VULVITIS Inflammation of the vulva.

W

WART Common, infectious, but harmless growths on the skin caused by viruses. Often found on the hand, where they form small swellings. Plantar wart is a wart on the sole of the foot.

WASSERMANN REACTION Formerly the most commonly used blood test to detect evidence of previous infection with syphilis.

WASTING Loss of muscle substance due to illness or prolonged lack of use, especially in cases where the nerve supply to the muscle has failed.

WEANING The gradual substitution of solid foods for milk in an infant's diet.

WEIL'S DISEASE *See* leptospirosis.

WHIPLASH INJURY An injury to the neck that is often sustained in car accidents, where sudden deceleration causes the neck to jerk backward and forward violently.

WHITLOW Infection of the nail bed, resulting in a collection of pus in the nail fold. Also called paronychia.

WHOOPING COUGH An infectious disease of the airways that is common in children who have not been vaccinated against it. There is a characteristic whooping sound after the cough. Also called pertussis.

WOMB *See* uterus.

XYZ

X CHROMOSOME A sex chromosome. Females carry a pair of X chromosomes, whereas males carry one X chromosome and one Y chromosome.

X RAY A method of passing electromagnetic radiation through the various tissues of the body and projecting the resulting image onto photographic film. Those tissues that are more radiopaque (allow fewer X rays to pass through them), such as bone, show up as shadows on the film. Used for diagnostic purposes.

Y CHROMOSOME *See* X chromosome.

YEAST Types of fungi, some of which can cause infections of the skin or mucous membranes. The most common disease-causing yeast is *Candida albicans*.

YELLOW FEVER A serious viral disease that is spread from person to person by mosquitoes, causing fever and jaundice.

Further reading and research

General

American Medical Association, Leikin, Jerrold B., and Lipsky, Martin S. *American Medical Association Complete Medical Encyclopedia*. New York, NY: Random House, 2003.

Griffith, H.W. *Complete Guide to Symptoms, Illness, and Surgery Edition 4*. New York, NY: G. P. Putnam's Sons, 2000.

Mayo Clinic. *Mayo Clinic Family Health Book*. 3rd edition. New York: HarperCollins, 2003.

Warrell, David A., et al. *Oxford Textbook of Medicine*. 4th edition. New York, NY: Oxford University Press, 2004.

Accidents, emergencies, and first aid

American Medical Association Staff. *American Medical Association Handbook of First Aid and Emergency*. Chicago: American Medical Association, 1999.

American Medical Association. *Handbook of First Aid and Emergency Care*. New York, NY: Random House, 2000.

American Red Cross and Handal, K. A. *The American Red Cross First Aid and Safety Handbook*. New York, NY: Little, Brown and Company, 1992.

Alternative and complementary medicines

Navarra, Tova. *The Encyclopedia of Complementary and Alternative Medicine (Library of Health and Living)*. New York, NY: Facts on File, 2004.

Acupuncture

Hecker, Hans-Ulrich, et al. *Color Atlas of Acupuncture: Body Points, Ear Points, Trigger Points*. New York, NY: Thieme Medical Publishers, 2001.

Saul, Helen. *Healing with Acupressure*. Lincolnwood, IL: NTC Publishing Group, 2001.

Aromatherapy

Richardson, Jo (Editor). *Aromatherapy*. Lansing, MI: Thunder Bay Press, 2001.

Herbal

Chevalier, Andrew. *Natural Health Encyclopedia of Herbal Medicine*. New York, NY: DK Publishing, 2000.

Joiner, Thomas Richa. *Chinese Herbal Medicine Made Easy: Effective and Natural Remedies for Common Illnesses*. Alameda, CA: Hunter House, 2001.

Homeopathy

Ullman, Dana. *Essential Homeopathy: What It Is and What It Can Do for You*. Novato, CA: New World Library, 2002.

Osteopathy

McKone, Walter LLewellyn. *Osteopathic Medicine: Philosophy, Principles and Practice*. Malden, MA: Blackwell Publishers, 2001.

Scott-Conner, Carol E., and Ward, Robert C., Contribution by American Osteopathic Association. *Foundations for Osteopathic Medicine*. Hagerstown, MD: Lippincott Williams & Wilkins, 2002.

Reflexology

Kunz, Barbara, and Kunz, Kevin. *Reflexology: Healing at Your Fingertips*. New York, NY: DK Publishing, 2003.

Shiatsu

Ohashi, Wateru, and Lindner, Vicki. *Do-It-Yourself Shiatsu*. New York, NY: Penguin, 2001.

Yoga

Belling, Noa. *The Yoga Handbook*. New York, NY: Barnes & Noble Books, 2001.

Groves, Dawn. *Yoga for Busy People*. New York, NY: Barnes & Noble Books, 2002.

Iyengar, B. K. S. *Yoga: The Path to Holistic Health*. New York, NY: DK Publishing, 2001.

Anatomy and physiology

Avraham, Regina. *Digestive System*. Langhorne, PA: Chelsea House Publishers, 2000.

Baron-Faust, Rita, et al. *The Autoimmune Connection*. New York, NY: McGraw-Hill Companies, 2003.

Burkey, John M., et al. *Hearing Better: Understanding Your Hearing and Ear Care Options*. Boca Raton, FL: Upublish.com, 1999.

Cohen, Barbara Janson, and Wood, Dena Lin. *Memmler's Structure and Function of the Human Body*. 7th edition. Hagerstown, MD: Lippincott Williams & Wilkins, 2000.

Fray, Henry, and Carter H. V. (Illustrator). *Gray's Anatomy*. New York, NY: Barnes & Noble Books-Imports, 2000.

Gallo, Fred, and Vincenzi, Harry. *Energy Tapping*. Oakland, CA: New Harbinger Publications, 2000.

Goldsby, David A., et al. *Immunology*. New York, NY: W. H. Freeman Company, 2002.

Handin, Robert I. I., Stossel, Thomas P., and Lux, Samuel E. *Blood: Principles and Practice of Hematology*. Hagerstown, MD: Lippincott Williams & Wilkins, 2002.

Harding, Richard, Pinkerton, Kent, and Plopper, Charles (Editors). *The Lung: Development, Aging, and The Environment*. Burlington, MA: Academic Press, 2003.

Kopf-Maier, Petra (Editor). *The Color Atlas of Human Anatomy*. New York, NY: Barnes & Noble Books, 2003.

Lancraft, Thomas M. *Interactions: Exploring the Functions of the Human Body, Disease Resistance: The Lymphatic, Integumentary and Immune Systems*. Indianapolis, IN: John Wiley & Sons, 2003.

Marieb, Elaine N., Mallatt, Jon, and Hutchinson, Matt. *Human Anatomy and Physiology*. San Francisco, CA: Benjamin-Cummings Publishing Company, 2003.

McMahon, T. A. *Muscles, Reflexes, and Locomotion*. Princeton, NJ: Princeton University Press, 1984.

Millen, James Knox. *Your Nose Knows: A Study of the Sense of Smell*. Lincoln, NE: iUniverse, 2000.

Moorcroft, William H. H., and Belcher, Paula. *Understanding Sleep and Dreaming*. Boston, MA: Kluwer Academic Publishers, 2002.

Olsen, Wayne. *Mayo Clinic on Hearing: Strategies for Managing Hearing Loss, Dizziness, and Other Ear Problems*. New York, NY: Kensington Publishing Corporation, 2003.

SparkNotes Editors. *Muscular System (SparkCharts)*. New York, NY: Spark Publishing, 2002.

Walker, Pam, and Wood, Elaine. *Skeletal and Muscular System*. Farmington Hills, MI: Gale Group, 2003.

West, John B. *Respiratory Physiology: The Essentials*. 7th edition. Hagerstown, MD: Lippincott Williams & Wilkins, 2004.

Wolsey, Thomas A. A., Hanaway, Joseph, and Gado, Mokhtar H. *Brain Atlas: A Visual Guide to the Human Central Nervous System*. Indianapolis, IN: John Wiley & Sons, 2002.

Children's health and development

Broer, Ted. *A.D.H.D.—Attention Deficit Hyperactivity Disorder: A Natural Approach to Help and Heal a Hyperactive Child*. Lake Mary, FL: Strang Communications Company, 2002.

Children's Hospital Boston and Brazelton, T. Berry (Introduction). *Children's Hospital Guide to Your Child's Health and Development*. New York, NY: Perseus Publishing, 2002.

Fox, Jane A. *Primary Health Care of Infants, Children, and Adolescents*. San Diego, CA: Elsevier Science, 2002.

Markel, Howard, and Oski, Frank A. *The Practical Pediatrician: The A–Z Guide to Your Child's Health, Behavior, and Safety*. New York, NY: W. H. Freeman and Company, 1996.

Pruitt, David B. (Editor). *Your Adolescent: Emotional, Behavioral, and Cognitive Development from Early Adolescence through the Teen Years*. New York, NY: HarperCollins Publishers, 2000.

Wiseman, Lisa. *Pediatric Home Companion*. St. Louis, MO: Quality Medical Publications, 1997.

Death

Lippincott Williams & Wilkins and Wijdicks, Eelco F. (Editor). *Brain Death: A Clinical Guide*. Hagerstown, MD: Lippincott Williams & Wilkins, 2001.

Dental health and hygiene

Community Oral Health. Tempe, AZ: Scholargy Custom Publishing, 2000.

Langlais, Robert P. P., and Miller, Craig S. *Color Atlas of Common Oral Diseases*. Hagerstown, MD: Lippincott Williams & Wilkins, 2002.

Sutton, Amy (Editor). *Dental Care and Oral Health SourceBook: Basic Consumer Health Information about Dental Care, including Hygiene, Dental Visits, Pain Management, Cavities, Crowns, Bridges, Dental Implants, and Fillings, and Other Oral Health Concerns*. Detroit, MI: Omnigraphics, 2003.

Disability issues

Blanck, Peter David. *Employment, Disability, and the Americans with Disabilities Act: Issues in Law, Public Policy, and Research*. Chicago, IL: Northwestern University Press, 2000.

Lavin, Judith Loseff. *Special Kids Need Special Parents*. New York, NY: Berkley Trade, 2001.

Swanson, H., et al (Editors). *Handbook of Learning Disabilities*. New York, NY: Guilford Publications, 2003.

Szymanski, Edna (Editor), Parker, Randall, and Parker, Randall M. (Editor). *Work and Disability: Issues and Strategies in Career Development and Job Placement*. Austin, TX: PRO-ED, 2003.

Varga, Josie. *Footprints in the Sand: A Disabled Woman's Inspiring Journey to Happiness*. New York, NY: America House, 2004.

Environmental health

Capstone Editors and Petheram, Louise. *Acid Rain*. Mankato, MN: Capstone Press, 2002.

Fuchs, Jurgen, and Packer, Lester. *Environmental Stressors in Health and Disease*. New York, NY: Marcel Dekker, 2001.

Manufactured by Simon & Schuster. *Allergy Solutions*. New York, NY: Simon & Schuster, 2001.

Nadakavukaren, Anne. *Our Global Environment: A Health Perspective*. Long Grove, IL: Waveland Press, 2000.

Nordhaus, William D., and Boyer, Joseph. *Warming the World: Economic Models of Global Warming*. Cambridge, MA: MIT Press, 2003.

Schecter, Arnold, Gasiewicz, Thomas, and Gasiewicz, Thomas A. *Dioxins and Health*. New York, NY: John Wiley & Sons, 2003.

Shapiro, Jacob. *Radiation Protection*. Cambridge, MA: Harvard University Press, 2002.

Ethics

Jonsen, Albert R., Siegler, Mark, and Winslade, William. *Clinical Ethics: A Practical Approach to Ethical Decisions in Clinical Medicine*. 5th edition. New York, NY: McGraw-Hill Companies, 2002.

Kittredge, Mary, and Thurman, Sandra; Koop, C. Everett (Introduction). *Organ Transplants*. Langhorne, PA: Chelsea House Publishers, 2000.

Munson, Ronald. *Intervention and Reflection: Basic Issues in Medical Ethics*. Florence, KY: Wadsworth, 2003.

Pence, Gregory. *Classic Cases in Medical Ethics: Accounts of Cases That Have Shaped Medical Ethics, with Philosophical, Legal, and Historical Backgrounds*. New York, NY: McGraw-Hill Companies, 2003.

Stock, Gregory. *Redesigning Humans: Choosing Our Genes, Changing Our Future*. Boston, MA: Houghton Mifflin Company, 2003.

Eyes and eye care

Cassel, Gary H., Billig, Michael D., and Randall, Harry G. *Eye Book: A Complete Guide to Eye Disorders and Health*. Baltimore, MD: Johns Hopkins University Press, 2000.

Lavine, Jay B., and Barnard, Neil. *Eye Care SourceBook*. Lincolnwood, IL: NTC Publishing Group, 2001.

Fitness

Barough, Nina. *Walking for Fitness: The Low-Impact Workout That Tones and Shapes*. New York, NY: DK Publishing, 2003.

Carmichael, Chris, and Rutberg, Jim. *Chris Carmichael's Food for Fitness*. New York, NY: Putnam Adult, 2004.

Juba, Kelvin. *Swimming for Fitness*. Guilford, CT: Lyons Press, 2002.

Kolata, Gina. *Ultimate Fitness: The Quest for Truth about Exercise and Health*. New York, NY: Farrar, Straus, and Giroux, 2003.

Food, nutrition, and eating disorders

American Dietetic Association and Duyff, Roberta Larson. *American Dietetic Association Complete Food and Nutrition Guide*. New York, NY: John Wiley & Sons, 2002.

Dole Foods (Editor), and University of California at Los Angeles. *Encyclopedia of Foods: A Guide to Healthy Nutrition*. San Diego, CA: Elsevier Science, 2001.

Jantz, Gregory L. *Hope, Help, and Healing for Eating Disorders*. Colorado Springs, CO: WaterBrook Press, 2002.

Lutz, Carroll A. A., and Przytulski, Karen Rutherford. *Nutrition and Diet Therapy*. 3rd edition. Los Angeles, CA: F. A. Davis, 2001.

Trueit, Trudi Strain. *Eating Disorders*. New York, NY: Scholastic Library Publishing, 2004.

Weil, Andrew. *Eating Well for Optimum Health*. New York, NY: Knopf Publishing Group, 2000.

Wong, Dominic W. S. *Food Enzymes: Structure and Mechanism*. Westport, CT: Chapman & Hall, 1999.

Genetics and heredity

Cefrey, Holly. *Cloning and Genetic Engineering*. New York, NY: Scholastic Library Publishing, 2001.

Heyman, Bob, and Henriksen, Mette. *Risk, Age, and Pregnancy: A Case Study of Prenatal Genetic Screening and Testing*. New York, NY: Palgrave Macmillan, 2001.

Iannucci, Lisa. *Birth Defects*. Berkeley Heights, NJ: Enslow Publishers, 2000.

Mueller, Robert F., Emery, Alan E. H., and Young, Ian. *Emery's Elements of Medical Genetics*. San Diego, CA: Elsevier Science, 2001.

Mulunsky, Aubrey (Editor). *Genetic Disorders and the Fetus: Diagnosis, Prevention, and Treatment*. Baltimore, MD: Johns Hopkins University Press, 2004.

Petchesky, Rosalind Pollack. *Global Prescriptions: Gendering Health and Human Rights*. New York, NY: Zed Books, 2003.

Yount, Lisa. *Biotechnology and Genetic Engineering*. New York, NY: Facts on File, 2000.

Zurayk, Huda. *Gender, Development, and Health*. Oxford U.K.: Oxfam Publishing, 2001.

Geriatric health

Gosden, Roger G., et al. *Cheating Time*. New York, NY: W. H. Freeman Company, 1999.

Hazzard, William R., et al. *Principles of Geriatric Medicine and Gerontology*. 5th edition. New York, NY: McGraw-Hill Companies, 2003.

Rosenfeld, Isadore. *Live Now, Age Later: Proven Ways to Slow Down the Clock*. New York, NY: Warner Books, 2000.

Illnesses, conditions, and impairments
AIDS

Barnett, Tony, and Whiteside, Alan. *AIDS in the Twenty-First Century: Disease and Globalization*. New York, NY: Palgrave Macmillan, 2003.

Bartlett, John G., and Finkbeiner, Ann K. *Guide to Living with HIV Infection: Developed at the Johns Hopkins Aids Clinic*. Baltimore, MD: Johns Hopkins University Press, 2001.

Levenson, Jacob. *The Secret Epidemic: The Story of AIDS and Black America*. New York, NY: Pantheon Books, 2004.

Snodgrass, Mary Ellen. *World Epidemics: A Cultural Chronology of Disease from Prehistory to the Era of SARS*. Jefferson, NC: McFarland & Company, 2003.

Alcoholism

Goodwin, Donald. *Alcoholism—The Facts*. New York, NY: Oxford University Press, 2000.

Alzheimer's disease

Molloy, William. *Alzheimer's Disease: Everything You Need to Know*. Ontario: Firefly Books Ltd., 2003.

Anemia

Ross, Allison J. *Everything You Need to Know about Anemia*. New York, NY: Rosen Publishing Group, 2000.

Wick, Manfred, Pinggera, W., and Lehmann, P. *Clinical Aspects and Laboratory: Iron Metabolism, Anemias*. New York, NY: Springer-Verlag, 2003.

Arthritis

Brewer, Earl J., and Angel, Kathy Cochran. *The Arthritis Sourcebook*. New York, NY: McGraw-Hill Companies, 2000.

Asthma

Fanta, Christopher H., et al. *The Harvard Medical School Guide to Taking Control of Asthma*. New York, NY: Simon & Schuster Trade, 2003.

Navarra, Tova. *Encyclopedia of Asthma and Respiratory Disorders*. New York, NY: Facts on File, 2002.

Blindness

Jeffrey, Laura S. *All About Braille*. Berkeley Heights, NJ: Enslow Publishers, 2004.

Mogk, Lylas G., and Mogk, Maria. *Macular Degeneration: The Complete Guide to Saving and Maximizing Your Sight*. New York, NY: Ballantine Books, 2003.

Sardegna, Jill, et al. *Encyclopedia of Blindness and Vision Impairment*. New York, NY: Facts on File, 2002.

Cancer

Dollinger, Malin, Tempero, Margaret (Editor), and Rosenbaum, Earnest H. (Editor). *Everyone's Guide to Cancer Therapy*. Kansas City, KS: Andrews McMeel Publishing, 2002.

Eyre, Harmon J., Morris, Lois B., and Lange, Dianne. *Informed Decisions: The Complete Book of Cancer Diagnosis, Treatment, and Recovery*. Atlanta, GA: American Cancer Society, 2001.

Quillin, Patrick, with Quillin, Noreen. *Beating Cancer with Nutrition: Combining the Best of Science and Nature for Full Spectrum Healing in the 21st Century*. Tulsa, OK: Nutrition Times Press, 2001.

Rossman, Martin L. *Fighting Cancer from Within: How to Use the Power of Your Mind for Healing*. New York, NY: Henry Holt & Company, 2003.

Cystic Fibrosis

Abramovitz, Melissa. *Cystic Fibrosis*. Farmington Hills, MI: Gale Group, 2003.

Orenstein, David. *Cystic Fibrosis: A Guide for Patient and Family*. Hagerstown, MD: Lippincott Williams & Wilkins, 2003.

Deafness

Dugan, Marcia B. *Living with Hearing Loss*. Bellingham, WA: Gallaudet University Press, 2003.

Gordon, Melanie A., and Gordon, M. A. *Let's Talk about Deafness*. New York, NY: Rosen Publishing Group, 2003.

Turkington, Carol, and Sussman, Allen E. *Encyclopedia of Deafness and Hearing Disorders*. New York, NY: Facts on File, 2003.

Diabetes

American Diabetes Association (Editor). *American Diabetes Association Complete Guide to Diabetes*. New York, NY: Bantam Books, 2003.

Down Syndrome

Cohen, William I. (Editor), National Down

Syndrome Society Staff, et al. *Down Syndrome: Visions for the 21st Century.* New York, NY: John Wiley & Sons, 2002.

Kumin, Libby. *Early Communication Skills for Children with Down Syndrome: A Guide for Parents and Professionals,* Vol. 1. Bethesda, MD: Woodbine House, 2003.

Epilepsy

Freeman, John M., et al. *Seizures and Epilepsy in Childhood: A Guide.* Baltimore, MD: Johns Hopkins University Press, 2002.

Gastrointestinal disorders

Kalibjian, Cliff. *Straight from the Gut: Living with Crohn's Disease and Ulcerative Colitis.* Sebastopol, CA: O' Reilly & Associates, 2003.

Minocha, Anil, and Carroll, David. *Natural Stomach Care: Treating and Preventing Digestive Disorders with the Best of Eastern and Western Healing Therapies.* Wayne, NJ: Avery, 2003.

Heart Disease

Bernstein, Jonathan Sackner, and Kelly, Kate. *Before It Happens to You: A Simple, Safe and Scientific Program to Reverse Heart Disease and Reduce the Risk.* Cambridge, MA: Da Capo Press, 2004.

Cooke, John P., and Zimmer, Judith. *The Cardiovascular Cure: How to Strengthen Your Self-Defense against Heart Attack and Stroke.* New York, NY: Broadway Books, 2003.

Superko, Robert, et al. *Before the Heart Attacks: A Revolutionary Approach to Detecting, Preventing, and Even Reversing Heart Disease.* New York, NY: Rodale Press, 2003.

Hemophilia

Britton, Beverly, and Sheen, Barbara. *Diseases and Disorders: Hemophilia.* Farmington Hills, MI: Gale Group, 2003.

Monroe, Dougald M., Hoffman, Maureane R., and Hedner, Ulla. *Hemophilia Care in the New Millennium.* Boston, MA: Kluwer Academic Publishers, 2001.

Hepatitis

Hollinger, F. Blaine (Editor), Purcell, Robert H., and Gerin, John L. *Viral Hepatitis.* Hagerstown, MD: Lippincott Williams & Wilkins, 2002.

Influenza

Manufactured by Health Publica Icon Health Publications. *Influenza—A Medical Dictionary, Bibliography, and Annotated Research Guide to Internet References.* San Diego, CA: ICON Health Publications, 2004.

Leukemia

Henderson, Edward S., Lister, T. Andrew, and Greaves, Mel F. *Leukemia.* Orlando, FL: Harcourt Health Sciences, 2002.

Malaria

Humphreys, Margaret. *Malaria in the United States: Poverty, Race, and Public Health.* Baltimore, MD: Johns Hopkins University Press, 2001.

Multiple sclerosis

Hill Beth. *Multiple Sclerosis Q & A: Reassuring Answers to Frequently Asked Questions.* New York, NY: Putnam Publishing Group, 2003.

Schapiro, Randall T. *Managing the Symptoms of Multiple Sclerosis.* Trenton, NJ: Demos Medical Publishing, 2003.

Parkinson's disease

Lieberman, Abraham N. *100 Questions and Answers about Parkinson's Disease.* Sudbury, MA: Jones & Bartlett Publishers, 2003.

Sickle-cell anemia

Gold, Susan Dudley, and McMahon, Lillian. *Sickle Cell Disease.* Berkeley Heights, NJ: Enslow Publishers, 2001.

Sacerdote, Alan, and Platt, Allan F. *Hope and Destiny: A Patient's and Parent's Guide to Sickle Cell Anemia.* Roscoe, IL: Hilton Publishing, 2001.

Spinal cord injuries

Landau, Elaine. *Spinal Cord Injuries.* Berkeley Heights, NJ: Enslow Publishers, 2001.

Tuberculosis

Leonard, Barry. *Improving Patient Adherence to Tuberculosis Treatment.* Collingdale, PA: Diane Publishing Company, 2000.

Yancey, Diane. *Tuberculosis.* Brookfield, CT: Millbrook Press, 2001.

Medical technology

Henry, John Bernard, Davey, M.D., and Woods, McPherson. *Clinical Diagnosis and Management by Laboratory Methods.* 20th edition. Newbury Park, CA: Sage Publications, 2001.

Leach, Donna, and Ryman, Denny. *Prentice Hall Health's Outline Review of Medical Technology/Clinical Laboratory Science.* Upper Saddle River, NJ: Prentice Hall, 2002.

Novelline, Robert A. *Squire's Fundamentals of Radiology.* 6th edition. Cambridge, MA: Harvard University Press, 2004.

Medication, drugs, and addiction

DiClemente, Carlo C. *Addiction and Change: How Addictions Develop and Addicted People Recover.* New York, NY: Guilford Publications, 2003.

Goozner, Merrill. *The $800 Million Pill: The Truth behind the Cost of New Drugs.* San Diego, CA: University of California Press, 2004.

Heymann, Philip B., and Brownsberger, William N. (Editors). *Drug Addiction and Drug Policy: The Struggle to Control Dependence.* Cambridge, MA: Harvard University Press, 2001.

Liska, Ken. *Drugs and the Human Body with Implications for Society.* Upper Saddle River, NJ: Prentice Hall, 2003.

Men's health

Grimm, Peter D., Sylvester, John, and Blasko, John. *The Prostate Cancer Treatment Book.* New York, NY: McGraw-Hill Companies, 2003.

Issa, Muta M., and Marshall, Fray F. *Contemporary Diagnosis and Management of Diseases of the Prostate.* Newtown, PA: Associates in Medical Marketing Company, 2000.

Simon, Harvey B., Greenfield, Harriet (Illustrator), and Buring, Julie E. *Harvard Medical School Guide to Men's Health.* New York, NY: Simon & Schuster Adult Publishing Group, 2002.

Pregnancy, abortion, and childbirth

Bowers, Nancy A. *The Multiple Pregnancy SourceBook: Pregnancy and the First Year with Twins, Triplets, and More.* New York, NY: McGraw-Hill Companies, 2001.

Carlson, Bruce. *Human Embryology and Developmental Biology.* San Diego, CA: Elsevier Science, 2004.

Cherry, Andrew L., et al. *Teenage Pregnancy: A Global View.* Westport, CT: Greenwood Publishing Group, 2001.

Dickason, Elizabeth J., Silverman, Bonnie L., and Schultz, Martha Olsen. *Maternal-Infant Nursing Care*. St Louis, MO: Mosby, 2002.

Knapp, Lynette. *Abortion Controversy*. Farmington Hills, MI: Gale Group, 2001.

Pinon, Ramon. *Biology of Human Reproduction*. Herndon, VA: University Science Books, 2002.

Simkin, Penny, Keppler, Ann, and Whalley, Janet. *Pregnancy, Childbirth, and the Newborn*. Minnetonka, MN: Meadowbrook Press, 2001.

Tsiaras, Alexander, and Werth, Barry. *From Conception to Birth: A Life Unfolds*. New York, NY: Doubleday & Company, 2002.

Winston, Robert. *The IVF Revolution*. East Mississauga, Ontario: Random House of Canada, 2000.

Psychology, psychotherapy, and mental health

Barry, Patricia D., Farmer, Suzette, and Barry, Dent. *Mental Health and Mental Illness*. Hagerstown, MD: Lippincott Williams & Wilkins, 2001.

Bourne, Edmund J. *The Anxiety and Phobia Workbook*. Oakland, CA: New Harbinger Publishers, 2000.

Campbell, Anne. *Men, Women, and Aggression: From Rage in Marriage to Violence in the Streets: How Gender Affects the Way We Act*. New York, NY: Basic Books, 2004.

Carlson, Trudy. *Learning Disabilities: How to Recognize and Manage Learning and Behavioral Problems in Children*. Duluth, MN: Benline Press, 2000.

Fawcett, Jan, Golden, Bernard, and Rosenfeld, Nancy. *New Hope for People with Bipolar Disorder*. New York, NY: Crown Publishing Group, 2000.

Maj, Mario, et al. *Phobias*. New York, NY: John Wiley & Sons, 2004.

Mondimore, Francis Mark. *Bipolar Disorder: A Guide for Patients and Families*. Baltimore, MD: Johns Hopkins University Press, 2004.

Wittig, Arno, F., and Sinnett, and Laura M. (Editor). *Schaum's Easy Outline of Introduction to Psychology*. New York, NY: McGraw-Hill Companies, 2002.

Public health

Isaacs, Stephen L., and Knickman, James R. *Generalist Medicine and the U.S. Health Care System (Public Health/Health Services Text Series)* New York, NY: John Wiley & Sons, 2004.

Rothstein, Wlliam G. *Public Health and the Risk Factor*. New York, NY: University of Rochester Press, 2003.

Scutchfield, F. Douglas, Keck, C. William (Editors), and Williams, Stephen J. (Introduction). *Principles of Public Health Practice*. Florence, KY: Delmar Learning, 2002.

Shi, Leiyu, and Singh, Douglas A. *Delivering Health Care in America: A Systems Approach*. Sudbury, MA: Jones & Bartlett Publishers, 2003.

Sex, sexuality, and sexual health

Ayer, Eleanor H. *It's Okay to Say No: Choosing Sexual Abstinence*. New York, NY: Rosen Publishing Group, 2000.

Carey, Michael P. *Sexual Dysfunction*. 2nd edition. New York, NY: Guilford Publications, 2001.

James M. Stanlie, and Robertson, Claire C. (Editors). *Genital Cutting and Transnational Sisterhood*. Champaign, IL: University of Illinois Press, 2002.

Maltz, Wendy, and Arian, Carol. *The Sexual Healing Journey: A Guide for Survivors of Sexual Abuse*. New York, NY: HarperCollins Publishers, 2001.

Sheinberg, Marcia, and Fraenkel, Peter. *The Relational Trauma of Incest*. New York, NY: Guilford Publications, 2000.

Skin and skin care

Connor, Steven. *Book of Skin*. New York, NY: Cornell University Press, 2003.

Fitzpatrick, Thomas B., et al. *Color Atlas and Synopsis of Clinical Dermatology, CD-ROM*. New York, NY: McGraw-Hill Companies, 2001.

McClay, Edward F., Smith, Jodie, and McClay, Mary-Eileen T. *100 Questions and Answers about Melanoma and Other Skin Cancers*. Sudbury, MA: Jones & Bartlett Publishers, 2003.

Pitts, Victoria L. *In the Flesh: the Cultural Politics of Body Modification*. New York, NY: Palgrave Macmillan, 2003.

Surgery

Barash, Paul G., Stoelting, Robert K., and Cullen, Bruce F. *Clinical Anesthesia*. Hagerstown, MD: Lippincott Williams & Wilkins, 2000.

Greenfield, Lazar J., et al. *Surgery: Scientific Principles and Practice*. Hagerstown, MD: Lippincott Williams & Wilkin, 2001.

Pfenninger, John L., and Fowler, Grant C. *Pfenninger & Fowler's Procedures for Primary Care*. 2nd edition. San Diego, CA: Elsevier Science, 2003.

Zollinger, Robert Jr., and Zollinger, Robert Sr. *Zollinger's Atlas of Surgical Operations*. New York, NY: McGraw-Hill Professional, 2002.

Viruses and germs

Coffin John M., Varmus, Harold E., and Hughes, Stephen H. (Editors). *Retroviruses*. New York, NY: Cold Spring Harbor Laboratory Press, 2002.

Sompayrac, Lauren, and National Safety Council Staff. *How Pathogenic Viruses Work*. Sudbury, MA: Jones & Bartlett Publishers, 2002.

Strauss, James H., and Strauss, Ellen G. *Viruses and Human Disease*. San Diego, CA: Elsevier Science & Technology, 2001.

Women's health

Banks, Martha E., and Kaschak, Ellyn (Editors). *Women with Visible and Invisible Disabilities: Multiple Intersections, Multiple Issues, Multiple Therapies*. New York, NY: Haworth Press, 2003.

Carlson, Karen J., Eisenstat, Stephanie A., and Ziporyn, Terra Diane. *The New Harvard Guide to Women's Health*. Cambridge, MA: Harvard University Press, 2004.

Eyler, Amy A. (Editor). *Environmental, Policy, and Cultural Factors Related to Physical Activity in a Diverse Sample of Women: The Women's Cardiovascular Health Network Project*. New York, NY: Haworth Press, 2003.

Lowdermilk, Deitra Lleonard, and Perry, Shannon E. *Maternity and Women's Health Care*. San Diego, CA: Elsevier Science, 2003.

McCloud, Melody T., and Ebron, Angela. *Blessed Health: The African-American Woman's Guide to Physical and Spiritual Well-Being*. New York, NY: Simon & Schuster Adult Publishing Group, 2003.

Northrup, Christiane. *Women's Bodies, Women's Wisdom: Creating Physical and Emotional Health and Healing*. New York, NY: Bantam Books, 2002.

Slater, Lauren, et al. *The Complete Guide to Mental Health for Women*. Boston, MA: Beacon Press, 2003.

Research tools and health-related Websites

The American Academy of Family Physicians
www.familydoctor.org
The academy has produced a Website with health information for the whole family. There is an A–Z index of conditions and diseases, as well as health tips, topical problems, and specific links for men, women, parents, kids, and seniors. There are also many topics on how the whole family can stay healthy.

American Cancer Society
www.cancer.org
A self-help Website for patients, family, and friends to learn about cancer, various treatment options and choices, clinical trials, and coping with the disease. There are links to connect patients with cancer survivors and support programs.

American Red Cross
www.redcross.org
This Website outlines the functions of the Red Cross, how people can help support them, safety tips, and news and current features about the work of the Red Cross at home and abroad.

Centers for Disease Control and Prevention
www.cdc.gov
A core reference title of government-compiled health information, including health statistics, research and development, and numerous links to other Websites.

Harvard School of Public Health
www.hsph.harvard.edu
Health information with an emphasis on awareness of public health and hence, prevention of disease. Education is the key with an aim of getting people to make healthier lifestyle choices.

Haubrich, William S. *Medical Meanings: A Glossary of Word Origins*. 2nd edition. American College of Physicians, 2003.
A glossary that explains the meaning of medical terms and their origins.

Information on clinical trials and human research studies
www.clinicaltrials.gov
Updated information gives details of federally and privately supported clinical research with human volunteers. The site gives information about the aims of a trial, who can take part, locations, and telephone numbers to obtain more details.

KidsHealth
www.kidshealth.org/kid
A site for kids, with features and interactive activities that deal with young people's feelings, illnesses, and health problems. A glossary of medical terms is also included.

KidsHealth (For parents)
www.kidshealth.org/parent
Kid's health from a parent's perspective. The site includes general health, emotions and behavior, growth and development, nutrition and fitness, doctors and hospitals, and first aid and safety.

MayoClinic
www.mayoclinic.com
A site produced by a collective of medical experts with a mission to help people manage their health. Information is up-to-date and all health issues are discussed.

MedHist: the guide to history of medicine resources on the Internet
www.medhist.ac.uk
MedHist provides resources covering all aspects of the history of health and development of medical knowledge. Recommended for students of the history of medicine or for interested laypeople.

MedlinePlus
www.nlm.nih.gov/medlineplus/databases.html
The Website provides several databases on different health topics, safety issues, and toxicology.

National Cancer Institute
www.cancer.gov/cancer_information
A comprehensive site that covers all aspects of suffering from cancer. All types of cancer are listed, and conventional treatments and complementary and alternative medicine treatments are outlined. There are links to prevention, genetics, and causes of cancer, as well as screening, testing, and strategies for coping with cancer.

National Institutes of Health (U.S. Department of Health and Human Services)
www.nih.gov
Health information with an A–Z index of NIH resources, clinical trials, health hotlines, and drug information. Also includes Medlineplus.

National Library of Medicine (PubMed)
www.ncbi.nlm.nih.gov/pubmed
This Website provides more than 14 million citations for medical articles spanning 50 years. Links to many sites access full text articles as well as other resources.

National Mental Health Information Center
www.mentalhealth.org
All aspects of mental health are covered on this site, which has links to a large spectrum of topics. Particularly useful is a drop-down menu that allows users to look for mental health and substance abuse services by state.

National Women's Health Information Center
www.4woman.gov/index.htm
Free, reliable health information for women. The site includes FAQs about women's health, educational campaigns, lists of resources, and special sections on pertinent topics.

Nutrition Source
www.hsph.harvard.edu/nutrition/source
A Website maintained by the Department of Nutrition at the Harvard School of Public Health, which aims to provide topical information for professionals and the public. All aspects of nutrition are covered, including healthy eating advice, news about diet, and other sources of information and links.

TeenGrowth
www.teengrowth.com
A free Website covering health information specifically for teens. Topics include weight loss, questions about sex and puberty, suicide, and skin cancer. Teens can ask questions and join in debates.

Health organizations

ABSTINENCE

Respect Incorporated
PO Box 349
Bradley, IL 60915-1349
Tel: (877) 673-7732
Website: www.sexrespect.com

ACCIDENT PREVENTION

Accident Prevention Corporation
11516 Country Club Road
Woodstock, IL 60098
Tel: (815) 337-7785
Website: www.safetyman.com

AGING

Administration on Aging
1 Massachusetts Avenue,
Suites 4100 and 5100
Washington, DC 20201
Tel: (202) 619-0724
Website: www.aoa.gov

American Geriatrics Society
Empire State Building
350 5th Avenue, Suite 801
New York, NY 10118
Tel: (800) 247-4779
Website: www.americangeriatrics.org

National Institute on Aging
Building 31, Room 5C27
31 Center Drive, MSC 2292
Bethesda, MD 20892
Tel: (301) 496-1752
Website: www.nia.nih.gov

National Council on the Aging
300 D Street, SW, Suite 801
Washington, DC 20024
Tel: (202) 479-1200
Website: www.ncoa.org

AIDS

AIDS Information Hotline
American Social Health Association
PO Box 13827
Research Triangle Park, NC 27709
Tel: (800) 342-2437
Website: www.ashastd.org/hotlines/index.html#

American Foundation for AIDS Research
733 3rd Avenue, 12th Floor
New York, NY 10017
Tel: (800) 392-6327
Website: www.amfar.org

Elizabeth Glaser Pediatric AIDS Foundation
41 Madison Avenue, 29th Floor
New York, NY 10010
Tel: (212) 448-6654
Website: www.pedaids.org

Foundation for Children with AIDS
1800 Columbus Avenue
Roxbury, MA 02119
Tel: (617) 442-7442
Website: www.caaf4kids.org

ALCOHOL/DRUG ABUSE

Alcohol and Drug Problems Association of North America Inc.
307 N. Main
St. Charles, MO 63301
Tel: (314) 589-6702
Website: www.adpana.com

Alcoholics Anonymous World Services
475 Riverside Drive, 11th Floor
New York, NY 10115
Tel: (212) 870-3400
Website: www.alcoholics-anonymous.org

Association for Addiction Professionals
901 N. Washington St., Suite 600
Alexandria, VA 22314
Tel: (703) 741-7686
Website: www.naadac.org

ALLERGIES/ASTHMA

American Academy of Allergy, Asthma, and Immunology
611 East Wells Street
Milwaukee, WI 53202
Tel: (414) 272-6071
Website: www.aaaai.org

Association of Asthma Educators
1215 Anthony Avenue
Columbia, SC 29201-1701
Tel: (888) 988-7747
Website: asthmaeducators.org

Asthma and Allergy Foundation of America
1233 20th Street NW, Suite 402
Washington, DC 20036
Tel: (800) 727-8462
Website: www.aafa.org

National Institute of Allergy and Infectious Diseases
Building 31, Room 7A-50
31 Center Drive MSC 2520
Bethesda, MD 20892-2520
Tel: (301) 496-5717
Website: www.niaid.nih.gov

ALTERNATIVE AND COMPLEMENTARY MEDICINE

Acupuncture Association of Washington
PO Box 2271
Gig Harbor, WA 98335-4271
Tel: (253) 851-4756
Website: www.acupuncturewashington.org

Alexander Technique International
1692 Massachusetts Ave., 3rd Floor
Cambridge, MA 02138
Tel: (888) 668-8996
Website: www.ati-net.com

Alternative Medicine Foundation
5411 W. Cedar Lane, Suite 205-A
Bethesda, MD 20814
Tel: (301) 581-0116
Website: www.amfoundation.org

American Academy of Medical Acupuncture
4929 Wiltshire Blvd., Suite 428
Los Angeles, CA 90010
Tel: (323) 937-5514
Website: www.medicalacupuncture.org

American Alternative Medicine Association
708 Madelaine Drive
Gilmer, TX 75644-3140
Tel: (888) 764-2237
Website: www.joinaama.com

American Chiropractic Association (ACA)
1701 Clarendon Boulevard
Arlington, VA 22209
Tel: (800) 986-4636
Website: www.amerchiro.org

American Herbalists Guild
1931 Gaddis Road
Canton, GA 30115
Tel: (770) 751-6021
Website: www.americanherbalistsguild.com

American Herbal Pharmacopoeia
Box 5159
Santa Cruz, CA 95063
Tel: (831) 461-6317
Website: www.herbal-ahp.org

American Institute of Homeopathy (AIH)
801 N. Fairfax Street, Suite 306
Alexandria, VA 22314
Tel: (703) 246-9501
Website: www.homeopathyusa.org

American Society of Alternative Therapists
PO Box 703
Rockport, MA 01966
Tel: (978) 281-4400
Website: www.asat.org

American Yoga Association
PO Box 19986
Sarasota, FL 34276
Tel: (941) 921-4844
Website: www.americanyogaassociation.org

International Chiropractors Association
1110 N. Glebe Road, Suite 1000
Arlington, VA 22201
Tel: (800) 423-4690
Website: www.chiropractic.org

National Association for Holistic Aromatherapy
2000 2nd Avenue, Suite 206
Seattle, WA 98121
Tel: (206) 256-0741
Website: www.naha.org

North American Society of Homeopaths
1122 East Pike Street
Seattle, WA 98122
Tel: (206) 720-7000
Website: www.homeopathy.org

ARTHRITIS

American College of Rheumatology
1800 Century Place, Suite 250
Atlanta, GA 30345-4300
Tel: (404) 633-3777
Website: www.rheumatology.org

Arthritis Foundation
1330 West Peachtree Street
Atlanta, GA 30309
Tel: (800) 283-7800
Website: www.arthritis.org

National Institute of Arthritis and Musculoskeletal and Skin Diseases
Information Clearinghouse
National Institutes of Health
1 AMS Circle
Bethesda, MD 20892-3672
Tel: (301) 495-4484
Website: www.niams.nih.gov

ATTENTION DEFICIT HYPERACTIVITY DISORDER

Children and Adults with Attention-Deficit/Hyperactivity Disorder
8181 Professional Place, Suite 150
Landover, MD 20785
Tel: (800) 233 4050
Website: www.chadd.org

AUTISM

Autism Society of America
7910 Woodmont Ave., Suite 300

Bethesda, MD 20814-3067
Tel: (301) 657-0881
Website: www.autism-society.org/site/PageServer

BEREAVEMENT

Association for Death Education and Counseling
432 North Main Street
West Hartford, CT 06117-2507
Tel: (860) 586-7503
Website: www.adec.org

Pregnancy and Infant Loss Center
1421 E. Wayzata Boulevard, #40
Wayzata, MN 55391
Tel: (612) 473-9372
Website: www.bloomington.in.
us/socserv/mit/PREGNANCY_AN
D_INFANT_LOSS_CENTER.html

Compassionate Friends Inc.
PO Box 3696
Oak Brook, IL 60522-3696
Tel: (630) 990-0010
Website: www.compassion
atefriends.org

BIRTH DEFECTS

Birth Defects Research for Children
930 Woodcock Road, Suite 225
Orlando, FL 32803
Tel: (407) 895-0802
Website: www.birthdefects.org

Cleft Palate Foundation
1504 E. Franklin Street, Suite 102
Chapel Hill, NC 27514-2820
Tel: (919) 933-9044
Website: www.cleftline.org

BLINDNESS

American Council for the Blind
1155 15th Street NW, Suite 1004
Washington, DC 20005
Tel: (800) 424-8666
Website: www.acb.org

American Foundation for the Blind Inc.
11 Penn Plaza, Suite 300
New York, NY 10001
Tel: (800) 232-5463
Website: www.afb.org

Association for Macular Diseases
210 East 64th Street, 8th Floor

New York, NY 10021
Tel: (212) 605-3719
Website: www.macula.org

Eye Care Foundation
115 East 61st Street
New York, NY 10021
Tel: (212) 832-7297
Website: www.eyecarefounda
tion.org

Prevent Blindness America
500 East Remington Road
Schaumburg, IL 60173
Tel: (800) 331-2020, ext. 322
Website: www.preventblindness.
org

BLOOD DONORS

American Association of Blood Banks
8101 Glenbrook Road
Bethesda, MD 20814-2749
Tel: (301) 907-6977
Website: www.aabb.org

BREAST-FEEDING

Academy of Breastfeeding Medicine
191 Clarksville Road
Princeton Junction, NJ 08550
Tel: (877) 836-9947, ext. 25
Website: www.bfmed.org

CANCER

American Association for Cancer Education
MD Anderson Cancer Center
1515 Holcombe Boulevard
Houston, TX 77030
Tel: (800) 392-1611
Website: www.aaceonline.com

Cancer Care Inc.
National Office, 275 7th Avenue
New York, NY 10001
Tel: (800) 813-4674
Website: www.cancercare.org

CancerNet
Building 31, Room 10A03
31 Center Drive MSC 2580
Bethesda, MD 20892-2580
Tel: (800) 422-6237
Website: www.cancernet.com

National Cancer Institute
NCI Public Inquiries Office,

Suite 3036A
6116 Executive Blvd., MSC8322
Bethesda, MD 20892-8322
Tel: (800) 422-6237
Website: www.cancer.gov

Leukemia and Lymphoma Society
1311 Mamaroneck Ave.
White Plains, NY 10605
Tel: (914) 949-5213
Website: www.leukemia.org

CELIAC DISEASE

Celiac Disease Foundation
13251 Ventura Blvd., #1
Studio City, CA 91604
Tel: (818) 990-2354
Website: www.celiac.org

CHILD ABUSE

Childhelp USA
15757 North 78th Street
Scottsdale, AZ 85260
Tel: (800) 422-4453
Website: www.childhelpusa.org

CHILDREN

Child Development Institute
3528 E. Ridgeway Road
Orange, CA 92867
Tel: (714) 998-8617
Website: www.cdipage.com

Child Find of America Inc.
PO Box 277
New Palz, NY 12561-0722
Tel: (845) 255-1848
Website: www.childfindofamer
ica.org

Children's Foundation
725 15th Street NW, Suite 505
Washington, DC 20005-2109
Tel: (202) 347-3300
Website: www.childrensfounda
tion.net

Starlight Children's Foundation
5900 Wilshire Blvd., Suite 2530
Los Angeles, CA 90036
Tel: (323) 634-0080
Website: www.starlight.org

The American Academy of Child and Adolescent Psychology
3615 Wisconsin Avenue, NW
Washington, DC 20016-3007

Tel: (202) 966-7300
Website: www.aacap.org

American Academy of Pediatrics
141 Northwest Point Boulevard
Elk Grove Village, IL 60007-1098
Tel: (837) 434-4000
Website: www.aap.org

CHRONIC FATIGUE SYNDROME

Chronic Fatigue Immune Dysfunction Syndrome Association of America
PO Box 220398
Charlotte, NC 28222-0398
Tel: (704) 365-2343
Website: www.cfids.org

CYSTIC FIBROSIS

Cystic Fibrosis Foundation
6931 Arlington Road
Bethesda, MD 20814
Tel: (800) 344-4823
Website: www.cff.org

DEAFNESS

Alexander Graham Bell Association for the Deaf
3417 Volta Place NW
Washington, DC 20007-2778
Tel: (202) 337-5220
Website: www.agbell.org

Deafness Research Foundation
575 5th Avenue, 11th Floor
New York, NY 10017
Tel: (212) 599-0027
Website: www.drf.org

National Association of the Deaf
814 Thayer Avenue
Silver Spring, MD 20910-4500
Tel: (301) 587-1788
Website: www.nad.org

DIABETES

American Diabetes Association
1701 North Beauregard Street
Alexandria, VA 22314
Tel: (800) 342-2383
Website: www.diabetes.org

International Diabetic Athletes Association
1647B Bethany Home Road
Phoenix, AZ 85015

Tel: (800) 898-4322
Website: www.diabetes-exercise.org

Juvenile Diabetes Foundation International
120 Wall Street
New York, NY 10005-3904
Tel: (800) 533-2873
Website: www.jdf.org

National Diabetes Foundation Clearinghouse
1 Information Way
Bethesda, MD 20892-3560
Tel: (301) 654-3327
Website: www.nlm.nih.gov

DIGESTIVE DISORDERS

Crohn's and Colitis Foundation of America
386 Park Ave. South, 17th Floor
New York, NY 10016-8804
Tel: (800) 932-2423
Website: www.ccfa.org

National Digestive Diseases Information Clearinghouse
2 Information Way
Bethesda, MD 20892-3570
Tel: (800) 891-5389
Website: digestive.niddk.nih.gov

United Ostomy Association
19772 MacArthur Blvd., Suite 200
Irvine, CA 92612-2405
Tel: (800) 826-0826
Website: www.uoa.org

DISABILITIES

Council for Disability Rights
205 West Randolph, Suite 1650
Chicago, IL 60606
Tel: (312) 444-9484
Website: www.disabilityrights.org

International Council on Disability
25 East 21st Street
New York, NY 10010
Tel: (212) 420-1500
Website: www.disabilityworld.org

Learning Disabilities Association of America
4156 Library Road

Pittsburg, PA 15234-1349
Tel: (412) 341-1515
Website: www.ldanatl.org

EATING DISORDERS

Eating Disorder Referral and Information Center
2923 Sandy Pointe, Suite 6
Del Mar, CA 92014-2052
Tel: (858) 792-7463
Website: www.edreferral.com

National Association of Anorexia Nervosa and Associated Disorders
Box 7, Highland Park, IL 60035
Tel: (847) 831-3438
Website: www.anad.org

FAMILY PLANNING/ PREGNANCY

American Society for Reproductive Medicine
1209 Montgomery Highway
Birmingham, AL 35216-2809
Tel: (205) 978-5000
Website: www.asrm.org

International Childbirth Education Association, Inc.
PO Box 20048
Minneapolis, MN 55420
Tel: (952) 854-8660
Website: www.icea.org

Maternity Center Association
281 Park Avenue South
New York, NY 10010
Tel: (212) 777-5000
Website: www.maternitywise.org

National Campaign to Prevent Teen Pregnancy
1776 Massachusetts Avenue NW, Suite 200
Washington, DC 20036
Tel: (202) 478-8500
Website: www.teenpregnancy.org

Planned Parenthood Federation of America
810 7th Avenue
New York, NY 10019
Tel: (800) 230-7526
Website: www.plannedparenthood.org

FEET

American Podiatric Medical Association
9312 Old Georgetown Road
Bethesda, MD 20814
Tel: (301) 571-9200
Website: www.apma.org

GENERAL HEALTH INFORMATION

American Academy of Family Physicians
11400 Tomahawk Creek Parkway
Leawood, KS 66211-2672
Website: www.familydoctor.org

American Association for World Health
1825 K Street NW, Suite 1208
Washington, DC 20006
Tel: (202) 466-5883
Website: www.thebody.com/aawh/aawhpage.html

American Health Care Association
1201 L Street NW
Washington, DC 20005
Tel: (202) 8420-4444
Website: www.ahca.org

American Health Foundation
320 East 43rd Street
New York, NY 10017
Tel: (212) 953-1900
Website: www.ahf.org

American Health Information Management Association
233 N. Michigan Ave., Suite 2150
Chicago, IL 60601-5800
Tel: (312) 233-1100
Website: www.ahima.org

American Medical Association
515 N. State Street
Chicago, IL 60610
Tel: (800) 621-8335
Website: www.ama-assn.org

American Red Cross
2025 E. Street, NW
Washington, DC 20006
Tel: (202) 303-4498
Website: www.redcross.org

National Institutes of Health
9000 Rockville Pike

Bethesda, MD 20814
Tel: (301) 496-4000
Website: www.nih.gov

GENETIC DISEASES

Genetic Alliance, Inc.
4301 Connecticut Ave. NW,
Suite 404
Washington, DC 20008-2369
Tel: (202) 966-5557
Website: www.geneticalliance.
org

HEART DISEASE

American Heart Association
7272 Greenville Avenue
Dallas, TX 75231-4596
Tel: (800) 242-8721
Website: www.americanheart.
org

Mended Hearts Inc.
7272 Greenville Avenue
Dallas ,TX 75231-4596
Tel: (214) 706-1442
Website: www.mendedhearts.
org

HEMOPHILIA

Committee of Ten Thousand
236 Massachusetts Avenue NE,
Suite 609
Washington, DC 20002
Tel: (800) 488-2688
Website: www.catalogueforphi
lanthropy.org/ma/1997/commit
tee_ten_355.htm

National Hemophilia Foundation
116 West 32nd Street, 11th Floor
New York, NY 10001
Tel: (212) 328-3700
Website: www.hemophilia.org

LIVER DISEASES

American Association for the Study of Liver Diseases
1729 King Street, Suite 200
Alexandria, VA 22314
Tel: (703) 299-9766
Website: www.aasld.org

American Liver Foundation
75 Maiden Lane, Suite 603
New York, NY 10038
Tel: (800) 465-4837
Website: www.liverfoundation.
org

MEN'S HEALTH

American Prostate Society
PO Box 870
Hanover, MD 21076
Tel: (800) 308-1106
Website: www.ameripros.org

Circumcision Resource Center
PO Box 232
Boston, MA 02133
Tel: (617) 523-0088
Website: www.circumcision.
org

MENTAL HEALTH

American Psychiatric Association
1000 Wilson Blvd., Suite 1825
Arlington, VA 22209-3901
Tel: (703) 907-7300
Website: www.psych.org

American Psychological Association
750 1st Street NE
Washington, DC 20002-4242
Tel: (292) 336-5500
Website: www.apa.org

Anxiety Disorders Association of America
8730 Georgia Ave., Suite 600
Silver Spring, MD 20910
Tel: (240) 485-1001
Website: www.adaa.org

Association for Advancement of Behavior Therapy
305 7th Ave., 16th Floor
New York, NY 10001-6008
Tel: (212) 647-1890
Website: www.aabt.org

Child and Adolescent Bipolar Foundation
1187 Wilmette Ave., PMB #331
Wilmette, IL 60091
Tel: (847) 256-8525
Website: www.bpkids.org

National Alliance for the Mentally Ill
Colonial Place Three
2107 Wilson Blvd., Suite 300
Arlington, VA 22201-3042
Tel: (800) 950-6264
Website: www.nami.org

National Mental Health Consumer Self-Help Clearinghouse
1211 Chestnut Street
Philadelphia, PA 19107
Tel: (800) 668-4226
Website: www.mhselfhelp.org

MENTAL RETARDATION

Association for Children with Retarded Mental Development
345 Hudson Street, 3rd Floor
New York, NY 10014
Tel: (212) 741-0100
Website: www.nyc.gov/html/
mopd/html/mrdd_reip.html

National Association for Down Syndrome
PO Box 4542
Oak Park, IL 60522-4542
Tel: (630) 325-9112
Website: www.nads.org

National Down Syndrome Society
666 Broadway
New York, NY 10012
Tel: (800) 221-4602
Website: www.ndss.org

NEUROLOGICAL AND MUSCULAR DISORDERS

Alzheimer's Association
919 N. Michigan Ave., Suite 1000
Chicago, IL 60611-1676
Tel: (800) 272-3900
Website: www.alz.org

Christopher Reeve Paralysis Foundation
500 Morris Avenue
Springfield, NJ 07081
Tel: (800) 225-0292
Website: www.apacure.com

Epilepsy Foundation of America
4351 Garden City Drive
Landover, MD 20785
Tel: (301) 459-3700
Website: www.apa.org/science/
efa.html

Huntington's Disease Society of America, Inc.
140 West 22nd Street, 6th Floor
New York, NY 10011-2420
Tel: (212) 242-1968
Website: www.hdsa.org

Myasthenia Gravis Foundation Inc.
5841 Cedar Lake Road, Suite 204
Minneapolis, MN 55416
Tel: (800) 541-5454
Website: www.myasthenia.org

National Aphasia Association
29 John Street, Suite 1103
New York, NY 10038
Tel: (800) 922 4622
Website: www.aphasia.org

National Ataxia Foundation
2600 Fernbrook Lane, Suite 119
Minneapolis, MN 55447
Tel: (763) 553-0020
Website: www.ataxia.org

National Spinal Cord Injury Association
8701 Georgia Avenue, Suite 500
Silver Spring, MD 20910
Tel: (800) 962-9629
Website: www.spinalcord.org

National Stroke Association
9707 E. Easter Lane
Englewood, CO 80112
Tel: (303) 649-9299
Website: 199.239.30.192/
NationalStroke/default.htm

Paralyzed Veterans of America
801 18th Street NW
Washington, DC 20006-3517
Tel: (800) 424-8200
Website: www.pva.org

Parkinson's Disease Foundation, Inc.
710 West 168th Street
New York, NY 10032-9982
Tel: (800) 457-6676
Website: www.parkinson.org

United Cerebral Palsy National
1660 L Street, NW, Suite 700
Washington, DC 20036
Tel: (800) 872-5827
Website: www.ucp.org

NUTRITION

American Dietetic Association
216 West Jackson Boulevard
Chicago, IL 60606-6995
Tel: (312) 899-0040
Website: www.eatright.org

American Society for Parenteral and Enteral Nutrition
8630 Fenton Street, Suite 412
Silver Spring, MA 20910-3803
Tel: (800) 727-4567
Website:
www.nutrition care.org

Council for Responsible Nutrition
1875 Eye Street NW, Suite 400
Washington, DC 20006-5194
Tel: (202) 872-1488
Website: www.crnusa.org

OSTEOPATHY

American Association of Colleges of Osteopathic Medicine (AACOM)
5550 Friendship Blvd.,
Suite 310
Chevy Chase, MD 20815-7231
Tel: (301) 968-4100
Website: www.aacom.org

American Osteopathic Association
142 East Ontario Street
Chicago, IL 60611
Tel: (800) 621-1773
Website: www.osteopathic.org

PAIN

American Academy of Pain Management
13947 Mono Way #A
Sonora, CA 95370
Tel: (209) 533-9744
Website: www.aapainmanage.org

American Chronic Pain Association
PO Box 850
Rocklin, CA 95677
Tel: (916) 632-0922
Website: www.theacpa.org

American Pain Society
4700 West Lake Avenue
Glenville, IL 60025
Tel: (847) 375-4715
Website: www.ampainsoc.org

PHARMACISTS

American Pharmacists Association
2215 Constitution Ave., NW
Washington, DC 20037-2985
Tel: (202) 628-4410
Website: www.aphanet.org

PHYSICAL FITNESS

Aerobics and Fitness Association of America
15250 Ventura Blvd., Suite 200
Sherman Oaks, CA 91403
Tel: (877) 968-7263
Website: www.afaa.com

PLASTIC AND RECONSTRUCTIVE SURGERY

American Academy of Facial Plastic and Reconstructive Surgery
310 S. Henry Street
Alexandria, VA 22314
Tel: (703) 299-9291
Website: www.facial-plastic-surgery.org

POLLUTION

U.S. Environmental Protection Agency
Clean Air Markets Division
1200 Pennsylvania Avenue, NW
Washington, DC 20460
Tel: (202) 343-9150
Website: www.epa.gov

SEXUAL HEALTH

CDC National STD Hotline
PO Box 13827
Research Triangle Park
Durham, NC 27709
Tel: (800) 221-8922
Website: www.ashastd.org/NSTD/index.html

Gay and Lesbian Medical Association
459 Fulton Street, Suite 107
San Francisco, CA 94102
Tel: (415) 255-4547
Website: www.glma.org

Sex Information and Education Council of the United States
130 West 42nd Street, Suite 350
New York, NY 10036-7802
Tel: (212) 819-9776
Website: www.siecus.org

SICKLE-CELL ANEMIA

American Sickle Cell Anemia Association
10300 Carnegie Avenue
Cleveland, Ohio 44106
Tel: (216) 229-8600
Website: www.ascaa.org

Sickle Cell Disease Association of America
200 Corporate Point, Suite 495
Culver City, CA 90230-8727
Tel: (800) 421-8453
Website: www.sicklecelldisease.org/default.htm

SKIN AND HAIR DISORDERS

American Academy of Dermatology
PO Box 4014
Schaumburg, IL 60168-4014
Tel: (847) 330-0230
Website: www.aad.org

American Burn Association
625 N. Michigan Ave., Suite 1530
Chicago, IL 60611
Tel: (312) 642-9260
Website: www.ameriburn.org

Vascular Birthmarks Foundation
PO Box 106
Latham, NY 12110
Tel: (877) 823 5665
Website: www.birthmark.org

SLEEP DISORDERS

National Sleep Foundation
1367 Connecticut Avenue, NW
Washington, DC 20036
Tel: (202) 347-3471
Website: www.sleepfoundation.org

SMOKING

Action on Smoking and Health (ASH)
2013 H Street NW
Washington, DC 20006
Tel: (202) 659-4310
Website: www.ash.org

American Lung Association
1740 Broadway
New York, NY 10019-4374
Tel: (800) 568-4872
Website: www.lungusa.org

Coalition on Smoking or Health
1150 Connecticut Avenue NW,
Suite 820
Washington, DC 20036
Tel: (202) 452-1184
Website: tobaccodocuments.org

SPORTS MEDICINE

American College of Sports Medicine
PO Box 1440
Indianapolis, IN 46206-1440
Tel: (317) 637-9200
Website: www.acsm.org

SUDDEN INFANT DEATH SYNDROME

American Sudden Infant Death Syndrome Institute
2480 Windy Hill Road
Marietta, GA 30067
Tel: (800) 232-7437
Website: www.sids.org

SURGERY

American College of Surgeons Professional Association
633 N. Saint Clair Street
Chicago, IL 60611-3211
Tel: (800) 621-4111
Website: www.facs.org

TRANSPLANTS

Organ Donors
PO Box 6725
Houston, TX 77265-6725
Tel: (800) 528-2971
Website:
www.multiline.com.au/~donor

URINARY SYSTEM DISORDERS

American Urological Association
1000 Corporate Blvd.
Linthicum, MD 21090
Tel: (866) 746-4282
Website: www.auanet.org

National Kidney Foundation
30 East 33rd Street, Suite 1100
New York, NY 10016
Tel: (212) 889-2210
Website: www.kidney.org

Renal Physicians Association
1700 Rockville Pike, Suite 220
Rockville, MD 20852
Tel: (301) 468-3515
Website: www.renalmd.org

Thematic indexes

The following thematic indexes reflect the five categories of articles in the encyclopedia: Human Body; Diseases and Other Disorders; Treatments and Cures; Prevention and Diagnosis of Disease; and Human Behavior. Included is a brief People Index, identifying scientists, researchers, physicians, and other figures mentioned in articles.

Boldface numbers indicate complete articles; **boldface** numbers preceding colons are volume numbers; numbers following colons indicate page numbers; *italic* page numbers refer to photographs and other illustrations.

HUMAN BODY

abdomen **1**:11–13
  ascites **4**:545; **11**:1533
    infertility investigation **7**:945;
      8:1033–1034
    knife wound to **11**:1534
    laparoscopy **4**:568, 569, 570, 571;
      8:1033–1034; **9**:1236; **11**:1459, 1520;
      15:2138
    laparotomy **8**:1035
    ligaments **8**:1069
    pain **1**:*11*–13; **6**:797; **11**:1475, 1520–1521,
      1578; **15**:2152
    swelling **15**:2148
    tuberculosis **16**:2290
    tumors **16**:2291
acetabulum **11**:1523
acetylcholine **2**:158; **6**:857; **9**:1266
  Alzheimer's disease and **1**:82, 83
  myasthenia gravis and **10**:1313
achalasia, of the esophagus **6**:787
acid-base balance **1**:26–27
acini **11**:1486–1487
ACTH *see* adrenocorticotropic
  hormone
Adam's apple **10**:1332, *1335*; **16**:*2213*
adaptation syndrome **15**:2099
adenoids **1**:40–41; **2**:281; **10**:1372, 1375;
  11:1557; **16**:2212–2213
    adenoidectomy **1**:41; **16**:2212
    snoring and **14**:*2005*
adenosine triphosphate (ATP) **5**:703
adipose tissue **8**:1079–1080
adrenal glands **1**:46–48; **9**:1246
  overactive **6**:858
  pituitary gland and **4**:567; **12**:1598
  underactive **6**:858
adrenaline (epinephrine) **1**:47; **4**:*566*;
  12:1724
  in the brain **2**:229
  effects **1**:*48*; **9**:1246; **15**:2085, 2099
    blushing **2**:244
    as a bronchodilator **1**:140
    dry mouth **9**:1262
    fat breakdown **5**:622
    glycogen breakdown **15**:2064
    on the heart **6**:781
    high blood pressure **1**:46
  too much **6**:858
  used as a drug **1**:47
adrenocorticotropic hormone (ACTH)
  12:1599, 1601
afterbirth *see* placenta
aging **1**:53–55

absentmindedness **4**:459
Alzheimer's disease **1**:82
antiaging treatment
  melatonin **9**:1186, 1187
  serums **9**:1273
arthritis **5**:691
  osteoarthritis **1**:*135–138*
balance and **2**:167; **11**:1581
blackouts **5**:691
cataracts **3**:326
causes **1**:53–54
cells and **1**:54–55; **3**:330
cystitis and **4**:450
deafness **4**:455; **5**:692–693
dementia **5**:692, 693
drowsiness **4**:523
eyesight and **5**:608; **10**:1412
fibrositis **5**:643
free radicals and **1**:101
frostbite and **5**:665–666
geriatric medicine **5**:691–694
  physical therapy and **11**:1581
glaucoma **2**:221; **5**:701
height loss **1**:53; **3**:324
hip fractures **6**:828, 830, 855
hypothermia **5**:693–694; **7**:900,
  901, 902
impairment of faculties **14**:1910
incontinence **5**:693
libido **1**:53
lower-back pain **5**:630
macular degeneration **2**:220, 222;
  8:1119; **13**:1811, 1812
malnutrition **8**:*1127*
memory and **9**:1190, 1192; **14**:1908,
  1909–1910
osteoporosis **5**:693; **6**:855;
  11:*1450–1451*
physical disabilities **6**:751
prostate enlargement **12**:1691
psychiatric disorders **14**:1910–1911
retirement and **8**:1067
sense of taste **16**:2169
skin **14**:*1970*, 1975
  age spots **8**:1090
  liver spots **8**:*1091*
  wrinkles **14**:*1970*; **15**:2127;
    17:2427–2428
strokes **5**:691–692
suicide in the elderly **6**:839
tiredness **5**:620; **16**:2229
weight gain **10**:1384
aldosterone **1**:47; **2**:238, *239*; **4**:*566*;
  6:858; **8**:1020
alimentary canal **1**:11, 67–69
  see also colon; digestive system;
    duodenum; stomach
alopecia *see* baldness
alpha-1 antitrypsin **4**:563, *564*; **5**:681
alpha-linoleic acid **10**:1382
altitudes, high
  people living at **6**:*847*
  training at **15**:2052
alveolar processes **16**:2175
alveoli (air sacs) **2**:281; **4**:*563*
  COPD and **3**:370, *371*
amino acids **4**:488; **12**:1701, *1702*
  dietary **10**:1381; **12**:1701–1702
amniotic sac **9**:1188, 1189
amylase (ptyalin) **4**:*494*, 495; **5**:702;
  8:1149; **9**:1149, 1261; **11**:1487, *1487*;
  13:1853; **15**:2063, *2064*

amyloid precursor protein (APP) **1**:83
anabolism **9**:1214
anal canal, hemorrhoids **6**:*807*–808
androgens **1**:48; **2**:169
  acne and **1**:32
  see also testosterone
angiotensin **2**:238, 239
ankles
  edema **4**:*544*, 545; **6**:790; **15**:2146
  fractured **5**:661
  ligaments **8**:1070
  osteoarthritis **10**:1437
  sprained **6**:764; **15**:*2057*, 2145
  stiffness **15**:2079
antibodies (immunoglobulins) **2**:165,
  227; **7**:908, 940; **8**:1113; **17**:2330
  allergies and **1**:72–73, 140
  antilymphocyte **7**:914
  antinuclear **8**:1107
  antiphospholipid **8**:1107
  classes of **7**:909
  from donated blood **2**:232
  treatment for Guillain-Barré
    syndrome **6**:*728*, 729
antidiuretic hormone (ADH) **4**:*566*,
  567; **5**:597; **6**:858; **7**:898–899;
  8:1018–1020; **12**:1599, 1601
anus **1**:102–103; **13**:1787
  bleeding from **1**:102
  boils **1**:*102*, 103
  damage to, and constipation **3**:405
  fissures **1**:*102*, 103; **6**:808
    treatment **6**:808
    use of laxatives and **8**:1046
  fistulas **1**:*102*, 103; **6**:808
    treatment **6**:808
  hemorrhoids **6**:807–808
    constipation and **3**:405
    during pregnancy **5**:637; **12**:1662,
      1675
    external (prolapsed) **1**:*103*; **6**:*808*;
      15:2095, *2096*
    strangulation of **15**:2095
    internal **1**:*103*; **6**:*808*; **15**:2096
    treatment **6**:808
    use of laxatives and **8**:1046
  itching **1**:103
  rectal prolapse **1**:*103*; **12**:1686, *1687*,
    1688
  skin tags **6**:*808*
aorta **1**:118; **3**:372, 419
  aneurysms **1**:121; **6**:803
  coarctation of the **9**:1289
  dissection of the **1**:121; **13**:1754
  valves **3**:320
apocrine glands **5**:*700*; **11**:1544; **14**:*1970*
appendix **1**:*109*, 110
  appendicitis **1**:109–111; **11**:1512
    peritonitis and **1**:111; **11**:1532,
      1534–1535
    symptoms **1**:110, 111; **11**:1535
  gangrenous **5**:669
  "grumbling" **1**:21, 109, 110
  on the left side **2**:252
  perforated/ruptured **1**:111; **11**:*1532*,
    1534
  removal **1**:110, 111; **11**:1512
    discharge from the scar **5**:644
    flatulence after **1**:109, 111
    as a preventative measure **1**:109
    scar **1**:109
appestat **1**:113

aqueous humor **5**:701
armpits, swollen lymph nodes
  8:**1109**, 1111
arms
  artificial **1**:127, 128; **12**:*1696*, *1697*, 1698
  bionic **2**:*191*
  body language and **2**:*247*
  broken, treatment **15**:*2048*,
    2049
  reattached **9**:1218
  stiffness **15**:2078
  swollen after lymph node removal
    8:**1109**, 1112
arteries and artery disease **1**:**118–121**
  arteries
    bleeding from **1**:18, 20; **6**:803
    bypassing blocked arteries
      9:1221; **10**:1403; **17**:2341, 2357
    clearing blocked arteries **3**:421;
      9:*1170–1171*, 1172
    fatty degeneration and
      hemorrhaging **6**:803, *804*
    grafting **5**:711
    pulse and **13**:*1753–1754*
    structure **1**:119, *121*
  atherosclerosis **1**:119; **2**:214; **3**:372, 419;
    10:1382; **16**:2215
  cholesterol and **1**:119–120; **3**:366;
    6:783
  coronary artery **1**:121; **3**:419–420
  development of **1**:*121*
  epileptic seizures and **5**:583
  gangrene and **5**:669
  men and **1**:118
  obesity and **10**:1385
  prevention **5**:600; **17**:2387
  smoking and **1**:118; **6**:783
  strokes and **1**:121; **15**:2107
  transient ischemic attacks and
    16:2261
  treatment **3**:345, 346
    coronary arteries and
      thrombosis **1**:118; **3**:419–421;
      6:783–784
    coronary artery surgery
      3:420–421; **10**:1403
    coronary disease **3**:421; **6**:789
    coronary thrombosis **3**:419–420;
      6:783–784; **16**:2215–2216,
      2217
    hardening & loss of elasticity
      (arteriosclerosis) **1**:119; **15**:2121
    limping and **8**:1075
    smoking and **1**:101, 118; **5**:669;
      6:783
arytenoid cartilages **17**:2389
ATP (adenosine triphosphate)
  5:703
atropine **2**:158
aura, color therapy and **3**:390
autonomic nervous system **2**:156–158;
  9:1268; **10**:*1345*
  labile **5**:612
  axons **10**:1344, 1347

babies
  abdomen **1**:11
  accident prevention **1**:23–25
  anxiety **1**:104
  appetite **1**:112
  balance **2**:167
  blue **2**:242–243; **6**:788

bonding with 2:204
burping 3:306
choking 1:135
colic 3:356; 4:444, 445; 5:702
constipation 1:69
convulsions 3:413
coordination 3:415
cradle cap 14:1972–1973
crying 4:444, 445; 6:758; 10:1366
dangers of shaking babies 11:1515
development 3:354–355, 356
diarrhea 1:69; 4:485, 486; 7:1004;
    13:1856
drooling 9:1262
of drug addicts 4:524
eczema 4:542, 543
erections 5:589
exchange transfusions 2:240; 7:992
eye color 5:639, 682
feces 4:486; 5:623
feeding
    breast milk 2:272–274; 4:486;
        9:1186
    cow's milk 4:494
    formula milk 4:494
    solid food 3:354
feet 5:626
fontanelles (fontanels) 2:257;
    14:1967
gastroenteritis 4:486; 5:671
gestational limits and viability
    10:1336
handicapped 6:749
head injuries 6:762
head lifting 10:1332
head shape 7:878
heat loss 7:900, 901, 902
hiccups 1:67
hygiene and 7:886
hypertonic 4:444
illness diagnosed in 15:2149
infantile acne 1:32
inherited immunity in 7:908;
    13:1763
meningitis 9:1196
middle-ear infection 11:1453
mouth
    putting things into 9:1260
    thrush (Candida) 17:2437, 2438
newborn
    begin to breath 8:1102–1103
    brain damage at birth 2:267
    can sense pain 10:1338
    with a caul 9:1188
    jaundice 3:336; 6:810; 7:990, 991,
        992; 8:1087
    oxygen therapy 2:266
    pediatrics and 11:1515–1516, 1517,
        1518
    PKU heel-prick test 11:1559
    screening 14:1893
    skeleton 14:1967
    sucking reflex 13:1789, 1792
    teeth already in the mouth
        16:2175
    tests for congenital diseases
        3:401; 11:1518, 1559; 14:1893
    vitamin K for 17:2385, 2386
overweight 4:488
period 17:2328
premature 2:204, 279; 7:933;
    10:1338; 11:1516, 1517;
    12:1666–1669
    giving oxygen to 11:1464, 1466
rashes 12:1685
    diaper rash 1:102, 103; 4:481–483;
        5:598; 14:1973, 2009; 17:2438
reflexes 13:1789, 1790, 1791, 1792

screening 14:1893
    eye tests 10:1407
    hearing tests 4:454
sense of touch 16:2239
shyness 3:356
skull 14:1967
sleep 3:354; 14:1976, 1980
sleeping position 15:2116, 2117
spitting out food 9:1262
    sudden infant death syndrome
        (SIDS) 15:2116–2117
suffocation 1:135
teeth 16:2175, 2176, 2177
teething 9:1262; 16:2177, 2178
temperature 15:2116
vaccinations, diphtheria 4:497
vision 11:1515
vomiting 1:67, 69
weaning, and flatulence 5:645
see also children; fetus
back and backache 2:159–163, 258
back injuries, hydrotherapy and
    7:883
causes of backache 2:160, 161–163;
    8:1094
    ankylosing spondylitis 1:126;
        2:163; 8:1094
    arthritis 2:163; 7:1002
    cancer 2:161; 8:1094
    chills 2:160
    crush fractures 8:1094
    fibrositis 5:643
    gallstones 2:161
    gynecological disorders 2:161
    muscular spasm 2:163; 5:643
    osteoporosis 2:163
    pregnancy 2:159, 163; 11:1526;
        12:1662
    psychosomatic 2:161
    sciatica 2:161–163; 8:1078, 1094,
        1095; 10:1349; 14:1885–1887, 1983
    shingles 2:161
    slipped disks 14:1983
    strains or sprains 2:160, 161;
        8:1072, 1094, 1095
    tuberculosis of the spine 2:161
    wear and tear 2:160–161
exercises to avoid backache
    2:162
humpback 11:1450, 1451
lower-back pain (lumbago) 2:160,
    161; 8:1094–1095
    treatment 2:163; 5:630
manipulation 8:1135
stiff back 15:2078
    heat treatment 15:2076
treatment of backache 2:163;
    8:1094, 1095; 13:1796
    heat 6:797, 798
    spinal fusion 7:1002
    yoga 17:2442
see also spine
backbone see spine
balance 2:167–168; 4:453, 454; 17:2364
    dizziness/vertigo and 4:502;
        17:2364–2365
    physical therapy and 11:1581
baldness (alopecia) 2:169; 5:709; 6:736;
    17:2387
    male pattern (androgenic alopecia)
        2:169; 6:737; 14:1969
    in patches (alopecia areata) 2:169;
        6:736; 14:1969
Bartholin glands 5:690; 7:964; 9:1269;
    17:2394
    abscess 6:733; 17:2335, 2394
    blocked 17:2333, 2335
    infection 17:2394

basal metabolic rate (BMR) 2:173;
    17:2401
basophils 2:227
belladonna 2:158
belly button, pierced 11:1515
bile 2:179–180; 3:366; 4:494; 5:597, 598,
    667; 7:991
    digestion of fats and 5:621
    gallstones and 5:667–668
    lack of 4:495
    vitamin K absorption and 17:2385
bile duct, common, obstruction 5:668
bilirubin 2:180; 5:598, 623
    jaundice and 7:990, 991; 11:1581
biliverdin 2:180
biological clocks 2:187–188; 9:1187
    jet lag and 7:993–994
    sleep and 14:1976, 1977
biorhythms 2:194–197; 8:1055
birth 2:200–205
    "baby blues" following 9:1247;
        12:1649
    biological clock and 2:187
    breathing exercises during 12:1679
    breech 2:205, 284–285; 3:342
    can men experience pain of? 11:1476
    cesarean 2:204–205; 3:340–342;
        7:931, 932
    development of PMS after 12:1671
    emergency delivery 2:205
    episiotomy 2:203, 285; 5:586;
        8:1030; 10:1322, 1324
    father at the 12:1676
    forceps delivery 2:201, 208
    lack of libido and difficulties with
        sex after 8:1062; 14:1921, 1928
    multiple 9:1277
    natural childbirth 2:200;
        10:1321–1325
    pain relief
        acupuncture 1:39
        drugs 10:1319, 1324
        epidural anesthesia 1:93; 2:201,
            285; 8:1093; 15:2041
        postnatal sessions 11:1580
    postpartum depression and
        psychosis 4:465; 8:1062; 9:1247;
        10:1322; 12:1648–1651
    puerperal sepsis following
        17:2338–2339
    umbilical-cord accidents 15:2094
    vaginal discharge after
        17:2338–2339
    vaginal lacerations 8:1031; 17:2333
    see also babies, newborn; labor
bladder and bladder problems
    2:216–218
    bladder capacity 17:2324
    bladder control 2:217–218
    cystoscopy 4:570; 9:1236
    problems
        cancer 3:316; 13:1776; 17:2325
        cystitis 2:217, 218; 3:409;
            4:449–450; 6:857; 7:886;
            17:2324
        incontinence 2:218; 5:693;
            7:925–926; 12:1687; 15:2040
        prolapse (cystocele) 7:925;
            12:1686, 1687
        stones 17:2325
        tumors 2:217
blind spot 5:606, 607; 10:1410
blinking 13:1789, 1792
blood 2:225–228
    "blue" 2:225
    clotting 1:17; 2:226, 227; 6:801–802
        thrombus formation 16:2214
    clotting disorders 2:228; 6:804

hemophilia 2:206, 228;
    5:685–686; 6:801–802; 7:922;
    10:1306
    purpura 2:228; 13:1756
    vitamin K deficiency 2:228;
        17:2385–2386
    von Willebrand's disease 17:2392
manufacture of blood cells 2:226,
    227–228
pH 1:26
plasma 2:227; 12:1611
    burns or scalds 2:227; 13:1867,
        1868
    transfusions 12:1611; 13:1867
    platelets 2:226, 227, 228; 3:298;
        13:1755
    red blood cells 2:225, 281
        anemia 1:88
        broken down 7:990–991
        sickle-cell anemia 14:1954, 1955
    sugar 15:2121
    tests 2:225; 4:475; 8:1029;
        15:2024–2025
    "tired" 2:225
    umbilical-cord 5:676, 677
    white blood cells 2:165, 225–227;
        7:946
        disorders 2:228
        inflammation 7:948
        leukemia 8:1059, 1060–1061
        see also eosinophils; lymphocytes
blood-brain barrier (BBB) 2:229–230;
    3:318–319
    cellular phones and 3:334
blood groups 2:233–235
    blood transfusions 2:234, 240, 241
    see also rhesus (Rh) factor
blood pressure 2:237–239; 3:373
    biofeedback techniques 2:183
    changes in a day 2:188
    control 2:239; 6:847
    low (hypotension) 2:237
        postural hypotension 2:215;
            17:2364
    measurement 1:119; 3:373; 15:2036
        in the heart 14:1945, 1947
    raised (hypertension) 1:46; 2:237;
        12:1724–1725
        effect on the kidneys 8:1017,
            1021
        headaches 6:759
        the heart 4:551
        hemorrhoids 6:807
        hypertensive retinopathy 13:1812
        "malignant" 8:1124
        salt and 13:1861
        self help for 2:238
        stroke 15:2107, 2111
        treatment 2:181, 183, 183–184, 237,
            239; 4:500; 5:611, 650; 9:1173
blushing 2:244; 14:1974
body mass index (BMI) 11:1577; 17:2399,
    2400, 2401
body odor 2:249
body structure 2:252–254
bones 2:257–260
    in the back 2:159
    bent 3:352
    cancer 2:161, 163, 260; 14:1966
        pain relief 8:1093; 12:1692
        in ribs 13:1834
        thermography and 16:2208
    chipped 5:662
    congenital diseases 2:259
    cracked 5:662
    cysts 4:447; 11:1503
    fractures 2:258, 259; 5:660–664;
        14:1964, 1968

avulsion 8:1072
Colles' 5:660; 17:2430
comminuted (crushed) 5:660, *661*, 664
compound 5:660, *662*; 10:*1432–1433*
dangers 5:663
first aid 4:556; 5:663; 10:1393
greenstick 5:660, *662*; 14:1964
hairline 15:2048
healing 5:660
infection 5:660
manipulation 8:1135
march 5:662
osteoporosis and 2:161; 3:310; 5:660; 6:828; 8:*1078*
pathological 5:660; 14:1964
Pott's 5:661
recovery 5:*664*
repair 2:260
simple 5:660, *661*
spontaneous 14:1964
sports 15:2050–2051, 2054
stress 15:2050–2051, 2054
treatment 5:663–664; 8:1135; 10:*1430–1433*; 15:*2048*, *2049*; 16:2253, *2254*, 2255
untreated 5:664
grafts 5:709, 711; 10:1430, 1432; 12:*1616*, 1617
growth 5:698, 717–*718*
gigantism or acromegaly 5:698
infections (osteomyelitis) 2:258, 260
movement and 9:1265
osteomalacia 2:259; 13:1835, *1836*
osteoporosis 2:258, 260; 3:310, 311; 5:693; 6:854, *855*; 9:1199; 11:**1450–1451**; 14:1968
backache and 2:161, 163
causing limping 8:1078
fractures and 2:161; 3:310; 5:660; 6:828; 8:*1078*
HRT and 2:260; 6:*855*, 856; 9:1199; 11:1450, 1451
immobilization 2:260
Paget's disease 2:260
tumors 2:258, 260
rib 13:1834
vitamin deficiencies and 2:260; 3:*311*; 13:1835, 1836
see also joints; skeleton
bowel 5:597
cancer 3:316
intussusception 5:624; 15:2095–2096
obstruction 11:1533; 15:2094
see also colon; small intestine
Bowman's capsule 8:1018
brain 2:262–264; 6:761; 10:1345
blood circulation, monitored 16:2208
cerebrospinal fluid circulation 7:*879*
circulation of cerebrospinal fluid 7:*879*
communication and 1:*108*
consciousness and 17:2318
coordination and 3:414, *415*
electroencephalograms (EEGs) 2:263, 266; 4:552; 10:1356; 14:*1892*
biofeedback and 2:183, *184*
epilepsy and 4:552; 5:*584*
unconsciousness and 3:394–*395*; 17:*2319*
layered, and flotation therapy 5:650
the mind and 9:1228
movement and 9:*1265*
pain and 11:*1475–1476*

scans 10:*1354, 1355*; 11:1547; 12:*1713*; 13:1869
speech and 15:2029
survival time without oxygen 4:555
temporal lobes, and epilepsy 5:*583*, 585
touch and 16:2241–2242
transplants 16:2263
visual cortex 5:606
waves 5:648–649
during meditation 9:1179
brain stem 2:263; 10:1345
damage to, and vertigo 17:2366
sleep-wakefulness center 14:1977, *1978*
unconsciousness and 17:2318–2319
vomiting and 17:*2391*
Braxton Hicks contractions 2:201
breastbone *see* sternum
breast feeding 2:272–274, 275–276; 3:311
allergies and 13:1750
eczema and 4:542, 543
foods to avoid while 4:485
lactation 8:*1032*
medications taken while 11:1461; 12:1648
passing on immunity and 7:908
premature babies 12:1668
when suffering from mastitis 9:*1158*, 1159
breasts 2:275–277; 8:*1032*
biopsies 2:*192*; 3:315; 8:1132, 1147; 9:1147
cancer 2:277; 3:316; 8:*1098*, 1130; 9:1187
deaths from 10:1399
family history of 8:1124
histopathology 11:1512–1513
hormone replacement therapy and 6:856; 7:875
mastitis and 4:446
risk of 8:1129–1130
screening for 8:*1129–1132*
self-checking for 12:*1680*
staging 8:1098–1099, 1132
thermography and 16:2208
treatment 2:176; 3:315; 8:1098–*1099, 1145–1148*; 9:*1145–1148*, 1172
changes in 2:276–277
cosmetic surgery 3:424, 425
cysts 2:277; 4:446, 447; 9:1159
effect of the Pill on 10:1417; 14:1956
examination 2:276, 277; 8:1098, 1147; 9:1147; 15:2148
external prostheses 8:1145, 1146, 1148; 9:1145, 1146, *1148*; 12:1698, *1699*
implants 12:1614, 1615, *1616*, 1700
following a mastectomy 8:*1145*; 10:1421; 12:1614, 1698
mastitis 9:1158–1159, 1284
chronic 2:276–277; 4:446
microcalcification 8:1131
pregnancy and 2:276; 12:1663, *1664*
prevention of mastitis 9:1159
problems 2:275, 276
reduction 12:1615, 1617
thermography 16:2207, 2208
tumors 2:277; 16:*2292*
unequal size 13:1739
breathing 2:279–283; 4:484; 8:1101–1102; 13:*1833*
deep 11:1578
how babies begin 8:*1102*–1103

hysterical overbreathing 3:311; 11:1504
problems, crooked nose and 10:1372
reflex 13:1790, 1792
tests 13:1752
through the mouth 1:40; 9:1262; 16:2209
breech birth 2:205, 284–285; 3:342
bronchi 2:281
wheezing and 17:*2407–2408*
bronchioles 4:*563*
bronchodilators, natural 1:139–140
burping 3:306

calories 5:655
daily intake 17:2401
used in everyday activities 4:490; 5:655–656; 9:*1214*–1215
weight loss and 4:492
capillaries 3:318–319
bleeding from 6:803
inflammation and 7:947–948
capitulum 4:*546*, 547
carbon dioxide
gas exchange and 8:1102
levels measured 5:598
poisoning 12:*1632*
pollution 1:59
removed from the body 2:*281*
carpals 6:745; 17:2429
cartilage 3:324–325; 14:1966
artificial 2:189
knee
removal 3:324, 325; 10:1432, 1436
torn 3:*325*; 8:1026–1027; 10:1432, *1434*; 15:2055
osteoarthritis and 1:123
catabolism 9:1214
Caucasians 2:253
caul 9:1188
cavities, body 2:252
cells 3:330–332
aging and 1:54–55; 3:330
cancer 3:312
division 3:331–332
aging and 1:55
membranes 9:1241
organelles 9:1240
types 3:*331*
cementum 6:730; 16:2175, *2178*
cerebellum 2:263; 10:1345
ataxia and 2:149
cerebrospinal fluid (CSF) 7:878, *879*
hydrocephalus and 7:878, 879
lumbar puncture and 8:1097
meningitis and 9:1195, *1197*
cerebrum 2:264
cerebral cortex 2:*264*; 10:1345
taste and 16:2171
touch and 16:2241
cerumen *see* earwax
cervix and cervical smears 3:337–339
cancer 3:316, 337, 338–339; 4:574; 6:733; 11:1488, 1489; 17:2327, 2368
circumcised men and 3:374
genital herpes and 6:825; 14:*1933*
see also cervix and cervical smears, Pap smear
cervical erosion 3:338; 6:733; 11:1488; 17:2327
cervicitis 3:337
dysplasias and carcinoma in situ 6:733; 11:1488, 1489; 17:2327
incompetent or abnormal cervix 3:338; 9:*1238*, 1239; 17:2326
mucus 9:*1203*, 1269
the rhythm method and 13:1829, *1830*

Pap smear (cervical smear) 3:313, 314, 337, *338*; 6:734; 7:*966*, 967; 8:*1126*; 11:**1488–1489**, 1513; 14:*1894*
after sterilization 15:2071
detecting infection 17:2336
during pregnancy 12:1676
polyps 13:*339*; 5:642; 6:733; 11:1488; 17:2327
chest 3:347–348
bandaging 4:519
barrel chest 3:295; 4:564
concavity 13:1832
infections, after flu 7:950
pains 3:347, 348; 15:2151
ECGs and 4:550
pleurisy and 12:1619–1620; 15:2151
pigeon chest 3:347; 12:**1590–1592**
steering-wheel injury to 4:556
strapping 13:1832
see also ribs; sternum
chewing *see* mastication
childbirth *see* birth
children
abdominal pain 1:*11*, 13, 111
accident prevention and 1:*23–25*
alimentary problems 1:69
allergies 1:70
aphasia 1:*107*, 108
appendicitis 1:111
attending funerals 4:457
attention deficit hyperactivity disorder (ADHD) 1:*86*; 2:151–152; 4:536; 8:1051
autism 2:153–155; 8:1051–1052
speech difficulties and 10:1308, 1309
avoiding vehicle sickness in 9:*1254*
bed-wetting 2:217–218; 7:925, 926
blindness 2:219–220
breath holding 1:132; 2:278; 3:413; 17:2320
bullied 12:1710
checkups 11:1518–1519, *1568*
child development 3:354–357; 11:1518–1519
speech 15:*2028*, 2030–2031
choking 1:132
clumsiness 3:414
constipation 1:69
convulsions 3:413; 5:583, 585, 641
cross-eye 8:1047; 10:1407
deafness 4:453
hearing tests 4:*454*
death of a child 4:458
diarrhea 1:69; 4:486; 7:1004
diet 4:488
milk 3:310
protein 4:489
spicy foods 4:494
dwarfism 4:*532*; 5:684
dyslexia 4:534–535, 536
dyspraxia 4:536
eczema 4:542, 543
educational psychology and 12:*1716*, 1717, 1718
emergency care of 4:560
emotional outbursts 7:*907*
exercise 5:600
eye tests 10:1407
fears 11:1563
feet 5:626
fever 5:641
flat feet 5:628
food 11:1516
fractures 5:660, *662*, 663, 664
gastroenteritis 5:671
giving medicines to 9:*1173*, 1175
grieving 5:712

growing pains 5:715, 716
growth 5:716–717; 9:1186–1187
hallucinations 6:742
handicapped 6:748, 749–751
heart murmurs 6:788; 9:1289
homesickness 6:848, 849
in hospitals 7:870, 871; 11:1516–1517, 1518
hydrocephalus 7:878, 879–880
incontinence 7:925, 926
independence 6:848
lead poisoning 8:1049
lethargy 8:1058
leukemia 8:1060, 1061
lisping 8:1081–1082; 11:1483; 15:2060
mastoiditis 9:1160, 1161
mentally retarded 9:1210–1213
middle-ear infection 11:1453
Munchausen syndrome by proxy and 9:1285, 1286
mutism 10:1307–1308, 1309
nosebleeds 10:1371
of one-parent families 3:397
overdose and 11:1460–1461, 1462
overweight 10:1383
personality 11:1538
pigeon toes 12:1593–1594
rheumatoid arthritis (Still's disease) 1:123
scarlet fever (scarlatina) **14:1878–1879**
screening 14:1893–1894
sex education 6:768, 769
sexual abuse of 3:353; 14:1926–1927
skeleton 14:1967
skin conditions 14:1972–1974
sleep 9:1186–1187
    needing little 1:85
    nightmares 4:511; 14:1978
    sleepwalking 14:1981
speech problems 8:1081–1082; 15:2028, 2030, 2032, 2033
    stammering and stuttering 15:2058–2061
    therapy for 15:2032, 2033
spitting out food 9:1262
squint 4:505
sunburn 15:2128, 2129
teeth 16:2176, 2177, 2178
temper tantrums 3:356, 413; 7:906
thumb sucking 7:1081
urination reflex 13:1791
vaccination/immunization 5:641; 11:1519
vomiting 1:69
worms 5:623
see also babies
cholecalciferol 17:2380
cholecystokinin 2:180; 11:1487
cholesterol 3:366
    in the body 1:120; 5:622; 7:991
        atherosclerosis and 1:119–120; 3:366; 6:783
    dietary 1:120; 3:366; 5:621–622
    reduction 17:2379
cholinesterase 10:1313
chordae tendineae 17:2341
chromosomes 3:331; 5:682
    abnormalities, and mutations 10:1305
    division 3:331–332
        aging and 1:55
    extra 5:676, 683; 10:1305
        Down syndrome and 3:368; 4:507, 508
    Philadelphia 8:1061
    sex and 3:331; 5:672, 683
    structure 3:332

chyme 1:67, 68, 69; 4:494; 15:2088
circadian clock 2:187–188; 7:993; 9:1187
circulatory system 3:372–373
    William Harvey and 17:2358
    see also arteries and artery disease; capillaries; heart; pulse; veins
climacteric 9:1198
clitoris 5:690; 7:964; 14:1919; 17:2393, 2394
clotting factors 6:804
coccyx 2:159; 11:1522
cochlea 6:777
    damage, and tinnitus 16:2228
cochlear implants 2:191; 6:780
collagen 14:1896–1897; 17:2378, 2427, 2428
    in skin creams 17:2427
collarbone, broken 14:1948–1949
colon and colitis 3:383
    colitis 3:383, 404; 15:2152
        acute 3:383
        chronic (ulcerative) 3:383; 4:443, 485; 17:2311
        treatment 3:383; 4:486; 15:2152
    colon
        cancer 3:386, 387; 4:442; 5:624; 15:2022
        colonic irrigation 3:384–385
        colonoscopy 3:386–387; 4:501, 570, 571; 12:1643
        colostomy 3:392–393; 5:644; 13:1787, 1788
        diverticulitis 3:384, 386; 4:501
            constipation and:404, 405
            halitosis and 6:741
            perforated 11:1535
        feces in 5:623
        polyps 3:386, 387; 12:1642, 1643
        sigmoidoscopy 4:501, 570; 14:1960
        spastic colon 15:2022–2023
        tumors 16:2291
        ulceration 3:387
colostrum 2:273, 276; 8:1032; 12:1663, 1664
conception 3:399–400; 5:634; 13:1828; 15:2035
    artificial methods of 1:129–131
        in vitro fertilization (IVF) 1:129, 131; 7:971–974; 11:1520
    lovemaking positions and 14:1916
    menstruation and 9:1201
    unlikely while breast-feeding 12:1600
connective tissue, massage 8:1144; 9:1144
contractions 2:201
    Braxton Hicks 2:201
coordination 3:414–415
    dyspraxia and 4:536
cornea 3:416; 5:604
    grafting 3:416; 4:504; 5:710, 711; 10:1407
        passing on rabies 13:1766
    inflammation 5:607
    laser surgery on 8:1043–1044
    ulcers 13:1758
corpus callosum 2:264
corpus luteum 5:593; 9:1202; 11:1458, 1459, 1548
Corti, organ of 6:777
cortisol 1:47–48; 6:858
cortisone 4:566; 12:1598, 1601
    treatment using 1:46
COX (cyclo-oxygenase) 10:1369
creatinine 8:1020
cyclic AMP 6:859; 15:2085

cytokines 7:946; 8:1113, 1121–1122
cytoplasm 3:330, 331

dendrites 10:1347
dentine 16:2175, 2178
dermatomes, shingles and 14:1938, 1939
dextrocardia 2:252
diaphragm 2:281; 4:484; 8:1102
    hiccups and 6:826, 827
    stitch and 15:2087
digestion 1:67–69; 4:487
    aids to 1:68
    drowsiness and 4:523
    of fruit and vegetables 1:67
    of starch 15:2063
    see also digestive system
digestive system, stomach, cancer 6:741; 15:2090; 16:2292
digestive system 4:494–495
    appendicitis 1:109–111; 11:1512
        peritonitis and 1:111; 11:1532, 1534–1535
        symptoms 1:110, 111; 11:1535
    celiac disease 1:71–72; 3:329; 4:485
    colitis 3:383, 404; 15:2152
        acute 3:383
        chronic (ulcerative) 3:383; 4:443, 485; 17:2311
        treatment 3:383; 4:486; 15:2152
    constipation 3:385, 404–405; 5:596, 619, 624
        in babies 1:69
        before menstruating 9:1201
        causing anal fissures 1:102
        in children 1:69
        during pregnancy 3:404; 8:1045; 12:1662, 1675
        flatulence and 5:645
        hemorrhoids and 6:807
        spurious diarrhea and 7:925
        treatment 3:404, 405; 4:572; 8:1045–1046; 15:2132, 2133, 2152
    Crohn's disease 4:442–443
        fistulas and 5:644
    diverticulitis 3:384, 386; 4:501
        constipation and 3:404, 405
        halitosis and 6:741
        perforated 11:1535
    duodenal (intestinal) ulcers 4:495, 530, 531
        bleeding from 6:803–804; 8:1042
        body weight and 15:2090
        excess salivation and 13:1854
        kissing ulcers 17:2313
        pain 17:2313
        perforated 11:1534, 1535; 17:2313
        treatment 2:157, 158; 4:531; 8:1042; 15:2138; 17:2340
    fistula 5:644
        anal 1:102, 103; 6:808
        for dialysis 8:1015
        from the bowel 4:443
        urinary 7:925
    food poisoning 5:657–659, 670; 7:928
        botulism 2:261; 4:485; 5:657, 659
        diarrhea 4:485; 5:657–658
        from irradiated foods 7:979
        prevention 5:658; 7:886
        reactive arthritis and 13:1785, 1786
        salmonella and 5:657, 659; 7:928; 13:1855, 1856–1857
        staphylococcus and 5:657, 659; 7:928; 15:2062
        treatment 4:486; 5:657–659
        vomiting and 4:531; 5:657–658

gastritis 5:670, 671; 9:1269; 15:2088, 2089
    viral 15:2090
gastroenteritis (gastric flu; summer flu) 4:485, 495, 573; 5:670–671; 15:2089, 2152
    in babies 4:486; 5:671
    prevention 5:671
    treatment 5:671; 15:2151
indigestion 7:929–930; 9:1189, 1269; 10:1331
    on eating fatty foods 5:667
    hiatus hernia and 4:484
    persistent 15:2090
    treatment 7:929; 9:1177
intestinal obstruction 3:405
irritable bowel syndrome (IBS) 4:501; 7:980; 15:2022
    spastic colon 15:2022–2023
membranes 9:1269
peritonitis 1:111; 4:501; 9:1189; 11:1532, 1533–1535
problems 4:495
stomach (gastric) ulcers 1:11; 4:495; 5:581; 15:2088, 2089–2090; 17:2313, 2314
    aspirin and 1:122; 11:1479
    asymptomatic 17:2312
    biopsy 2:192
    bleeding from 6:803–804; 8:1042; 14:1945
    body weight and 15:2090
    causes 15:2089; 17:2313
    gastroscopy and 4:570, 571; 8:1042
    stomach or arm pain and 14:1948
    treatment 2:157, 158; 5:581; 8:1042; 15:2090
    see also alimentary canal; colon; duodenum; stomach
DNA 3:331, 332; 5:682–683; 9:1240–1241
    mutations in 10:1304
    size 9:1240
dopamine 11:1507
    amphetamines and 1:85–86
    antipsychotic drugs and 12:1720; 13:1737
drowsiness 4:523
    after a meal 2:156; 5:618
    biological clock and 2:187
ductus arteriosus 8:1102, 1103
ductus venosus 8:1102
duodenum 1:68; 4:494–495, 530–531
    ulcers 4:495, 530, 531
        bleeding from 6:803–804; 8:1042
        body weight and 15:2090
        excess salivation and 13:1854
        kissing ulcers 17:2313
        pain 17:2313
        perforated 11:1534, 1535; 17:2313
        treatment 2:157, 158; 4:531; 8:1042; 15:2138; 17:2340

eardrums 4:453
    perforated 4:456; 11:1453; 15:2156
    caused by syringing 15:2157
ears 6:778; 11:1452
    balance and 2:167–168; 4:454
    bionic (cochlear implants) 2:191; 6:780
    coordination and 3:414
    loud noises and 4:453, 455, 456; 6:777; 10:1365–1366
    piercing 2:250, 251
        keloid scars and 14:1880
    plastic surgery 12:1612
    "popping" 9:1262
    problems 2:168

heart *(cont'd)*
    tiredness and 16:2231
    treatment 13:1861; 15:2083, 2151
  fitness and the 11:1576–1577
  heartbeat 6:781
    control 6:782; 9:1267, *1268*
    exercise and 7:997
    pulse and 13:1754
    rate decrease during meditation
      9:*1178*
    smoking and 10:1360, *1361*
    sneezing and 14:2002
    see also pulse, rate
  holes in the 2:242, *243*; 3:402;
    9:1289; 10:1401; 17:2342
    closing on their own 6:788
    surgery 10:1402
  murmurs 8:1103; 9:1287–1289;
    15:2074
    in children 6:788; 9:1289
  muscle 9:1266, 1267, 1290, *1293*
  pacemaker
    artificial 2:*190*; 3:*421*; 6:788;
      11:*1472–1473*
    natural (sinoatrial node) 6:*782*;
      9:1267; 11:1472
  pain, radiation of 15:2149
  pericarditis
    pain 3:348
    tuberculous 16:2289
  stops, and time before permanent
    damage 13:1807
  strangulation of 15:2096
  stress and the 7:997
  stroke volume 11:1576–1577
  surgery
    physical therapy after 11:1581
    ventricular fibrillation and
      17:2359
  see also valves
height 2:252; 5:716
  aging and 1:53; 3:324
  gigantism 5:*697–698*, 718; 12:1601
  heredity and 6:817
  inferiority complexes and 3:397
  tallest man 14:*1964*
    ever 5:697
  see also growth
hemoglobin 2:225; 11:1464; 14:1954
  broken down 7:990–991
  deficiency, and anemia 1:88
  sickle-cell anemia and 14:1954
  thalassemia and 16:*2200*
heparin 2:227
hepatic portal system 17:2358
hepatocytes 8:1084
heredity 6:816–818
  nature versus nurture 6:817–818
  see also genetics
hexosaminidase 16:2174
hip 6:828–830
  arthritic 1:*122*; 10:*1436*, 1437
  bandaging 4:*518*
  damage, and limping 8:*1077*
  dislocation 4:498, 499
    congenital 3:402; 4:499;
      6:829–830; 10:1434; 15:2048;
      16:*2254*
    traction for 16:2253
  fractures 5:660–661, 693; 6:828,
    830, 855; 9:1199; 17:2424
    osteoporosis and 11:1450
  ligaments 8:*1071*
  pain 11:1578
  Perthes' disease 6:830; 8:1076; 11:**1546**
  replacement 1:*122*; 2:*189*; 6:829, 830;
    7:998, *999*, 1000; 10:*1438*;
    12:1696, 1699

fitting a new 12:1696
  hydrotherapy and 7:883
  rehabilitation after 13:1798
  see also pelvis
histamine 1:72, 73; 6:756, 831
  producing itches 7:988
HLA-B27 13:1785, 1786
homeostasis 6:846–847; 7:898
hormones 6:847, 857–859
  hormonal disorders 4:567
    Addison's disease 1:48; 2:237;
      6:747; 7:896; 9:*1181*; 13:1862;
      15:2150
    Cushing's syndrome 1:46; 12:1601;
      15:2152
    diabetes 4:471–473
    dwarfism 4:532
    gigantism 5:697–698
    goiter 5:704; 10:1334; 16:*2224*,
      2225, 2226
    hyperparathyroidism 11:1504,
      1505
    hypoglycaemia 7:896; 15:2121
    hypothyroidism *see* thyroid,
      underactive
    thyroid gland tumors 4:567
    thyrotoxicosis *see* thyroid,
      overactive
  moods and 9:1246
  substitutes 5:699
  see also endocrine system
human chorionic gonadotropin (HCG)
  3:400; 15:2024
Human Genome Project 5:678
hunger 1:112; 6:846
hymen 5:690; 7:*889*; 17:2367, 2368,
  2393–2394
  imperforate 17:2335
hypertrophy, muscle 11:1577
hypothalamus 2:263; 6:847;
  7:897–899
  appetite and 1:113; 7:897–898
  body temperature and 5:640, 641;
    7:897, *898*; 9:*1264*; 14:*1941*, 1942;
    16:2182–2183
  effect on the pituitary gland 6:859;
    7:897
  heart rate and 9:1268
  narcolepsy and 7:897, *899*
  water balance and 7:898–899;
    16:2209

ileum 4:495
ilium 11:1522–1523
immune system 7:908–909, 940;
  17:2330–2331
  allergies and 1:72–73
  cellular immunity 17:2330–2331
  Crohn's disease and 4:442
  deficiency
    causes 10:1409
    opportunistic infections and
      10:1409; 16:2220
  inherited immunity 7:908; 13:1763
  natural immunity 2:227
  thymus and 16:2221, 2222
  UV radiation and 11:1470–1471
  see also antibodies; lymphocytes
immunoglobulins *see* antibodies
inferior vena cava 3:373
inhibitory factors (releasing factors)
  7:899
insulin 4:471–473; 6:858; 7:896, **960**;
  9:1215; 11:*1487*; 15:*2064*, 2121
  administered 4:472–473; 7:960
    genetically engineered 5:679
    overdose 3:395
    transdermal delivery 16:2260

made by the body 4:*472*, *566*;
  5:*702–703*; 7:*960*; 10:1368
resistance 10:1368
intercourse 7:963–965; 14:*1918*–1919
  abstinence 1:22, 45
  bleeding during or after 11:1488,
    1489
  conception and 3:399
  during adolescence 1:43
  during pregnancy 5:634; 7:963;
    12:1661, 1675
  lack of interest in
    after menopause 9:1200
    since taking the Pill 7:963
  painful (dyspareunia) 4:568; 7:965;
    8:1034; 9:1269; 14:1924–1925,
    1929
  salpingitis and 13:1860
  positions, and conception 14:1916
interleukin-2 7:914
interpubic disk 11:1523
intestines 9:*1268*
  enteritis 5:670
  intussusception 15:2095–2096
  obstruction 3:405
  peristalsis 1:*69*; 15:2023
  polyps 12:1642, 1643
  strangulation 15:2094–*2095*
  tumors 13:1774
    removal 15:2136
  see also bowel; colon; small
    intestine
intrinsic factor 1:89; 11:1536
iodine, deficiency 8:1128
iris 5:605
  iridology and 7:975–976
islets of Langerhans 7:*960*; 11:*1486*,
  1487

jaw
  cancer of 14:*1998*
  osteoarthritis 7:1002
  wiring 10:1386
joints 2:259; 7:1000–1003;
  9:1265–1266; 10:1435; 14:1968
  being "double jointed" 7:1002;
    13:1819
  chiropractic and 3:363
  effects of hydrotherapy on 7:882
  injections into 15:2078
  ligaments 8:1069, 1070, *1071*
  problems
    bleeding (hemathrosis) 6:802
    bursitis 3:*307–309*; 4:*547*; 6:799;
      7:1002; 8:1025, 1027; 9:1189
    clicking 3:324
    cysts 4:447
    dislocation 4:498–499; 8:1069;
      15:2055
    locked joints 8:1135
    loose bodies in 8:1025, 1136
    osteoarthritis 1:123, *123*; 3:325;
      5:691; 10:1435–1438; 11:1581
      14:1968
    rheumatoid arthritis 1:122–123
      126; 3:323; 7:1002, 1003; 11:1581;
      13:1820–1824; 16:2207, 2208
    sports injuries 1:50; 15:2054–2055
    sprains 6:764; 8:1072; 15:2048,
      2051, 2055, **2056–2057**,
      2145
    stiffness 8:1136; 15:2076,
      2077–2079
  replacement 7:998–999, 1003;
    10:1434, 1438
    hips *see* hip, replacement
    knees 7:*998*, 999; 10:1430
  synovial membranes 9:1188, *1189*

keratin, in the skin 14:1970
keratinocytes 8:1090
kidneys and kidney diseases
  5:596–597; 8:**1017–1021**; 17:2324
  abscesses 17:2325
  birth- and congenital defects 2:207;
    17:2325
  blood pressure and 2:238, *239*;
    8:1017
  cancer 17:2325
    hormone production 11:1504
    treatment 13:1772, 1776
  cysts 4:450
    polycystic kidneys 2:207; 4:447;
      8:*1018*; 17:2325
  function tests 8:1020
  glomerulonephritis 8:1020; 15:2097;
    17:2325
  gout and 5:707
  infections 8:1018, 1020–1021
  kidney failure 8:1020; 12:1701
    drugs and 14:1958
    kidney dialysis 2:190; 5:598;
      8:**1014–1016**, 1020; 17:*2322*
  multicystic kidneys 17:2325
  nephrectomy 10:**1339**
  nephritis 5:707; 17:2325
  nephrosis 17:2325
  pain 2:161
  pyelonephritis 17:2325
  salt levels controlled 13:*1862*
  stones (calculi) 2:217; 3:311; 4:450;
    6:786; 8:1018, *1020*, 1021; 11:1505;
    17:2325
    gout and 5:708
    kidney removal for 10:1339
    treatment 8:1020, *1021*
  uremia 15:2150; 17:**2322**
  X rays 17:2432
kilocalories 5:655; 9:1214
  see also calories
knee 7:1001–*1002*; 8:**1025–1027**
  arthritic 1:*123*, 124, 125; 10:*1436*, 1437
  arthrograms of 17:2432
  "baker's cyst" 1:122
  bandaging 4:*520*
  bursitis 3:*307*, *309*; 7:1002; 8:1025
  cartilage
    removed 3:324, 325; 10:1432, 1436
    torn 3:*325*; 8:1026–1027; 10:1432,
      1434; 15:2055
  fluid in (knee effusion) 8:1025, *1026*
  kneecap (patella) 8:1026
    dislocation 8:1027, *1136*
    manipulation 8:1135
  knee-jerk reflex 8:1025; 9:1266, *1267*;
    13:*1791*
  knock knees 5:628
  ligaments 8:*1071*
  limping and 8:1075
  loose bodies in 8:1024, 1136
  osteoarthritis, hydrotherapy and
    7:883
  replacement 7:998, 999; 10:1430
  stiffness 15:2079
  twists and sprains 8:1026
Kupffer's cells 8:1086

labia, inner and outer 5:690; 17:*2393*
labor 2:200, 201–204; 5:639
  accelerated 2:201
  breathing exercises 12:1679
  dry 7:932
  enema during 4:572
  induced 2:201; 7:931–934; 10:1322
  obstetricians and 10:1390
  premature 17:2326
  see also birth

lachrimal glands 4:444, 445; 5:700
lactation 8:1032; 12:1598
 see also breast-feeding
lactic acid 1:49, 50; 11:1576; 15:2076
lactose, intolerance 15:2023
large intestine *see* colon; rectum
larynx and laryngitis 8:1036–1039
 laryngitis 7:946; 8:1038, *1039*;
  10:1335; 14:2011, *2013*; 16:2212;
  17:2389
  acute 8:1036, 1037–1039
  in children 16:2211
  chronic 8:1036, 1037, 1039
 larynx 16:2212
  blocked 10:1333; 16:2213
  cancer 3:316; 6:832; 8:1036, 1037,
   1038, 1039; 10:1335; 16:2212, 2213
  cartilage 3:325
  diphtheria and 8:1037, 1039
  gastroesophageal reflux and
   6:786
  hoarseness and 6:832; 8:1039
  injury to 8:1037
  laryngotracheobronchitis (croup)
   2:282; 8:1037, 1038, 1039
  puberty and 13:1742; 17:2389
  removal 8:1036; 16:2251–2252;
   17:2389
  stenosis 15:2067
  vocal cord nodes or polyps 6:832;
   8:1037, 1039; 10:1335; 17:2389
 see also vocal cords
lateral geniculate body 10:1410
left-handedness
 correction, and stammering
  15:2060
 dyslexia and 4:534
legs
 artificial (prosthetic) 1:127;
  12:1696–1698
 blood clots in the veins
  15:2146–2147; 16:2218; 17:2357
 cramps 4:437
 edema 4:544, 554
 fractures 5:661, 664
  blood loss 6:805
  leading to other problems 11:1581
  leg shortening and 10:1430;
   11:1448
  limping after plaster removal
   8:1076
  osteoporosis following 11:1450
  treatment 10:1430, *1431*–1432,
   1433; 15:2048, *2049*; 16:2253;
   17:*2433*
 movements 6:828–829
 one shorter than the other 5:664,
  709; 11:1448
  causing spinal curvature 14:1890
 paralysis 11:1490, 1492
 pins and needles 12:*1597*
 rickets and 13:*1836*
 stiffness 15:2079
 ulcers 1:17; 17:*2310*, 2312
leptins 1:113; 10:1384
leukotrienes 1:139
Leydig cells 16:2195
LH *see* luteinizing hormone
libido 8:1062–1063; 14:1920–1921, 1922
 aging and 1:53
 the Pill and 7:963; 10:1414;
  14:1920–1921
 pituitary gland and 12:1598
Lieberkuhn, crypts of 4:495, *530*
ligaments 8:1069–1072; 9:1266
 peridontal 6:730, 731
 sprained 15:2056–2057
limbic system 2:262, *263*, 264

limbs
 bleeding
  control 17:2422
  tourniquets and 16:2245–2246;
   17:2422
 cramps 4:437
 fractured 5:663
  physical therapy and 11:1580
 growing pains 5:715
 paralysis 11:1490, 1492
 reattached 5:709; 9:1218, 1219–1221
 stiff 15:2076
 see also arms; legs
linoleic acid 10:1382
lipase 4:*494*, 495; 11:1487
lipoproteins
 HDL 3:366
 LDL 3:366; 5:656
liposomes, used in gene therapy 5:680
lips 9:*1260*
 bleeding from 9:1260
 blood blisters 13:*1756*
 blue 4:555, 564; 11:1463, 1464
 cheilosis 9:1263
 cleft 3:376, 401; 11:*1485*; 12:1612–1613,
  1614
 tattooing pigments to 16:2173
 ulcers 17:2311, *2312*
liver and liver diseases 5:597;
  8:1084–1087
 diseases and disorders
  abscesses 13:1757
  cancer 6:811; 8:1087; 10:1399
  cirrhosis 2:228; 3:375; 6:727; 7:968,
   991; 8:*1087*
  cysts 4:*446*, 447
  hepatitis 6:*810*, 811; 8:1087
  lacerations 8:1031
  liver failure 8:1087; 13:1755;
   14:1958
  liver fluke 8:1088–1089
  rupture 5:663
  shoulder or arm pain and 14:1948
  the spleen and 15:2046
 liver
  biopsies 2:192, 193
  blood clotting and 2:228
  glycogen storage 15:*2064*, 2120
  jaundice and 7:991
  removal of part of 10:1421
  transplants 4:*504*; 8:1084;
   16:2263, 2265, *2266*
lung and lung diseases 2:281; 3:347;
  8:1100–1104
 abscesses 12:1625
 adult respiratory distress syndrome
  (ARDS; shock lung; wet lung)
  14:1943, 1946
 asbestosis 1:136; 12:*1639*; 13:1751
 asthma 1:139–141; 8:1103–1104;
  11:1464; 13:1751
  avoidance of beta-blockers 3:419,
   420
  breast-feeding and 13:1750
  causes 1:59, 60, 140, 141; 7:888;
   8:1100, 1103; 15:2050
  eczema and 4:542
  pigeon chest and 12:1590,
   1592
  pneumonia and 12:1622
  prevention 1:73, 141
  symptoms 1:73, 140–141; 2:282;
   3:348; 11:1560; 17:*2407*, 2408
  treatment 1:73, 74, 141; 2:157, 158,
   282; 7:*953*–954; 8:1103; 15:2072;
   17:2408
 bronchiectasis 6:741; 12:1623–1624,
  13:1750, 1751

bronchitis 3:294–296, 348; 12:1623
 acute 2:282; 3:295, 296; 13:1751;
  15:2151
 chronic 2:282; 3:294, *295*, 296;
  8:1103; 11:1464; 13:1751; 15:2151
 open windows and 2:279
 wheezing and 17:2407, 2408
cancer 2:282; 3:294, 314; 6:727, 832;
  8:1103, 1104, *1125*; 13:1751
 asbestos-related 1:136
 in cities 12:1639
 deaths from 10:1399
 exposure to radon and 13:1839
 hormone production 11:1504
 smoking and 2:279, *283*; 3:314;
  8:1067, 1104; 13:1749; 14:1996,
  1997–*1998*, *1999*
 symptoms 3:316; 13:1751
 treatment 2:282; 13:1751, 1776
collapsed lung 13:1751
cystic fibrosis and 4:448
emphysema 3:295; **4:563–564**;
  11:1464; 13:1752
 smoking and 2:279; 3:294, 296;
  4:563–564; 8:1103
 treatment 2:282; 5:681; 13:1752
 types 4:*563*, 564
as excretory organs 5:596
fibrosing alveolitis 13:1751, 1752
forced expiratory volume (FEV)
  3:296, 371
gaseous irritants and 7:981
lung function tests 3:296; 13:1752
occupational hazards, from dusts
  10:1391, 1394; 14:*1961*
pleural effusions 12:1618
pleurisy 2:281, 282; 3:426; 9:1189;
  12:1618–1620; 13:1751, 1752
 pain 3:348
 pneumonia and 12:1625
 treatment 12:1620; 15:2151
pneumoconiosis 2:282; 4:564;
  12:1621; 13:1752
pneumonia 2:282; 3:347, 348; 7:*937*,
  938, 940; 8:1103, 1104;
  12:1622–1625; 13:1752
 aspiration pneumonia 12:1624,
  1625, 1631
 bronchopneumonia 8:1104;
  12:*1623*, 1624–1625
 a complication of other diseases
  3:350; 9:1165; 12:1625
 double 12:1622
 lobar 8:1104; 12:1622, *1623*, *1624*,
  1625
 pneumonic plague 12:1607
 prevention 12:1624
 secondary drowning 4:522
 treatment 2:282; 8:1103; 12:1624,
  1625; 13:1752
pneumothorax 13:1751, 1752
pulmonary embolism 13:1751, 1752;
  16:2215
removal of a lung 10:1421
shoulder or arm pain and 14:1948
small lungs 2:279
transplants 4:*504*; 13:1750
tuberculosis 16:2287–*2289*, 2290
wheezing 17:2407–2408
luteinizing hormone (LH) 9:*1200*, *1202*;
  11:1459; 12:1599–1600; 16:2195
lymph 8:1109
lymphatic system 8:1109–1112
 blockage 8:1111–1112
  elephantiasis 4:554; 8:1112; 11:1501;
   16:*2282*; 17:2419, *2420*
 cancer spread and 3:313; 10:*1400*
 lymphangitis 8:1111, 1112

lymphatic vessels 8:1109, *1111*
lymph nodes 3:313; 8:1109, *1111*, 1130
 removal in breast cancer 8:1098,
  1109, *1146*, 1147
 secondary tumors in 16:2292
 swollen 5:*699*; 6:*833*; 8:1109, 1114;
  10:1335; 15:2145, 2148
lymphoma 8:1110, 1112, **1114–1115**
 B-cell 5:588
  Burkitt's 5:588; 7:935
  Hodgkin's disease 3:317;
   6:*833*–834; 8:1114
  non-Hodgkin's 6:*833*; 8:1114
  the tonsils and 16:2237
 see also adenoids; tonsils
lymph nodes *see* lymphatic system,
 lymph nodes
lymphocytes 2:226, 227, 228;
  8:1109–1110, 1113
 B lymphocytes 7:908, 909;
  8:1109–1110, 1113; 16:2222
 T4, AIDS virus and 1:57
 T lymphocytes 7:908, *909*;
  8:1109–1110, *1113*; 16:2222
lymphokines 7:914; 8:1113
lysosomes 3:331; 9:1240

macula 13:1811, *1812*
mast cells 1:72; 6:756; 14:2003
mastication (chewing) 1:67, 68; **8:1149**
meconium 4:486; 5:623
meiosis 3:331–*332*; 5:683
melanin 6:736; 8:1090; 9:1180–1181;
  11:1468, 1564–*1565*; 14:1971, *1972*;
  15:2127
melanocytes 8:1090, 1091; 9:1180,
  1182–*1183*; 14:*1971*; 15:2127
melanocyte-stimulating hormone
  (MSH) 9:*1181*
melatonin 2:188; 9:1186–1187; 14:1898,
  1899
membranes 9:1188–1189
 cell 9:1241
 mucous 9:*1188*, 1189, 1269
 serous 9:1189
 synovial 7:1002; 9:1188, *1189*
memory 2:262, 264; 9:1190–1193, 1229;
  10:1345
 absentmindedness 4:459
 aging and 9:1190, *1192*; 14:1908,
  1909–1910
 dementia and 4:459
 false memory syndrome 7:923, 924;
  13:1734
 sense of smell and 14:1993
meninges 9:*1189*
 meningitis and 9:*1195*–1196
menopause 9:1198–1200
 acne rosacea 14:1975
 age at start of 9:1200
  inherited 6:816
 anxiety during 1:105
 atheroma and 1:118
 breast changes 2:276–277
 contraception and 6:732
 cystitis and 4:450
 disappearance of PMS 12:1672
 emotional changes 6:859
 endometriosis during 4:569
 estrogen and 5:593; 6:854–855;
  17:2326
 exercise 5:601
 hair loss 2:169
 hormone replacement therapy
  (HRT) 4:566; 5:594; 6:854–856;
  7:875; 9:1199; 11:1450
 hot flashes 4:496; 6:855–856;
  7:874–875; 9:1198–1199

menopause *(cont'd)*
  acne rosacea and **14**:1975
  menstruation stops **17**:2326
  osteoporosis and **2**:260; **3**:310, 311;
    6:854, 855, 856; **9**:1199
  the ovaries and **11**:1458
  risk of breast cancer **6**:856
  risk of heart disease **9**:1200
  sterilization and **15**:2070; **16**:2286
  sweats **11**:1544
  symptoms **6**:855–856
  tiredness **16**:2230
  the vagina and **17**:2334
    post-menopausal discharge
      17:2339
    vaginal atrophy **5**:593; **6**:856;
      9:1198, 1199
menstrual cycle **2**:188, 194; **7**:*944*;
    9:1201–1203; **12**:1671–1672; **17**:2328
  the breasts and **2**:276
  conception and **3**:399
  cramps **5**:601
  during puberty **13**:1741
  fluid retention and **4**:500;
    12:1672–1673, 1674
  hormones and **4**:567; **9**:*1200*
    estrogen **5**:*593*, 594
  lethargy **8**:1058
  libido and **14**:1921
  mid-cycle abdominal pain **1**:13
  pimples and **1**:32; **14**:1970
  premenstrual syndrome (PMS)
    6:859; **8**:1056; **9**:1201, 1202;
    12:*1671–1674*
    headaches **6**:758
    treatment **12**:*1674*; **14**:1898
  swollen abdomen and **15**:2148
  weight gain during **1**:112; **12**:1672
menstruation **5**:594; **9**:1201–1205;
    12:1671; **17**:2329
  cessation at menopause **17**:2326
  contraceptives and **3**:407, 410
  disorders **9**:1204, *1205*
    failure to menstruate **17**:2335
    heavy periods (menorrhagia)
      4:496; **5**:642; **9**:1202, 1204, 1205
    period pains **9**:1202–1205
  during puberty **13**:1739–1740
  exercise during **1**:49; **15**:2052
  first period **11**:1458; **13**:1739
  hair condition during **6**:737
  newborn babies and **17**:2328
  use of tampons, and toxic shock
    syndrome **16**:2247, 2248
  see also menstrual cycle
meridian lines **1**:35, *37*, 38, 117; **6**:776;
    8:1144; **9**:1144
mesenteries **1**:11
mesomorphs **2**:*253*
metabolism **9**:1214–1215
  aerobic **1**:49–50
  anaerobic **1**:49
  basal metabolic rate **2**:173; **17**:2401
  heat of **16**:2182
metacarpals **6**:745
mind **9**:1226–1229
  alters with age **14**:1909–1910
  over matter **9**:*1226*, 1228, 1229
  subconscious **9**:1228; **15**:2114–2115
  see also memory
mitochondria **3**:331; **9**:1240, *1241*
  in muscle cells **11**:1577
mitosis **3**:331, *332*
Mongoloid race **2**:252, *253*
monoamine oxidase enzymes **9**:1223
monocytes **2**:227, 228
mouth **9**:1260–1263
  breathing through **1**:40; **9**:1262

problems **9**:1263
  accident to the palate **11**:1485
  acidic diet **9**:1263
  aphthous stomatitis (aphthous
    ulcers) **9**:1263; **17**:*2311*
  cancer **3**:316
  cleft palate **2**:207; **3**:376, 401;
    11:1483, 1484, *1485*; **12**:1612–1613;
    15:2030
  cold sores **2**:223; **3**:382; **4**:543;
    6:825; **9**:1263; **14**:1970, 2008
  drooling **9**:1262, 1263
  dry mouth **9**:1262; **13**:1852
  halitosis (bad breath) **4**:460;
    6:740–741; **9**:1263; **12**:1608
  irritants **7**:981
  pyorrhea and gingivitis **4**:461;
    6:731, 740, 759; **9**:1263; **12**:1610;
    13:*1759–1761*
  salivary duct stones **9**:1263;
    13:*1854*
  stomatitis **9**:1263
  thrush **9**:1263; **16**:*2219*
  ulcers **9**:1260, 1263; **14**:2008;
    16:2234; **17**:2310–2312
  yeast infection **9**:1263; **11**:1484;
    17:2436
  pyorrhea and gingivitis **13**:*1759–1761*
    gingivitis **6**:731; **9**:1263;
      13:*1759–1761*
    halitosis and **6**:740
    pyorrhea (peridontal disease)
      4:461; **6**:731, 759; **12**:1610;
      13:1759–1760, 1761
  speech and **9**:*1262–1263*
  see also lips; teeth and teething;
    tongue
movement **9**:1264–1268
  ligaments and **8**:1071; **9**:1266
  muscles and **9**:1264, *1265*, 1294
MSH *see* melanocyte-stimulating
    hormone
mucus **9**:1188, **1269**; **11**:1560
  cervical **9**:*1203*, 1269
    the rhythm method and **13**:1829,
      1830
  nasal, and smell **14**:1991, *1994*
Müllerian ducts **17**:2328–2329
multiple births **3**:400; **9**:**1274–1277**
  fertility drugs and **7**:942; **9**:1274,
    1275
  from IVF **1**:129
  see also twins
muscles **9**:1290–1294
  anerobic metabolism **1**:49
  biceps and triceps **4**:546; **9**:1265
  building up **12**:1701
  disorders **9**:1292; **12**:*1724*
    cramp **1**:50; **4**:437, 437; **5**:599;
      6:796; **11**:1544; **12**:1662; **13**:1764,
      1861
    enzyme defects **9**:1292
    fibrositis **5**:643
    hamstring injuries **6**:743–744
    hot and cold treatment **6**:797,
      799
    hyperkalemic paralysis
      9:1292
    hypokalemic paralysis **9**:1292
    muscular dystrophy **9**:1292;
      10:**1301–1303**; **11**:*1490*
    myalgia **10**:**1310–1311**; **16**:2248
    myasthenia gravis **5**:619, 620;
      10:**1312–1313**; **11**:1491
    myopathies **9**:1292, 1294
    myositis **9**:1292, 1294
    paralysis **11**:1491
    polymyalgia rheumatica **9**:1292

pulled or strained muscles **6**:799;
    9:1292, 1294; **13**:*1747–1748*;
    15:*2051*, 2054
  stiffness **15**:2054, 2076–2077
  torn muscles **9**:1290, 1292
exercise and **5**:599; **9**:1290, 1294
fitness and **11**:1577
injections into **7**:955, 956
intercostal, and stitch **15**:2087
movement and **9**:1264, *1265*,
    1294
postural **16**:2182–2183
spasms
  around joints **7**:1000
  in the back **2**:163; **5**:643
  traction and **16**:2253
sports injuries, first aid **1**:50
structure **9**:1291–1294
types **9**:1290
  cardiac (heart) **9**:1266, 1267, 1290,
    1293
  smooth (involuntary) **9**:1266,
    1267, *1268*, 1290, *1293*
  striated (voluntary) **9**:1290, *1291*,
    1293
see also diaphragm; tendons
musculoskeletal system **14**:1966
myelin **9**:1280; **10**:1347
myofibrils **9**:1265, *1293*
myoglobin **11**:1463

nails **10**:**1314–1318**; **14**:1970–1971
  athlete's foot affecting **2**:150;
    13:1837, 1838
  biting **10**:1314, 1315–*1318*
  bruises under **3**:*298*; **10**:1314
  care **10**:*1316–1317*, 1318
    cutting toenails **5**:627; **10**:*1317*
  dermatologists and **4**:469
  flaky **10**:1315
  ingrown toenails **7**:**951–952**; **10**:1315,
    1318; **12**:1626
  iron deficiency and **7**:977;
    10:1315
  koilonychia **6**:747
  leukonychia **6**:747
  loss **10**:1314
  onycholysis **6**:747
  psoriasis and **12**:1708
  ridges **10**:1315
  ringworm **10**:1315
  splinter hemorrhages **16**:2277
  thrush (*Candida*) **16**:2220; **17**:*2437*,
    2438
  white spots **10**:1315
  whitlow (paronychia) **6**:747; **10**:1314;
    17:**2411**, 2438
nasopharynx **11**:1555–1557
nature versus nurture (inherited
    versus acquired) **6**:817–818;
    11:1539–1540
navel, umbilical hernia **6**:819, *821*
neck **10**:**1332–1335**
  Adam's apple **10**:1332, *1335*
  arthritis **10**:1335
    osteoarthritis **1**:122
    vertigo and **17**:2366
  broken **10**:1332, *1334*; **15**:2040
  bull neck **4**:497
  cervical ribs **13**:1832
  dislocation **4**:498
  glands in *see* parathyroid glands;
    thyroid
  goiter **5**:704; **10**:1334; **16**:2224, 2225,
    2226
  pain and spasm, heat treatment
    6:799
  stiff **10**:1332; **15**:2078, *2079*

swollen lymph nodes **5**:*699*; **6**:*833*;
    8:*1109*, 1114; **10**:1335
  whiplash injury **10**:1334, *1335*;
    13:*1747–1748*; **17**:**2409–2410**
  see also larynx and laryngitis;
    pharynx; throat; vocal cords
nephrons **8**:1017, 1020; **17**:*2325*
nervous system **10**:**1343–1347**
  autonomic *see* autonomic nervous
    system
  central **2**:262; **10**:1344–1345, *1346*
    see also brain; spinal cord
  disorders **10**:1347
  function tests **10**:1355–1356
  nerves
    cells (neurons) **2**:157; **9**:1256;
      10:1343, 1344, 1345–1347
    cranial **10**:1344
    facial **16**:2169, 2171
    glossopharyngeal **16**:2169, 2171
    growth **9**:1221
    Guillain-Barré syndrome and
      6:728, 729
    junction with muscles **10**:*1313*;
      11:1491, *1492*
    microsurgery and **9**:1218, 1219,
      1221
    multiple sclerosis and **6**:728;
      9:1280–1281
    numbness and **10**:*1376–1378*
    olfactory **16**:2169
    optic **2**:220; **5**:606; **10**:**1410–1411**
    paralysis and **11**:1491–1493
    pinched **10**:1344
    polio and **6**:728
    severed **1**:20; **8**:1030
    spinal **10**:1344; **15**:2042
    ulnar **10**:1344; **11**:1491;
      12:1595
    vagus **11**:1487
  pain from the **11**:1476–1477
  parasympathetic **2**:156, 158
  peripheral **10**:1343–1344, *1346*
  somatic **10**:1343, 1344, *1345*
  sympathetic **2**:156, 158
  neurons (nerve cells) **2**:157; **9**:1256;
    10:1343, 1344, 1345–1347
  of the spinal cord **15**:2042
neurotransmitters
  Alzheimer's disease and **1**:83
  myasthenia gravis and **10**:*1313*
neutrophils **2**:225, *227*
nipples
  extra **6**:726
  prenatal care **12**:1675
nocturnal emissions (wet dreams)
    5:589; **14**:1906
noradrenaline (norepinephrine) **1**:47;
    2:158, 198–199; **5**:622; **12**:1724
normality **6**:817
nose **10**:**1371–1375**
  adenoids **1**:40–41; **2**:281; **10**:1372,
    1375; **11**:1557; **16**:2212–2213
    adenoidectomy **1**:41; **16**:2212
    snoring and **14**:*2005*
  broken **10**:1372, 1374
  changing shape of (rhinoplasty)
    3:424, 425; **12**:*1613*
  cocaine and **3**:381
  common cold **10**:1374
  congestion **10**:1371, 1372, 1374
  cosmetic surgery to **3**:424, 425
  crooked **10**:1372
  foreign bodies **10**:1375; **14**:1962, 2003
  gaseous irritants and **7**:981
  hay fever **10**:1374
  nasal discharge **14**:1962
  nasal passages **2**:*279–281*

nosebleeds 4:568; 6:803; 10:1371
  treating 10:1374
  picking 10:1371
  polyps in 10:1372, 1375; 12:1642, 1643
  rhinitis 11:1560; 13:1825–1826;
    14:2002, 2003
    vasomotor 14:2003
  sinusitis 6:741; 9:1269; 10:1375;
    13:1826; 14:1962–1963
    headaches and 6:758, 759; 15:2150

old age see aging
olecranon 4:546
olfactory cells 14:1991
omentum 11:1532, 1533, 1534, 1535
optic disks 5:607
optic nerve 2:220; 5:606; 10:1410–1411
orgasm 7:964–965; 10:1423–1424
  female 7:964–965; 10:1423;
    14:1918–1919, 1921; 17:2394
    multiple orgasms 14:1916
    problems 10:1424; 14:1929
  male 5:590; 7:965; 14:1919, 1921
    problems 10:1423–1424
  simultaneous 7:963
oropharynx 11:1557
ossification 3:324
osteoid 13:1836
out-of-body experiences 9:1229
ova see eggs
ovaries 3:399; 5:594; 11:1458–1459
  cancer 11:1459
    laparoscopy and 8:1034
    treatment 7:905
  cysts 4:446, 447, 568, 569; 6:733;
    11:1459; 16:2195
  as endocrine glands 11:1459
  endometriosis of 4:568, 569
  one removed 10:1422; 11:1458
    pregnancy and 6:732; 10:1421
  oophoritis 9:1284
  salpingitis and 13:1860
  sterilization involving the 15:2069,
    2071; 16:2286
  tumors 8:1124
ovulation 5:594; 7:945; 11:1459
  cervical mucus and 13:1829
  failure 7:943
  pain on 1:13
  the rhythm method and 13:1827,
    1828, 1829, 1830
oxygen 11:1463–1465, 1574–1575
  carried around the body 2:281;
    11:1464
  cycle 11:1465
  debt 11:1463
  gas exchange and 8:1102
  hyperbaric 3:302; 11:1466, 1467
  liquid 11:1467
  transtracheal 11:1464
  uptake during exercise 11:1573,
    1575–1576
oxytocin 2:273; 4:566, 567; 6:857, 859;
    12:1599, 1605
  induced labor and 7:933, 934;
    10:1322
  nicotine and 10:1361

Paget's disease 2:260
palate 9:1260; 11:1483–1485
  accident to 11:1485
  cleft 2:207; 3:376, 401; 11:1483, 1484,
    1485; 12:1612–1613
    speech and 15:2030
  excessively concave 11:1485
  "falling" 11:1483
pancreas and disorders 5:700;
    11:1486–1487

cancer 5:624; 7:992; 11:1487
  cystic fibrosis affecting 11:1487
  diabetes and 4:471–472; 7:960;
    11:1487
  digestive function 4:495; 5:700;
    11:1486, 1487
  hemochromatosis affecting 11:1487
  injuries 11:1486
  pancreatitis 9:1283; 11:1486
  removal 11:1486, 1487
  shoulder or arm pain and 14:1948
  sugar levels and 7:960; 11:1486
  transplants 16:2264
  tumors 7:960
parathyroid glands 5:700; 10:1335;
    11:1503–1505
  bones and 2:259; 11:1505; 13:1836
  overactive 11:1504, 1505
  removal 11:1503, 1504
  tumor 3:311; 11:1505
  underactive 11:1504, 1505
parathyroid hormone (PTH;
    parathormone) 2:259; 3:310, 311;
    4:566; 6:858; 8:1020; 11:1504
  chelation therapy and 3:345
parotid glands 9:1261; 13:1853
patella see knee, kneecap
pelvis 11:1522–1526
  fractured 11:1526
  see also hip
penetrance 6:818
penis and disorders 5:690; 11:1530–1531
  disorders
    balanitis 10:1368; 11:1531; 17:2437
    cancer 11:1530; 17:2325
    discharge 11:1530, 1531
    hypospadias 2:207; 12:1613;
      17:2323
    impotence 1:130; 5:590;
      7:919–920; 11:1531; 14:1924
    pain 5:690
    paraphimosis 11:1531
    phimosis 3:374; 11:1531
    urethritis 11:1531
  penis
    circumcision 3:374; 5:688; 14:1918
    prosthesis 12:1700
    size 14:1920
  see also erection and ejaculation
pepsin 4:494, 531; 5:581
peridontium 6:730
perineum 11:1525
period see menstruation
periosteum 8:1070
peristalsis 1:69; 3:404, 405; 5:592;
    15:2023
peritoneum 1:11; 11:1532–1535
  dialysis through 8:1014, 1016; 17:2322
  peritonitis 1:111; 4:501; 9:1189; 11:1532,
    1533–1535
peroxisomes 9:1240
perspiration (sweat) 2:249; 5:597–598,
    699; 11:1543–1545; 14:1941–1942;
    15:2130–2131; 16:2183
  prickly heat and 12:1685
Peyer's patches, typhoid and 16:2295,
    2297
phagocytes 1:17–18; 3:319; 7:946, 948
phalanges 6:745
pharynx 11:1555–1557; 16:2211–2212
  cancer 16:2213
  pharyngeal web 16:2211
  pharyngitis 11:1556, 1557; 14:2011
  see also throat
phenylalanine 11:1558, 1559
phonation 15:2029
pineal gland 2:187–188; 5:700; 9:1186,
    1187; 14:1899

pituitary gland 4:567; 12:1598–1601
  direct influence 6:859
    antidiuretic hormone secretion
      6:859; 12:1599
    on growth 4:532; 5:697–698
    oxytocin secretion 6:857, 859;
      12:1599
    prolactin secretion 6:859; 8:1032;
      12:1598, 1600
  effect of hypothalamus on 6:859;
    7:897; 12:1598–1599; 13:1740
  effect on other glands 4:566, 567;
    6:859
    adrenal glands 4:567; 12:1598
    pancreas 5:699
    sex glands 11:1459
    thyroid gland 4:567; 6:847;
      12:1599; 16:2224
  failure 12:1598
  hormones 5:593; 7:899;
    9:1201–1202; 12:1599–1600
  tumors 5:607; 7:899; 10:1411;
    12:1598, 1600–1601
    gigantism or acromegaly and
      5:697–698
    menstrual disorders and 9:1204
pituitary portal system 12:1599
placenta 2:204; 8:1102; 12:1604–1605
  D & C and 4:496
  placenta previa 3:341; 9:1277; 12:1605
plasma 2:227; 12:1611
plasma cells 8:1113
platelets 2:226, 227, 228; 3:298; 13:1755
  deficiency 3:298
polygenes 6:817, 818
polymorphs 2:225–227
posture 12:1656–1658; 14:1948
  Alexander technique and 1:65, 66
  during pregnancy 12:1656, 1677, 1678
  ligaments and 8:1069, 1072
  massage and 8:1144
  working with computers 13:1804,
    1846
pregnancy 12:1661–1665
  alcohol taken during 5:633; 15:2080
  anemia 1:88
  ankles, swollen 15:2146, 2147
  blood samples during 11:1511
  "blossoming" during 12:1662
  breasts 2:276; 12:1663, 1664
    colostrum production 12:1663
    prevention of mastitis 9:1159
  calcium during 3:310, 311; 12:1678
  cancer during 13:1774
  carpal tunnel syndrome and 3:322,
    323
  cervical incompetence 3:338
  chicken pox and 3:350
  constipation 3:404; 8:1045; 12:1662,
    1675
  cramp 4:437; 12:1662
  cystitis 4:450
  dangers of parasites during 11:1498
  diabetes during 7:960
  diagnostic techniques 12:1664–1665
    amniocentesis 1:84
    chorionic villus sampling 2:207;
      3:367–368; 5:638; 7:877
    ultrasound 2:207, 285; 4:477, 479,
      480; 12:1664; 13:1869, 1870;
      14:1893, 1894; 17:2315, 2316–2317
    X rays 12:1664–1665, 1676; 17:2431
  diet 2:206; 3:402; 4:491; 8:1127, 1128;
    10:1379; 12:1662, 1665, 1675, 1678
    to avoid listeriosis 8:1083
  driving and 5:638
  drugs (medicines) taken during
    1:99; 3:401; 9:1170

antibiotics 1:99
  painkillers 11:1478
  thalidomide 2:206; 3:402; 6:749;
    9:1170; 11:1550; 16:2202–2204
ectopic 1:14; 4:541, 571; 6:733; 11:1521
  after hysterectomy 7:903
  after sterilization 15:2068, 2069,
    2070; 16:2286
  the Pill and 10:1417
  salpingitis and 13:1860
edema 4:544; 12:1662–1663; 17:2399
estrogen levels 5:593
fainting in 5:611, 612; 12:1662
fatigue 5:618
fetal alcohol syndrome and 5:633
first signs of 12:1661
flatulence 5:645
fluoride taken during 5:651
food fads 1:113
frights during 3:401; 5:634
goiter 5:704
gonorrhea and 5:705
gum disease and 6:731
hair during 6:735
heartburn 5:592; 6:786, 787; 12:1661,
    1662, 1675
hemorrhoids (piles) 5:637; 12:1662,
    1675
hepatitis during 6:809, 810
high-risk 13:1839
increased urination 12:1662
intercourse during 5:634; 7:963;
    12:1661, 1675
itches 7:988
lethargy in first few weeks 8:1056
lupus and 8:1105, 1106
malaria during 8:1122
manipulation of the fetus 8:1136
marijuana taken during 8:1137
mole changes during 9:1242
moods during 9:1246–1247
morning sickness 5:636, 645; 6:857;
    9:1248–1249; 17:2391
multiple see multiple births
multiple births detected 12:1676
occupational hazards and 10:1394
older women and 1:84; 5:682; 6:749,
    750
the pelvis and 11:1522, 1524
phantom 11:1548–1549
PKU sufferers and 11:1558, 1559
placenta previa 3:341; 9:1277; 12:1605
preeclampsia (preeclamptic
    toxemia; PET; proteinuric
    hypertension) 3:322; 7:931;
    8:1106; 12:1659–1660; 17:2399
rhesus (Rh) factor and 2:234–235;
    12:1604; 13:1815–1816; 15:2081
risk of birth defects 2:206; 4:506;
    6:749, 750
slipped disks 14:1982
smoking during 5:638; 10:1361;
    12:1604, 1665; 14:1995; 15:2080
snoring 14:2004
STDs and 12:1675; 14:1932, 1933, 1935
stretch marks 9:1276; 12:1661, 1662,
    1679; 15:2105, 2105
swelling and puffiness 12:1659
sympathetic 1:13
tests for 12:1661; 15:2024
trimesters 5:634–639
trying to become pregnant 6:732
vaccinations during 2:206;
    16:2284
vaginal discharge 12:1662
varicose veins 5:637; 12:1662,
    1675–1676; 17:2344
weight after 10:1384

pregnancy (cont'd)
  weight during 9:1248; 15:2105
  while breast-feeding 8:1032
  yeast infections 5:634
  see also conception; fetus; labor;
    placenta
progesterone 4:566
  breast development and 2:275
  the menstrual cycle and 9:1202;
    11:1459
  in the Pill 17:2326
  pregnancy and 2:276
    morning sickness 6:857
  the skin and 8:1091; 14:1900
  to treat premenstrual syndrome
    12:1674
prolactin 2:276; 4:566; 6:858, 859;
  7:899; 8:1032; 12:1598, 1600
prolactin-inhibiting factor 7:899
prostaglandins 6:758; 7:948; 12:1689
  NSAIDs and 10:1369, 1370
  aspirin 1:137; 12:1689
  used in abortions 1:14, 15, 16
  used to induce labor 7:933–934;
    10:1322; 12:1689
prostate gland 5:590, 690; 12:1690–1695
  cancer 3:316; 5:690; 9:1187; 12:1691,
    1694
    treatment and outlook
    12:1694–1695; 13:1776
  enlargement 2:217, 218; 5:690;
    12:1690, 1691–1692
    tests for 8:1020
  prostatitis 5:690; 9:1284;
    12:1690–1691
  rectal examination 12:1694
  surgery 10:1423; 12:1695
    removal 7:925; 10:1421; 12:1690,
    1692, 1693–1694, 1695
  uremia and 17:2322
protein 12:1701–1702
  dietary 4:488–489; 6:772, 773;
    10:1380; 12:1701
    during pregnancy 12:1678
  genetically engineered 5:679
  genetics and 12:1702
  processed in the liver 8:1084–1086
  synthesis in the cell 5:683, 685
prothrombin 2:228; 17:2385
ptyalin see amylase
puberty 13:1739–1742
  acne and 1:31; 13:1739
  breastlike swellings in boys 2:275
  chubbiness 13:1739
  delayed, in boys 16:2195, 2196, 2250
  estrogen and 11:1459
  failure to menstruate 17:2335
  the larynx 13:1742; 17:2389
  stretch marks 15:2105
  testosterone and 13:1742;
    16:2195–2196
puerperium 10:1390
pulse 3:373; 13:1753–1754
  rate
    fitness and 1:50; 11:1572, 1574
    irregular 6:781
    taking the 13:1753
      difficulty 17:2429
    see also heart, heartbeat
purines, and gout 5:707
pyrogen 5:641

race 2:252–253
radius 4:546, 547
rapid eye movement (REM) sleep 4:511,
  512; 7:957; 13:1781; 14:1978–1980
rectum 13:1787–1788
  cancer 13:1787, 1788

fistula connecting to the vagina
  5:644
  polyps 13:1787
  prolapse 1:103; 12:1686, 1687, 1688;
    13:1787
reflexes 2:262; 3:364; 9:1264–1265,
  1266; 10:1345; 13:1789–1792;
  15:2040, 2041
  absence 13:1789, 1792
  behavioral 13:1792
  blinking 13:1789, 1792
  breathing 13:1790, 1792
  conditioned 9:1253; 13:1789, 1792
  coordination and 3:414
  coughing 3:426
  knee-jerk 8:1025; 9:1266, 1267;
    13:1791
  light 10:1410
  Moro 13:1791
  orientation reflexes 13:1791
  shivering 9:1264
  testing 4:475, 476; 11:1519
  vomiting 17:2391
releasing factors (inhibitory factors)
  7:899
renin 2:238, 239
repression 9:1192
respiratory system
  health 2:283
  mucous membranes 9:1189, 1269
  phlegm and 11:1560
  see also breathing; lung and lung
    diseases
reticular formation 17:2318, 2319
retina and retinal disorders
  13:1811–1812
  disorders
    cotton wool spots 13:1812
    detached retina 2:220, 222;
      5:608–609; 13:1811, 1812
    deterioration with Tay-Sachs
      disease 16:2174
    diabetic retinopathy 5:609;
      13:1811, 1812
    hypertensive retinopathy 13:1812
    macular degeneration 2:220, 222;
      8:1119; 13:1811, 1812
    retinal artery occlusion 2:222
    retinal vein thrombosis 2:222
    retinitis pigmentosa 2:222;
      13:1811, 1812
  retina 5:606; 13:1811
    artificial sight and 2:191
    laser sugery on 2:221; 8:1041, 1042
    light-sensitive cells 10:1362, 1410;
      13:1811
    night vision and 10:1362
retinol 17:2373
rhesus (Rh) factor 2:233, 234–235;
  12:1604; 13:1815–1816; 15:2081
rheumatoid factor 13:1821
Rh factor see rhesus (Rh) factor
rhodopsin (visual purple) 10:1362;
  13:1812; 17:2373
ribosomes 3:331; 5:685; 9:1240
  effect of tetracyclines on 16:2199
ribs 13:1831–1834
  ankylosing spondylitis and 13:1834
  cervical 13:1832
  cracked 3:347; 13:1834
  dislocated 13:1834
  floating 13:1832
  fractured 3:347; 13:1832–1834
  joints 7:1002, 1003
  osteoid bumps 13:1836
  tumors in 13:1834
rigor 14:1942
rigor mortis 4:458

RNA
  messenger (mRNA) 5:683, 685
  transfer (tRNA) 5:685

sacrum 2:159; 11:1522
saliva 1:67; 4:494; 5:702; 8:1149 1261,
  1269; 13:1852–1854
  excess 13:1854
  lack of 4:495; 8:1149; 9:1149; 13:1854
    nervousness and 9:1262; 13:1852,
      1854
salivary ducts 13:1852
  stones in 9:1263; 13:1854
salivary glands 13:1852–1853
  mumps and 9:1283–1284; 13:1854
  tumors 13:1854
scabs 2:226; 14:1881, 1972
sclera 5:604
scrotum 11:1530
sebaceous glands 5:700;
  14:1900–1901, 1971
  acne and 1:32
  cysts 4:446, 447; 6:726; 14:1900;
    15:2147, 2148
  sties and 15:2112
sebum 1:32; 6:735; 14:1900, 1901
secretin 6:857–859; 11:1487
secretion 5:598
semen (seminal fluid) 3:399; 5:589,
  590, 690; 14:1906–1907; 15:2035
  see also sperm
semicircular canals 2:167; 17:2391
seminal fluid see semen
seminal vesicles 14:1906–1907, 1919;
  15:2035
seminiferous tubules 5:689; 16:2191,
  2194; 17:2347
serotonin (5-HT) 2:198; 7:875; 9:1222;
  16:2258
sex flush 5:590
sex hormones 12:1598
  reduced 6:858
  see also estrogen; progesterone;
    testosterone
sexual intercourse see intercourse
shape, body 2:253–254
shivering 9:1264; 14:1940–1942;
  16:2183
shoulder 14:1948–1949
  bandaging 4:518
  bursitis 3:308
  dislocated 4:498–499; 8:1069, 1135;
    10:1433; 14:1948
  exercise 14:1949
  frozen 1:124; 6:799; 14:1949, 1968;
    15:2076
  hydrotherapy and 7:883
  impingement syndrome 3:308
  injury to, affecting the elbow 4:546
  ligaments 8:1071
  osteoarthritis 10:1437
  painful 11:1475
    treatment 6:764; 11:1580
  "rounded" 14:1948
  stiff 14:1949; 15:2076, 2078, 2079
sight see eyes and eyesight
sinews see tendons
sinoatrial node (pacemaker) 6:782;
  9:1267; 11:1472
sinuses 5:644; 10:1372, 1373; 14:1962,
  1963
  radiation of pain from 15:2149
sinusoids 17:2358
situs inversus 2:252
skeleton 9:1265; 14:1964–1968
  backache and 2:258
  see also bones; cartilage; joints
Skene's glands 17:2394

skin and skin diseases 14:1969–1975
  dermatology 4:469–470
  disorders
    acne and pimples 1:31–34, 75;
      2:255; 7:885; 14:1880, 1970, 1974,
      1975
    Addison's disease 9:1181
    albinism 5:684, 686; 6:735; 7:921,
      922; 9:1181; 10:1304, 1305
    allergic reactions 1:71, 73; 4:467,
      468, 487, 542, 543; 6:747, 795;
      14:1974; 16:2172, 2173
    athlete's foot 2:150; 7:886, 937;
      13:1763, 1837; 14:1975; 17:2436
    birthmarks 2:208–209; 12:1613;
      14:1972, 1974
    blackheads (comedones) 1:31, 32;
      14:1901
    blisters 2:223–224; 3:300, 304,
      382; 7:918; 13:1756
    boils 2:255–256; 13:1757
    bruises (contusions) 3:298, 319;
      17:2422, 2423, 2424
    calluses 3:417, 418; 12:1627; 17:2362
    cancer 2:192, 208; 3:316; 4:573,
      574; 6:726; 8:1125, 1126;
      9:1182–1185; 11:1468, 1470;
      13:1776; 14:1975; 15:2024, 2127–2128
    in children 14:1972–1974
    corns 3:417–418; 12:1627; 17:2362
    cradle cap 14:1972–1973
    cysts 4:446–447
    dandruff 4:451–452; 15:2112
    dermatitis 1:71, 73; 4:467–468,
      481, 482; 7:946, 948; 13:1782
      14:1974, 2009
    eczema 2:224; 4:467–468,
      542–543; 14:1969, 1974–1975
    hives (urticaria) 6:831
    impetigo 2:223, 224; 7:918
    keloids 7:1005; 14:1880, 1881
    melanoma 9:1182–1185, 1242, 1243;
      11:1470; 14:1975
    moles 2:209; 6:726; 9:1182, 1183,
      1184, 1242–1243; 11:1511; 14:1972,
      1974, 1975
    photosensitivity 11:1564–1565;
      15:2126, 2129
    psoriasis 4:469; 6:739; 7:989;
      12:1706–1708; 16:2173
    purpura 2:228; 3:318; 13:1755–1756
    ringworm 7:938, 939; 10:1315;
      13:1837–1838; 14:1974
    rosacea 1:34; 7:875
    scleroderma (systemic sclerosis)
      14:1888–1889; 15:2148
    seborrhea (seborrheic dermatitis)
      1:32; 4:468, 482, 483; 7:988, 989;
      13:1783
    stretch marks 9:1276; 12:1661,
      1662, 1679; 15:2105–2106
    sunburn 2:223; 3:303; 6:831;
      11:1470; 15:2126–2129; 16:2272
    swellings 15:2147–2148
    thrush 16:2220
    treatment 4:469–470
    verruca (plantar wart) 3:418;
      5:625; 7:886; 12:1627;
      17:2361–2363, 2395
    vitiligo 9:1181; 14:1975; 17:2388
    warts 6:726; 14:1975; 17:2395–2397
    whitlow (paronychia) 6:747;
      10:1314; 17:2411, 2438
  skin
    aging 14:1970, 1975
    care 14:1975
    chemicals spilled onto 7:981
    cosmetics 3:422–423

dry 14:*1901*
excretion through 5:597–598
glands *see* glands, apocrine; glands, sweat; sebaceous glands
grafts 3:*302,* 304; 5:*709, 710–711;* 9:1221; 12:1612, 1615–1616
greasy 14:*1900, 1901*
hardening the 2:223
pigmentation (color) 6:817; 9:1181, 1183; 11:1468; 14:1971, *1972*
specimens 15:2024
structure 14:1969–1970, *1971*
synthetic 2:190
temperature 16:2208
touch receptors 16:2239–*2240*
wound healing 6:*765;* 14:1971–1972
wrinkles 14:*1970;* 15:2127; **17:2427–2428**
see also hair; melanin; nails
skull 6:760
bony lumps on 2:257
fractured 5:*662, 663;* 6:760
replacement surgery 10:1354, *1355,* 1356
suture joints 7:1000
small intestine 1:68
celiac disease and 3:*329*
Crohn's disease 4:*442–443*
digestion in 4:*494–495,* 530–531
duodenum 1:68; 4:*494–495,* **530–531**
ileum 1:68
jejunum 1:68
typhoid in 16:*2295,* 2297
smegma 11:1531
smell 14:**1990–1994**
disorders 14:1993
loss (anosmia) 14:1993; 16:2169, *2170*
emotions and 2:262; 14:1993
taste and 14:1992; 16:2169, *2170,* 2171
sodium
deficiency 8:1128
pump 13:1861–*1862*
somatotropin *see* growth hormone
somatrophin 2:252
sperm 3:399–400; 5:589, 689; 14:*1906;* **15:2034–2035;** 16:*2194*
analgesic and 1:137
chromosomes 5:683
first produced 15:2034
infertility and 1:129, *130;* 7:943; 14:1907; 16:2194
life span 3:399; 6:732; 7:945; 13:1827–1828
low sperm count 1:131; 3:399; 5:689; 7:943; 15:2034, 2035
IVF and 7:974
production 15:*2034,* 2035
tested 9:1238
for in vitro fertilization 7:*971*
see also semen
spermatic cord 16:2192; 17:2347
sphincter(s)
cardiac 1:67
pyloric (pylorus) 1:68; 15:2088
spinal canal 6:761
spinal cord 6:*761;* 10:1344–1345; 15:*2040–2043*
analysis of touch and pain in 16:2240–2241
multiple sclerosis and 9:*1280*
paralysis and 11:*1492,* 1493; 15:2043
problems 15:2041–2043
damage 11:*1492,* 1493; 15:2040, 2043
myelitis 15:2040, 2043

spine (backbone)
chiropractic and 3:*362, 363*
curvature 11:1448; 14:1968
lordosis (swayback) 13:*1848*
osteoporosis and humpback 11:*1450, 1451*
scoliosis 8:1078; 11:1448; 14:*1890–1891*
injuries, rehabilitation 13:1795
osteoarthritis 5:691; 10:1437
osteopathy and 11:1448, 1449
osteoporosis 11:*1451*
section through 10:*1346*
spinal anesthetics 8:1093
spinal traction 16:2255
see also back and backache
spleen 15:**2044–2046**
enlarged 8:1109; 15:*2045–2046*
feeling the 15:2045
lacerations 8:1031
multiple (polysplenia) 6:*805;* 15:2044
removal 8:1030, 1114; 15:2044, 2046
ruptured 5:663; 8:1030; 15:2044, 2046
stem cell 15:**2065–2066**
cloning and 3:378
embryonic 15:2065, 2066
stercobilin 5:623
sternum (breastbone) 12:*1591*
pigeon chest 3:347; 12:*1590–1592*
steroids, produced in the body 6:859; 15:2072
stomach 1:67–68; 15:**2088–2090**
cancer 6:741; 15:*2090;* 16:2292
cramps 5:599
gastritis 5:670, 671; 9:1269; 15:*2088,* 2089
mucous membrane 9:*1188*
removal 15:2088
"rumbling" 1:11
size 15:2088
stapling the walls of 10:1386
tumors 15:2090
ulcers (gastric ulcers) 1:11; 4:495; 5:581; 15:*2088,* 2089–2090; 17:*2313, 2314*
aspirin and 1:122; 11:1479
asymptomatic 17:2312
biopsy 2:192
bleeding from 6:803–804; 8:1042; 14:1945
body weight and 15:2090
causes 15:2089; 17:2313
gastritis and 5:671
gastroscopy and 4:570, 571; 8:1042
stomach or arm pain and 14:1948
treatment 2:157, 158; 5:581; 8:1042; 15:2090
subconscious 9:1228; 15:**2114–2115**
sublingual glands 9:1261; 13:*1853*
submandibular glands 13:1853
superior vena cava 5:373
suprachiasmic nucleus 2:187
swallowing 1:67; 5:592; 9:1261, 1262; 10:1334; 11:1484, *1556,* 1557
difficulty in, pharyngeal web and 16:2211
sweat *see* perspiration
synapses 2:157, *158;* 10:1344
synovial fluid 3:325; 4:547; 8:1025

T3 (triiodothyronine) 16:2225
T4 *see* thyroxine
taste 13:1853; 16:**2169–2171,** 2232–2233
appetite and 1:113
smell and 14:1992; 16:2169, *2170,* 2171

taste buds 16:*2169,* 2171, 2232, 2233
tear ducts 10:1373–1374
tears 4:*444–*445
teeth and teething 8:1149 **16:2175–2178**
abscesses 1:21; 13:1758
absence of teeth 16:2178
bridges 4:463
broken teeth 16:2176
brushing 6:*730,* 731; 12:1608; 13:1761
canines 16:2175–2177
impacted 7:*916*
capped 4:462
color 16:2178
crowned 4:462, *463*
decay (caries) 12:1609
halitosis and 6:740; 12:1608
deciduous (milk or baby) teeth 16:2175, *2176, 2178*
filling 16:2176
delayed teeth 16:2178
dental care 4:460–461; 6:740
anesthetics 1:92–93; 8:*1092;* 10:1378
avoiding plaque 4:461; 12:1610
during pregnancy 12:1676
fluoride 4:461; 5:651–652; 12:1636; 16:2176
gums and gum diseases 4:461, 462; 6:*730–731*
heart murmurs and 9:1287
orthodontics 10:*1425–1429;* 16:2175, *2177*
while wearing orthodontic appliances 10:1425, 1426
dentures 4:*462–463;* 8:1149
dietary sugar and 15:2120, 2121
impacted teeth 7:*915–917;* 14:*2012;* 16:2175
incisors 16:2175, *2176,* 2178
loss 6:730, 731
molars 16:*2176, 2178*
mottling 5:*651–652*
overlapping or crooked 6:730; 13:*1759*
pain, radiation from sinuses 15:2149
permanent teeth 16:2176
premolars 16:2175, *2176*
smoking and 4:460; 14:*1999*
stained by tetracyclines 16:2178, 2199
structure of a tooth 16:*2178*
teething 9:1262; 16:2176, 2177
transplants 10:1426
wired together 10:*1384*
wisdom 16:2177–2178
impacted 7:*915,* 916; 16:2175, 2177
infection and 15:*2148*
quinsy and 14:2012
X rays 17:*2434*
see also gums and gum diseases
telomeres 1:55
temperature 16:**2181–2184**
basal metabolic rate and 17:2401
changes in a day 2:*188*
core 16:2181
exercise and 16:2181
fertility and 7:945
fevers 5:*640–641;* 6:759; 9:1214; 11:1545; 15:2150
shivering with 14:1940, 1942
treatment 5:641; 9:1177; 15:2150
heat loss and 6:762; 16:2183
normal 5:640; 6:795; 14:1940–1941; 16:2181
regulation 3:319; 6:847; 7:897, *898;* 14:1940–1942; 15:2130; 16:*2182–2183*

biofeedback and 2:*183*
goose pimples 6:735; 14:1942
perspiration (sweat) 11:1543–*1545;* 15:2130–2131; 16:2183
shivering 14:1940, *1941,* 1942; 16:2183
the rhythm method and 13:1828–1829, *1830*
skin surface, and thermal imaging 16:2207, *2208*
taking 16:2181, 2183–2184
tendons 8:1069; 9:1265; 16:**2185–2186**
Achilles 5:626; 10:1433
cut through 16:2185
dislocated 16:2185
grafting 5:711
ruptured 10:1433
severed 1:20; 16:2185, 2186
sports injuries 15:2054
tenosynovitis 5:629; 8:1105; 16:2185, 2186; 17:2430
testes (testicles) 5:689; 16:**2191–2194;** 17:2347
cysts 4:447; 16:2191, 2193–2194
hydrocele 16:*2192,* 2193–2194
descended 5:689
enlargement 16:2192
infection and inflammation
epididymitis 16:2193
orchitis 9:1284; 16:2193
infertility and 16:2194
one removed 16:2191
prosthetic 12:1700
removal 16:2192, *2193*
temperature 16:2035
torsion or twisting 16:2191, 2192, 2193
tumors 16:2192, 2194
undescended 16:2192, 2195
varicocele 7:943–944; 16:2194
vasectomy and 16:2191
testosterone 1:48; 8:1062; 16:**2191–2192, 2195–2196**
deficiency 16:2196
excess
in men 16:2196
in women 16:2196
puberty and 13:1742; 16:2195–2196
sebaceous gland activity and 14:1901; 16:2196
transdermal patches 16:2260
tetraiodothyronine *see* thyroxine
thalamus 2:263
epilepsy and 5:*583*
pain and 11:1475
the sense of taste and 16:2171
the sense of touch and 16:2241, 2242
thirst 16:**2209–2210**
symptom of diabetes 15:2152; 16:2209, 2210
throat 14:*2011;* 16:**2211–2213**
cancer 3:316
diphtheria and 4:497
infections, causing ear pain 16:2212
obstruction 11:*1557;* 16:2211, 2213
sore throat 11:1555, 1557; **14:2010–2013**
laryngitis 7:946; 8:1036, 1037–*1039;* 10:1335; 14:2011, *2013;* 16:2212; 17:2389
strep 11:1555, *1556,* 1557; 15:2097; 16:*2212*
wartlike growths 17:2395
see also pharynx
thromboplastin 16:2214
thumb
double 3:*401*
great mobility 7:1002

thumb *(cont'd)*
  sucking 8:1081
thymus 5:700; 8:1113; 9:1187;
  16:2221–2222
  tumors 16:2222
thyroid 10:1334–1335; **16:2223–2226**
  cancer 5:704; 6:832; 13:1774; 15:2096;
    16:2225
    thermography and 16:2208
  effect of the pituitary on 4:567;
    6:847; 12:1599; 16:2224
  goiter 5:704; 10:1334; 16:2224, 2225,
    2226
  growth and 4:532
  metabolic rate and 16:2182; 17:2401
  overactive (thyrotoxicosis;
    hyperthyroidism) 5:704; 6:857;
    10:1332; 11:1450, 1503; 15:2150;
    16:2223–2224, 2226
    Graves' disease 16:2225–2226
    heat production and 16:2182
    treatment 13:1774; 15:2150;
      16:2223, 2224
    tremor and 16:2275
  radionuclide scans 4:477, 480
  removal 10:1332, 1421, 1422; 16:2225
  shivering and 14:1941
  thyroiditis 5:704; 16:2224, 2226
  tumors 4:567
  underactive (hypothyroidism;
    myxedema) 3:323; 5:699, 704;
    8:1055; 9:1214; 16:2223–2224,
    2226
    coma and 3:395
    congenital (cretinism) 16:2226
    growth and 4:532
    hair and 16:2224
    Hashimoto's disease and 5:704
    heat production and 16:2182
thyroid hormone *see* thyroxine
thyroid-stimulating hormone (TSH)
  4:567; 6:847; 7:899; 12:1599
  16:2224
thyroxine (thyroid hormone; T4;
  tetraiodothyronine) 2:225, 226;
  4:566, 567; 6:847; 16:2224, 2250
  deficiency 4:532; 6:858; 10:1383
    causing postpartum depression
      12:1649
    goiter and 5:704
    too much 6:858
tiredness 15:2150; 16:2229–2231
  chronic fatigue syndrome 3:369;
    10:1353
  old age and 5:620; 16:2229
tissue fluid 3:319
tissues 2:254
tocopherols 17:2382, 2384
toenails *see* nails
toes
  "ballet dancer's toe" 1:122
  fractured 5:627
  gangrenous 5:669
  gout 5:707
  reattached 9:1219
  stiffness 15:2079
tongue **16:2232–2234**
  cancer 16:2234
  coating of fur on 16:2234
  inflammation due to food allergy
    7:947
  injuries to 16:2234
  piercing 2:250, 251
  sense of taste 16:2169, 2232–2233
  strawberry tongue 14:1879
  structure 16:2169, 2170, 2232, 2233
  swallowing the 15:2118; 16:2232
  ulcers 16:2234; 17:2311

tonsils 2:281; 11:1557; 16:2212, **2235–2237**
  enlarged 16:2236
  peritonsillar abscess (quinsy)
    14:2012–2013; 16:2236–2237
  removal (tonsillectomy) 8:1113;
    14:2012–2013; 16:2235, 2236, 2237
  tonsillitis 2:281, 282; 8:1112; 14:2010,
    2011–2012; 16:2212, 2235,
    2236–2237
  swollen lymph nodes and 8:1109
  tumors 16:2237
  viral infections 16:2237
touch **16:2239–2242**
  the brain and 2:264
trachea (windpipe) 10:1333
TRH (TSH-releasing hormone) 16:2224
triglycerides 5:621
triiodothyronine (T3) 16:2225
trochlea 4:546
trypsin 4:494, 495; 11:1487
trypsinogen 11:1487
TSH *see* thyroid-stimulating hormone
twins 9:1274, 1276
  birth 2:204, 284
  can feel each other's pain 11:1476
  detected during pregnancy 12:1676
  identical 3:330, 400; 9:1274, 1275;
    11:1539, 1540; 12:1604
  nonidentical (fraternal) 3:400;
    9:1274, 1275, 1277; 11:1540; 12:1604
    conception 13:1828
  the placenta and 12:1604, 1605
  tendency inherited 6:816
  see also multiple births
tyrosine 11:1558–1559

ulna 4:546, 547
umbilical cord 2:203, 205
  accidents 15:2094
  blood 5:676, 677
  prolapse 12:1687–1688
ureters 2:216; 17:2324
urethra 2:216–217; 5:690; 8:1017;
  11:1530; **17:2323**
  . birth defects 2:207
  ejaculation and 14:1907
  narrowing or obstruction 2:217, 218
  urethral syndrome 4:449
uric acid, and gout 5:707, 708; 10:1306
urinary tract and disorders
  17:2324–2325
  disorders
    birth defects 2:207; 17:2325
    cancer 17:2325
    cystitis 4:449
    infections 7:925; 8:1018; 17:2324,
      2325
  urinary tract 2:216–217, 252; 7:926
  see also bladder and bladder
    problems; kidneys and kidney
    diseases
urination
  acute retention 12:1692
  bed-wetting 2:217–218; 7:925, 926
  during cold weather 11:1543
  during the night 5:598; 12:1691
  during pregnancy 12:1662
  incontinence 2:218; 5:693;
    7:925–926
    spinal cord damage and 15:2040
    stress 7:925; 12:1687
  prostate problems and 12:1690,
    1691, 1692
  reflex 13:1791
urine 5:597
  bacteria in 8:1018
  blood in 6:803
  color 2:216, 217; 5:598

biliary colic and 5:668
  jaundice and 5:596; 7:992
  kidney failure and 8:1020
  protein in (proteinuria) 2:239;
    12:1659
  tests 4:475; 5:596; 8:1029; 12:1676;
    15:2024, 2025, 2026
    for ketones 7:1006
    in pregnancy 15:2024
    for protein 8:1018, 1020
uterus (womb) **17:2326–2329**
  conception and 3:399, 400
  dilatation and curettage (D & C)
    4:496; 5:642; 9:1202; 17:2329
  lining (endometrium) 4:568; 9:1203
  position 17:2326–2328
  pregnancy and 17:2326, 2328
  problems 17:2327
    abnormal bleeding from 17:2327
    abnormal location of lining
      6:733; 17:2327
    absence 17:2327
    cancer 3:316; 7:905; 9:1204;
      14:1934; 17:2327, 2329
    congenital malformation 17:2327,
      2328–2329
    endometrial hyperplasia 17:2327
    endometritis 17:2327
    fibroids 5:642; 6:733; 17:2327
    polyps 5:642; 12:1642, 1643;
      17:2327, 2329
    pregnancy outside the uterus
      4:541
    prolapse 2:161; 6:733; 7:904, 905;
      12:1686–1687, 1688; 17:2327, 2335
  trophoblastic disease 17:2327
  see also cervix and cervical smears
uvula 9:1260; 11:1483
  cleft 11:1485

vagina 5:690; **17:2333–2335**
  absent 17:2355
  Bartholin glands 5:690; 9:1269
    abscess 6:733; 17:2335
    blocked 17:2333, 2335
  carcinoma 17:2335
  discharge 6:733; 17:2333, 2334, 2335,
    2336–2339
    bloodstained 3:338; 5:642; 17:2339
    during pregnancy 12:1662
    Pap tests and 11:1489
    of STDs 14:1933–1934
    thrush (*Candida*; candidiasis)
      6:733; 16:2220; 17:2334, 2336
    trichomoniasis 14:1934; 16:2278,
      2279; 17:2336, 2337–2338
  douching 5:689
  fistula connecting to the rectum
    5:644
  lacerations 8:1031; 17:2333
  menopause and 5:593; 6:856;
    9:1198, 1199; 17:2334
  prolapse into 2:161; 6:733; 7:904,
    905; 12:1686–1687, 1688; 17:2327,
    2335
    by intestines 12:1686
  unexplained bleeding from 3:338;
    4:496; 5:642; 6:727; 9:1202
  vaginal wall prolapse 17:2335
  vaginismus 7:919, 965;
    14:1924–1925; 17:2334
  vaginitis 17:2336
    atrophic 4:496; 9:1202; 17:2334,
      2335
    of trichomoniasis 16:2278, 2279;
      17:2336
  yeast infection 7:937; 17:2436,
    2437–2438

valves 6:782; **17:2341–2342**
  aortic 17:2341, 2342
  congenital abnormalities 17:2342
  grafting 5:711
  heart murmurs and 9:1287–1289
  heart valve disease 2:215; 6:788,
    789; 9:1287–1289; 16:2215;
    17:2341–2342
  mitral 17:2341, 2342
    prolapsing 17:2341, 2342
  pulmonary 17:2341, 2342
  replacement 6:788; 10:1401,
    1402–1403; 12:1698, 1699–1700;
    17:2341
  rheumatic fever and 13:1817;
    15:2067; 16:2215, 2216
  "Ross Switch" 15:2136
  tricuspid 17:2341
vasa deferentia 3:400; 5:689; 11:1530;
  14:1906, 1907; 16:2191; 17:2347
veins 1:119; 3:373; **17:2357–2358**
  bleeding from 6:803
  blood clots 15:2146–2147; 16:2218;
    17:2357, 2358
  grafts 5:711
  hepatic 17:2358
  intravenous infusions 7:970
  intravenous injections 7:955–956
  portal 16:2292
  thread veins or spider veins 3:424;
    4:553
  valves 17:2357, 2358
  varicose 16:2216, 2218; **17:2343–2346**
    during pregnancy 5:637; 12:1662,
      1675–1676; 17:2344
    edema and 4:544
    hemorrhoids and 6:807
    obesity and 17:2344–2345
    the Pill and 10:1414
    in the scrotum (varicocele)
      7:943–944; 16:2194
    swollen ankles and 15:2146–2147
    thrombophlebitis and 16:2218
    thrombosis and 16:2216
    treatment 17:2343, 2345–2346
    ulcers and 17:2312, 2343
    varicose eczema 7:987; 17:2345
    venular flares and 17:2344
venules 17:2357
vertebrae 2:159
  cervical 6:761; 10:1332, 1335
  lumbar 14:1982
    strain on 14:1984
  osteopathic manipulation and
    11:1448, 1449
  osteoporosis 11:1451
villi 4:495; 9:1189
vision 2:220; 10:1411, 1412–1413
  double 4:505
  navigational 13:1811
  night 10:1362
  testing 10:1413
  tunnel 2:219; 13:1812
  see also eyes and eyesight
visual purple (rhodopsin) 10:1362;
  13:1812; 17:2373
vitreous humor 5:606
vocal cords 8:1036; 10:1333–1334;
  16:2212; 17:2389
  artificial 17:2389
  hoarseness and 6:832; 8:1039
  nodes or polyps on 6:832; 8:1037,
    1039; 17:2389
  see also larynx and laryngitis
voice 8:1037
  loss 10:1308
    through shock 10:1334
  puberty and 17:2389

voice box *see* larynx
von Willebrand factor (vWF) **17**:2392
vulva **5**:690; **17**:2393–2394
  problems **6**:733
    cancer **17**:2393
    inflammation **17**:2393, 2394
    pruritis vulvae **17**:2393
    warts **17**:2393

walking, and the feet **5**:625–*626*
wax *see* earwax
weight **17**:2398–2401
  charts **10**:*1383*
  chubbiness in adolescents **13**:1739
  gain
    during the menstrual cycle **1**:112
    stretch marks and **15**:*2105*, 2106
  loss **17**:2398, 2403
    cancer and **6**:727
    eating disorders and **1**:*94*–95, 96
    exercise and **1**:49; **5**:600
    flotation therapy and **5**:649
    in health spas **6**:774
    liposuction not recommended
      for **8**:1079
    as a symptom of a disorder
      17:2399–2400
    visualization techniques **9**:1232
  metabolic rate and **9**:1214; **17**:2401
  overweight
    children **10**:1383
    cholesterol and **3**:366
    the circulation and **3**:372
    the hips and **6**:828
    runs in families **6**:816; **10**:1383
    snoring and **14**:2005
  the Pill and **10**:1416; **17**:2398–2399
  unexplained loss of **15**:2152
windpipe (trachea) **10**:1333
womb *see* uterus
wrist **17**:2429–2430
  carpal tunnel syndrome **1**:124;
    3:*322*–323; **6**:747; **10**:1344, 1396;
    13:*1804*
  dislocation **17**:2430
  fractures **3**:323; **5**:660; **17**:2429–2430
  rheumatoid arthritis **13**:*1823*, *1824*
  stiffness **15**:2078
  tenosynovitis **5**:629; **17**:2430
  weak **17**:2429

DISEASES AND OTHER DISORDERS

abrasions and cuts **1**:17–20; **17**:*2422*,
  2423
  healing **6**:*765*
  treatment **1**:18, 20; **17**:2424
  see also lacerations
abruption, placental **15**:2081
abscess **1**:21; **5**:641; **13**:1758
  heat treatment **6**:797, 799; **13**:1757
  meibomian **15**:2113
  parapharyngeal **16**:2237
  peritonsillar (quinsy) **14**:2012–2013;
    16:2236–2237
  releasing the pus **13**:1757, 1758
    drainage **5**:644
  tooth **1**:21; **13**:1758
Acanthamoeba polyphaga **12**:1704
achondroplasia **4**:532; **7**:922; **10**:*1306*
acidosis
  metabolic **1**:26–27
  respiratory **1**:27
acne and pimples **1**:31–34; **2**:255; **7**:*885*;
  14:1974
  acne rosacea **14**:1975

menstrual cycle and **1**:32; **14**:1970
  scarring from **1**:31; **14**:1880
  treatment **1**:32–*34*, 75
acrodermatitis enteropathica **16**:2250
acromegaly **5**:697, 698; **12**:1601
actinomycosis, pulmonary **13**:*1749*
acute abdomen **15**:2152
ADD (attention deficit disorder) **2**:152;
  13:1738
addiction
  hospital or polysurgical *see*
    Munchausen syndrome
  psychological **14**:1905
  to drugs **11**:1554; **12**:1710; **17**:2416
    sedatives **14**:1902, 1905
    tranquilizers **16**:2256
  treatment, using flotation therapy
    5:649
  see also alcoholism
Addison's disease **1**:48; **2**:237; **6**:747;
  7:896; **9**:*1181*; **13**:1862; **15**:2150
  fatigue and **5**:619
  treatment **15**:2072
adenoids **1**:40–41; **2**:281; **10**:1372, 1375;
  11:1557; **16**:2212–2213
  adenoidectomy **1**:41; **16**:2212
  snoring and **14**:*2005*
adenomyosis **9**:1204; **17**:2327
adenosine deaminase (ADA)
  deficiency **5**:679, 680, 681
adenosis, sclerosing *see* mastitis,
  chronic
adenoviruses, used in gene therapy
  5:680
ADHD *see* attention deficit
  hyperactivity disorder
adhesions **11**:1533, 1534
  stiffness and **15**:2077
adult respiratory distress syndrome
  (ARDS; shock lung; wet lung)
  14:1943, 1946
agammaglobulinemia **7**:909
age spots **8**:1090
  see also liver spots
agoraphobia **10**:*1357*, 1358; **11**:1561, 1562,
  1563
AIDS **1**:45, 56–58; **7**:938
  after acquiring a tattoo **16**:2172, 2173
  AIDS hotline **1**:56
  an occupational hazard **10**:1395
  the blood-brain barrier and **2**:229,
    230
  incubation period **7**:928
  mouth ulcers, treatment **16**:2204
  pigeon droppings and **10**:1409
  pneumonia and **12**:1623
  prevention **1**:58; **7**:936
  statistics **14**:1935
  testing **1**:56, *58*
  thrush **16**:2219
  transmission **1**:57; **7**:936
    donated blood and **1**:56, 57;
      2:240
  treatment **1**:58
    visualization **9**:1231
  tuberculosis and **16**:2287
AIDS-related complex (ARC) **1**:57
airsickness *see* motion sickness
albinism **5**:684, 686; **6**:735; **7**:*921*, 922;
  9:1181; **10**:*1304*, *1305*
alcoholism **1**:61–64; **7**:969; **14**:1903,
  1904
  appetite and **6**:753
  cirrhosis of the liver and **3**:375
  pregnancy, fetal alcohol syndrome
    and **5**:*633*
  treatment **2**:176
    aversion therapy **2**:176, 177; **7**:969

flotation therapy **5**:649
  rehabilitation **13**:1796, 1798
  tremor and **16**:*2275*
  ulcers and **4**:531
  vision and **3**:388
  withdrawal symptoms **1**:61; **6**:742;
    17:2417, *2418*
alkalosis
  metabolic **1**:27
  respiratory **1**:26, 27
allergies **1**:70–74; **3**:396; **16**:2238
  acute colitis and **3**:383
  blood cells and **2**:227
  breast-feeding and **13**:1750
  causes of **1**:72–73
  causing anaphylactic shock **14**:1945
  causing asthma **1**:140
  causing rhinitis **13**:1826; **14**:2002
  causing swelling **15**:2145, 2147
  diagnosis **1**:72, 73–74; **14**:1913
  ear **1**:71
  eye **1**:71, 74
    conjunctivitis and **3**:403
  nose **1**:41, 71
  self-help **1**:74
  skin
    causing eczema **1**:71, 73; **4**:467,
      468, 487, 542, 543
    contact dermatitis **1**:71, 73; **4**:467,
      468; **6**:747; **14**:*1974*
    heat and **6**:795
    urticaria *see* hives
  to animals **1**:72
  to bandages **4**:513, 516
  to drugs and medicines **7**:893;
    9:1174; **14**:1959; **16**:2270
  to food **1**:71–72; **4**:485, 487, 562;
    5:657
    causing migraine **9**:1224
    fish **1**:72
    milk **1**:72
    monosodium glutamate **5**:653
    shellfish **15**:2145
    soy **5**:675
  to metal **4**:467, 468
    chrome **4**:467
    nickel **2**:251; **4**:467; **14**:1969
  to penicillin **1**:70, 99, 100; **11**:1527,
    1528, 1529; **14**:1959; **16**:2199
  to soap **7**:884
  total allergy syndrome **16**:2238
  to tattoo pigments **16**:2172, 2173
  treatment **1**:74
  vaccines **11**:*1551*
  see also hay fever; sensitization
alpha thalassemia **16**:2201
altitude sickness **2**:283; **4**:502
alveolitis, fibrosing **13**:1751, 1752
Alzheimer's disease **1**:82–83; **4**:459,
  552; **5**:693
  treatment **1**:82, 83
    development of smart drugs
      14:1989
amblyopia *see* lazy eye
amenorrhea **9**:1205; **12**:1601
amnesia **9**:1192
  post-traumatic **6**:762
  retrograde **6**:762
amoebas **11**:1510
amputation
  phantom pain and **11**:1477
  reattachment of body parts **5**:709;
    9:1218, 1219–1221; **12**:1614–1615
  severed fingers **6**:747
amyotrophic lateral sclerosis (ALS)
  9:*1256–1259*
Ancylostoma duodenale **6**:852, 853
anemia **1**:88–90; **2**:225; **9**:1205

aplastic **1**:89–90
  blood transfusions for **2**:241
  of chronic diseases **1**:89
  effects of hemorrhage with **6**:805
  Fanconi's **5**:676
  hemolytic **1**:89, 90; **15**:2045
    with hookworm infection **6**:852, 853
  iron deficiency **1**:88–89, 90; **7**:977
    detection **7**:978; **11**:1514
    during pregnancy **1**:88
    and Patterson Brown-Kelly
      syndrome **16**:2211
  leukemia and **8**:1061
  pernicious *see* pernicious anemia
  sickle-cell *see* sickle-cell anemia
  symptoms **1**:90
    blackouts **2**:215
    fatigue **5**:619, 620; **16**:2230
    in the hand **6**:747
  thalassemia **1**:88, 89, 90;
    16:2200–2201
    detection **3**:367
  vitamin B12 deficiency and **17**:2355
  vitamin deficiency **1**:88
anencephaly **2**:207; **3**:401; **10**:1350
anesthesia, "glove and stocking" **7**:907
aneurysms
  aortic **1**:121; **6**:803
  berry, in the brain **6**:804; **15**:2107
angina **1**:121; **3**:419–420; **6**:783, 790;
  15:2067; **16**:2217
  exercise and **11**:1577
  pain **3**:348, 419–420; **6**:784, 786;
    15:*2149*
  pins-and-needles and **12**:1597
  shoulder or arm pain and **14**:1948
  treatment **15**:2151
    angioplasty **3**:421
    bypass surgery **3**:421; **10**:*1403*
    drugs **2**:157, 158; **3**:420; **16**:2260
    transdermal patches **16**:2260
ankylosing spondylitis **1**:123; **2**:161, 163
  cause **1**:123, 126
  the ribs and **13**:1834
  symptoms **1**:126; **8**:1094
  treatment **1**:126
anodontia **16**:2178
anorexia and bulimia **1**:94–96
  anorexia nervosa **1**:94–96; **4**:487;
    6:846; **17**:2398
    constipation **3**:405
  bulimia **1**:94, 95, 96; **10**:1384; **17**:2391
anosmia (loss of sense of smell)
  14:1993; **16**:2169, *2170*
anthrax **1**:97
  a biological weapon **1**:97; **2**:185, 186
  vaccination **1**:97
antibiotic-resistant bacteria **1**:98, 100;
  2:164; **9**:1174; **11**:1527, 1529; **13**:1744;
  16:2199
  MRSA **1**:98; **11**:1508; **15**:2062
antifreeze poisoning **12**:1631
ant stings **2**:211
anxiety **1**:104–106; **10**:1343, *1357–1358*;
  12:*1713*; **15**:2150
  disorders **10**:*1357–1358*
  nervous breakdown and
    10:1341–1342
  reactive **10**:1357
  symptoms **1**:106; **10**:1357; **12**:1724
    cold sores **3**:382
    dry mouth **9**:1262; **13**:1852, 1854
    gastrointestinal problems
      7:980
    insomnia **7**:959
    stomachache **1**:11, 13
    tremor **16**:2275
    ulcers **4**:531

anxiety *(cont'd)*
treatment 2:*176*; 9:1178;
13:1737–1738; 14:1905; 15:2150;
16:2256
see also hypochondria; obsessive-
compulsive disorder; phobias;
stress
anxiety complex 3:398
aphasia 1:107–108; 10:1308; 15:2030
apnea
in babies 15:2117
sleep 16:2236
appendicitis 1:109–111; 11:1512
"left-sided" *see* diverticulitis
peritonitis and 1:111; 11:1532, 1534–1535
symptoms 1:110, 111; 11:1535
appendix mass 11:1535
arboviruses 17:2406, 2439
ARDS (adult respiratory distress
syndrome; shock lung; wet lung)
14:1943, 1946
Arnold-Chiari malformation 7:*879*
arrhythmias 2:215; 3:421; 11:1472
sinus 6:781
arteriosclerosis 1:119; 15:2121
arteriovenous anomaly 15:2108
arteriovenous malformation 6:804
arteritis
temporal 15:2150
treatment 15:2073
arthritis 1:**122–126**
in the back 2:163; 7:1002
dysentery and 4:533
the feet and 12:1628
fibrositis and 5:643
flitting 13:1818
fractures and 5:662
from gonorrhea 5:*705*, 706
from Lyme disease 8:1108
from rubella 1:124
from tuberculosis 1:124
help available 1:*124*, 126
reactive *see* reactive arthritis
rheumatoid *see* rheumatoid
arthritis
septic 1:124
traumatic 1:123–124
treatment 1:124–126
heat 6:797, 799
hydrotherapy 7:881, 882
meditation 9:1178
rehabilitation 13:1795, *1798*, 1799
splints 15:2049
see also gout; osteoarthritis
asbestos 12:*1639*
an occupational hazard 10:1391, 1395
asbestosis 1:136; 12:*1639*; 13:1751
ascariasis 11:1501; 17:2419
Ascaris 11:1499, *1500*, 1501; 17:*2420*
ascites 4:545; 11:1533
Asperger's syndrome 4:536
asphyxia 1:132–135
asthma 1:**139–141**; 8:1103–1104; 11:1464;
13:1751
avoidance of beta-blockers 3:419, 420
breast-feeding and 13:1750
causes 1:140, 141; 8:1103
air pollution and 1:59, 60; 15:2050
anxiety as a trigger 8:1100
eczema and 4:542
pigeon chest and 12:1590, *1592*
pneumonia and 12:1622
prevention 1:73, 141
symptoms 1:73, 140–141; 2:282; 3:348
phlegm 11:1560
wheezing 17:*2407*, 2408
treatment 1:73, 74, 141; 2:157, 158,
282; 8:1103; 17:2408

desensitization 14:1913
herbal remedies 6:814
inhalants 7:953–954
steroids 7:953, 954; 15:2072
astigmatism 1:*142*; 4:505; 5:608;
10:1413
after cataract removal 3:328
ataxia 2:149; 3:*335*, 336
veganism and 17:2355
atheroma 1:118, 119–120; 3:419, 421;
6:783; 16:2215
atherosclerosis 1:119; 2:214; 3:372, 419;
10:1382; 16:2215
cholesterol and 1:119–120; 3:366;
6:783
coronary artery 6:783–784; 10:1403
angina and 3:419–420
heart attack and 1:121
development of 1:*121*
epileptic seizures and 5:583
gangrene and 5:669
men and 1:118
obesity and 10:1385
prevention
exercise 5:600
using antioxidants 17:2387
smoking and 1:118; 6:783
strokes and 1:121; 15:2107
transient ischemic attacks and
16:2261
treatment
chelation therapy 3:345, 346
surgery 3:346
athetosis 3:335, *336*
athlete's foot 2:150; 7:886, 937; 13:1763,
1838; 14:1975
affecting nails 2:150; 13:1837, 1838
Candida as cause of 17:2436
treatment 2:150; 13:1838
atopy (atopic syndrome) 1:70; 4:542;
6:756; 14:1975
atrial fibrillation 4:551
atrophic vaginitis *see* vaginitis,
atrophic
attention deficit disorder (ADD) 2:152
attention deficit hyperactivity
disorder (ADHD) 1:86; 2:**151–152**;
4:536; 8:1051
autism 2:**153–155**; 8:1051–1052
speech difficulties and 10:1308, 1309
autoimmune diseases 8:1113
Crohn's disease as 4:442
diabetes as 4:472
Guillain-Barré syndrome 6:728
lupus 8:**1105–1107**; 11:1565
pernicious anemia as 11:1536–1537
rheumatoid arthritis 1:122; 7:1002
scleroderma 14:*1888–1889*; 15:2148
treatment, immunosuppressive
drugs 7:914; 8:1113
vitiligo 17:2388
see also glomerulonephritis;
myasthenia gravis
avascular necrosis, of the head of the
femur *see* Perthes' disease
azoospermia 1:130

baby blues 9:1247; 12:1649
see also postpartum depression
and psychosis
bacilli 2:164; 5:*670*
Bacillus anthracis 1:97
bacteria 2:**164–166**; 7:935, 936–939
antibiotic-resistant 1:98, 100; 2:164;
9:1174; 11:1527, 1529; 13:1744;
16:2199
antibiotics and 1:99–100
causing fever 5:641

infections, incubation period 7:928
intestinal, and vitamin K 17:*2385*
toxins 7:936–939, 940
"baker's cyst" 1:122
Balamuthia mandrillaris 12:1703
balanitis 10:1368; 11:1531; 17:2437
balantidiasis 12:1704
"ballet dancer's toe" 1:122
Bartholinitis 17:2394
bedbugs 2:174, 175
bedsores (decubitus ulcers) 2:175;
11:1490, 1494; 14:*2008–2009*;
17:2310, 2314
bed-wetting (enuresis) 2:**217–218**;
7:925, 926
bee stings 2:210, 211–212
Behçet's disease 17:2311–2312
belle indifférence, la 7:907
Bell's palsy 3:403; 5:610
the sense of taste and 16:2171
Bell's phenomenon 5:610
bends 2:178
benzene poisoning 10:1393
beriberi 17:2375, 2376
beta thalassemia 16:2200–2201
bilharzia *see* schistosomiasis
bilious attacks 5:596
bipolar disorder 2:**198–199**; 9:1207,
1209, 1247; 12:1713
hypochondria and 7:895
treatment 2:198, 199; 9:1209;
12:1710, 1720; 13:1738
bird fancier's lung 13:1751
birth defects 2:**206–207**; 4:574
of the brain and spine (neural tube
defects) 2:207
anencephaly 2:207; 3:401;
10:1350
hydrocephalus 2:207; 7:**878–880**;
9:1197; 10:*1350*
meningocoele 10:1351; 15:2037,
2039
myelomeningocoele 10:1351
see also spina bifida
clubfoot 2:207; 3:*379*; 12:1594
detection 2:207
amniocentesis 1:84
chorionic villus sampling 2:207;
3:**367–368**; 5:638; 7:877
ultrasound 2:207, 285; 4:477, 479,
480; 12:1664, 1676; 13:1869, 1870;
14:1893, *1894*; 15:*2143*; 17:2315,
2316–*2317*
eye 2:207
genetic *see* genetic diseases and
disorders
heart 2:206–207, 242–*243*
hip dislocation 3:402; 4:499;
6:829–830
thalidomide and 2:206; 3:402;
6:749; 9:1170; 11:1550;
16:2203–2204
of the urinary tract 2:207
see also cleft palate; congenital
disorders
birthmarks 2:**208–209**; 12:1613; 14:1972,
1974
see also moles
bites and stings 2:**210–212**; 7:887;
15:*2145*, 2147
ants 2:211
bedbug 2:174, 175
bee 2:210, 211–212
blisters and 2:223, 224
dog 2:210, 211, 236
first aid 2:210, 211; 4:556
fleas 2:211; 5:**646–647**
itching 7:*988*, 989

jellyfish and similar creatures 2:210,
211; 16:2272
lice 2:211; 8:1065
mosquito 2:210, 211; 5:646; 12:*1703*;
16:2272
rabies and 13:1766–1767
sea urchin 2:212; 16:2272
snakebites 2:212; 14:**2000–2001**;
16:2280
ticks 2:211
wasp 2:210, 212
Black Death 12:1606, 1607
black eye 2:213; 5:604; 17:2424
blackheads (comedones) 1:31, *32*; 14:1901
blackouts 2:**214–215**
in the elderly 5:691
see also fainting; unconsciousness
blackwater fever 8:1123; 12:1704
bleach, swallowed 4:562; 5:592
bleeding *see* hemorrhage
blindness and braille 2:**219–222**
blindness 10:1411
color 3:**388–389**; 5:606
glaucoma and 5:701
hallucinations and 6:742
hearing and 6:777
hysterical 7:906, 907
night 10:1362; 17:2373, 2374
the senses and 14:1990,
1993–1994; 16:2239, 2242
toxins and 10:1411
braille 2:220, 221–222; 16:*2242*
blisters 2:**223–224**
blood 13:*1756*
cold sore 3:382
from burns 3:304
from impetigo 7:*918*
over bunions 3:300
blood poisoning 2:236; 14:1914
blue baby 2:**242–243**; 6:788
boils 2:**255–256**; 13:1757
Bordella pertussis 17:2412, 2414
Borrelia vincentii 2:166
botulism 2:261; 4:485; 5:657, 659
a biological weapon 2:185, 186
brachydactyly 5:684
braille 2:220, 221–222; 16:*2242*
brain damage and disease 2:**265–268**
aphasia 1:**107–108**; 10:1308; 15:2030
ataxia and 2:149
at birth 2:267
blood clots 2:266, 271; 6:759
brain damage, causing mental
illness 9:1206, 1208, 1209
cancer 2:268, 271
coma and 3:395
concussion 2:266, 267; 6:762;
17:2318, 2321
Creutzfeldt-Jakob disease 2:231;
4:438–439; 12:1709
embolisms 1:107; 15:2107–2108
fracture of the skull 2:267; 5:663;
6:760
from head injuries 6:760
hemorrhage 1:107; 2:266–267, 271;
3:395; 4:457; 6:803; 15:2108,
2109
hydrocephalus and 7:879
subarachnoid 8:1097
herniation of the brain 15:2096
hydrocephalus 2:207; 7:**878–880**;
9:1197; 10:1350
injuries 2:266–267, 268
life support and 2:266
memory loss and 2:267
psychiatric brain disorders 12:1712
recoveries from 2:268
speech difficulties 10:1308, 1309

symptoms 2:268
tests for 2:266
thrombosis in the arteries 1:107;
   15:2107
transient ischemic attack
   16:2261–2262
tumors 2:222, 268, 271; 6:727;
   10:1347, 1356
   coma and 3:395
   dementia and 4:459
   headaches and 6:758; 15:2150
   hydrocephalus and 7:879
   see also Alzheimer's disease; brain
      death; cerebral palsy; dementia;
      encephalitis; epilepsy;
      meningitis; multiple sclerosis;
      Parkinson's disease; stroke
brain death 2:265, 269–270; 3:394;
   4:503, 504; 10:1356
   organ donation and 4:503, 504;
      16:2264
breath
   bad see halitosis
   shortness of 13:1751–1752
breathlessness 15:2151
Briquet's syndrome 10:1357
bronchiectasis 6:741; 12:1623–1624;
   13:1750, 1751
bronchitis 3:294–296, 348; 12:1623
   acute 2:282; 3:295, 296; 13:1751;
      15:2151
   chronic 2:282; 3:294, 295, 296;
      8:1103; 11:1464; 13:1751; 15:2151
   colds and 7:936
   emphysema and 4:564
   smoking and 2:279; 3:294, 426
   treatment 13:1751; 15:2151
   open windows and 2:279
   wheezing and 17:2407, 2408
bronchopneumonia 8:1104; 12:1623,
   1624–1625
Brucella spp. 3:297
brucellosis (Malta fever; undulant
   fever) 3:297
bruises (contusions) 3:298, 319;
   17:2422, 2423, 2424
   black eyes 2:213; 17:2424
   treatment 3:298; 17:2424
   see also purpura
bulimia 1:94, 95, 96; 10:1384;
   17:2391
bullae 2:223
   on the lung surface 4:564
bull neck 4:497
bunions 3:299–300; 12:1627
   corns over 3:417, 418
Burkitt's lymphoma 5:588; 7:935
burns 2:224; 3:303–305
   chemical 7:981; 10:1393
   severity 3:301, 303–304
   shock and 3:304, 305; 6:806;
      13:1867, 1868; 14:1943, 1944
   treatment
      first aid 3:304; 4:556; 10:1393
      hospital 3:304–305; 12:1614
      physical therapy 11:1581
      skin grafts 3:302, 304
      vitamin C and 17:2379
   see also scalding; sunburn
bursas, prepatellar 3:307
bursitis 3:307–309; 9:1189
   of the elbow 3:307; 4:547; 6:799
   of the knees 3:307, 309; 7:1002;
      8:1025, 1027
   semimembranous 3:307

cadmium poisoning 10:1392, 1395
café-au-lait patches 2:209

calculus (tartar) 12:1609; 13:1761
calluses 3:417, 418; 12:1627; 17:2362
camptodactyly 6:818
cancer 3:312–317; 16:2291
   bladder 3:316; 13:1776; 17:2325
   bone 2:161, 163, 260; 14:1966
      pain relief 8:1093; 12:1692
      in ribs 13:1834
      thermography and 16:2208
   bowel 3:316
   brain 2:268
   breast 2:277; 3:316; 8:1098, 1130;
      9:1187
      deaths from 10:1399
      family history of 8:1124
      histopathology 11:1512–1513
      hormone replacement therapy
         and 6:856; 7:875
      mastitis and 4:446
      risk of 8:1129–1130
      screening for 8:1129–1132
      self-checking for 12:1680
      staging 8:1098–1099, 1132
      thermography and 16:2208
      treatment 2:176; 3:315;
         8:1098–1099, 1145–1148;
         9:1145–1148, 1172
   causes 3:313–314
      mutations 10:1304
   cervical 3:316, 337, 338–339; 4:574;
      6:733; 11:1488, 1489; 17:2327, 2368
      circumcised men and 3:374
      genital herpes and 6:825; 14:1933
   colon 3:386, 387; 4:442; 5:624;
      15:2022
      Crohn's disease and 4:442
   colorectal 3:386
   cure 13:1776
   deaths from 8:1125; 10:1399; 14:1998
   diagnosis 3:315; 11:1514
   during pregnancy 13:1774
   elephantiasis and 4:554
   encephalitis and 4:565
   endometrial 6:855; 17:2339
   Epstein-Barr virus and 5:587, 588
   esophageal 3:316; 5:591
   fallopian tubes, treatment 7:905
   gout and 5:707
   head and neck 3:333
   hereditary 3:314
   jaw 14:1998
   kidney 17:2325
      hormone production 11:1504
      treatment 13:1772, 1776
   laryngeal 3:316; 6:832; 8:1036, 1037,
      1038, 1039; 10:1335; 16:2212, 2213
   liver 6:811; 8:1087; 10:1399
   lung 2:282; 3:294, 314; 6:727, 832;
      8:1103, 1104, 1125; 13:1751
      asbestos-related 1:136
      in cities 12:1639
      deaths from 10:1399
      exposure to radon and 13:1839
      hormone production 11:1504
      smoking and 2:279, 283; 3:314;
         8:1067, 1104; 13:1749; 14:1996,
         1997–1998, 1999
      symptoms 3:316; 13:1751
      treatment 2:282; 13:1751, 1776
   lymph node involvement 8:1111, 1130
   malignant cysts 4:446, 447
   mouth 3:316
   nasopharyngeal 5:587, 588
   oncology 10:1399–1400
   outlook 3:317
   ovarian 11:1459
      laparoscopy and 8:1034
      treatment 7:905

pain, treatment 6:861
   pancreatic 5:624; 7:992; 11:1487
   penis 11:1530; 17:2325
   pharyngeal 16:2213
   physical therapy and 11:1581
   pleural effusion and 12:1619
   prostate 3:316; 5:690; 9:1187; 12:1691,
      1694
      treatment and outlook
         12:1694–1695; 13:1776
   protection against 8:1110; 10:1400
      garlic 6:814
   purpura and 13:1755
   rates 10:1399
   rectal 13:1787, 1788
      in the ribs 13:1834
   screening 3:314–315; 14:1892
   skin 2:192, 208; 3:316; 4:573, 574;
      6:726; 8:1125, 1126; 9:1182–1185;
      11:1468, 1470; 13:1776; 14:1975;
      15:2024, 2127–2128
   spread 3:313; 8:1126, 1130; 10:1400;
      16:2291–2292
   stomach 6:741; 15:2090; 16:2292
   stress and 3:314
   throat 3:316
   thyroid
      5:704; 6:832; 13:1774; 15:2096;
      16:2225
      thermography and 16:2208
   tiredness and 16:2231
   tongue 16:2234
   treatment 8:1126; 10:1400;
      13:1774–1775, 1776
      blocking hormone action 3:317
      bone marrow transplants 3:317
      chemotherapy 3:312, 314, 316–317,
         317; 8:1145; 9:1145; 10:1400;
         13:1775
      drug trials and 9:1172
      gene therapy 10:1400
      immunotherapy 10:1400
      integrative oncology 10:1399
      radioactive implants 3:316;
         10:1400; 12:1693; 13:1774
      radiotherapy 13:1772–1776
      side effects 3:317
      surgery 3:315; 13:1775
   urinary tract 17:2325
   uterine 3:316; 7:905; 9:1204; 14:1934;
      17:2327, 2329
   vulva 17:2393
   see also leukemia; lymphoma;
      malignancy
Candida see thrush
candidiasis see thrush
carbon monoxide poisoning 1:59;
   3:395; 12:1630, 1637–1638; 17:2320
carbuncles 2:255, 256
carcinoma 3:312; 16:2291
   basal cell 8:1124
   nasopharyngeal 5:588
   squamous cell 16:2237
carcinoma-in-situ 3:339
cardiac arrest
   cardiac massage and 1:134, 135;
      3:320–321
   hospital crash teams and 13:1810
   signs of 3:320
cardiomyopathy
   congestive 6:789
   dilated 16:2231
   hypertrophic 6:789
carpal tunnel syndrome 1:124;
   3:322–323; 6:747; 10:1344, 1396;
   13:1804
   treatment 3:323; 13:1846
carsickness see motion sickness

cataracts 2:219, 220, 222; 3:326–328;
   5:609; 11:1470, 1471
   congenital 2:207, 219; 3:326
   treatment 3:326, 327–328; 5:609;
      10:1408; 13:1811
catatonia 14:1882
cauda equina 8:1076
celiac disease 1:71–72; 3:329; 4:485
cellulitis 2:236
cerebral atrophy 1:83
cerebral palsy 2:267; 3:335–336; 15:2022
   ataxia 2:149
   physical therapy for 11:1578
   speech difficulties and 10:1308
cervical intraepithelial neoplasia (CIN)
   3:339
cervical spondylosis 2:214; 10:1437
cervicitis 3:337
Chagas' disease 12:1704
cheilosis 9:1263
chemical pathogens 11:1510
Chernobyl disaster 4:574; 6:821; 8:1110
chicken pox 3:349–350; 6:825; 7:927,
   938; 13:1814
   in adults 7:935
   rash (blisters) 2:223, 224; 3:349;
      13:1782, 1783
   Reye's syndrome and 13:1814
   scars 2:223, 224; 3:349; 13:1782, 1783
   shingles and 3:349, 350; 6:825;
      14:1938
   vaccination 3:350; 7:912
chilblains 6:746; 7:988, 989; 12:1596;
   14:1973
chlamydia 1:22; 2:161; 11:1520, 1531
   causing STDs 14:1931–1933, 1935;
      16:2192
   vaginal discharge and 17:2338
   Chlamydia psittaci 12:1705
   reactive arthritis and 13:1786
chloasma 8:1090, 1091; 11:1564
chloracne 1:32
choking 1:132, 135; 16:2212, 2252
cholecystitis 5:668; 15:2152
cholera 3:365; 4:485, 573; 5:624;
   16:2285; 17:2320–2321
   vaccination 3:365; 16:2272, 2282,
      2285
chromium, dangers of working with
   10:1392–1393, 1395
chronic fatigue syndrome (CFS) 3:369;
   5:619; 10:1311, 1353
chronic obstructive pulmonary
   disease (COPD) 3:370–371
   oxygen therapy for 11:1465, 1467
   see also emphysema
circulation, poor
   biofeedback and 2:183
   cramps and 4:437
   gangrene and 5:669
   massage to treat 8:1142; 9:1142
   numbness and 10:1378
   pins-and-needles and 12:1596, 1597
circumoral pallor 14:1878
cirrhosis 2:228; 3:375; 6:727; 7:968, 991;
   8:1087
   hemochromatosis and 6:800; 7:978
CJD see Creutzfeldt-Jakob disease
clang associations 12:1722
claudication 8:1075–1076
   intermittent 8:1075; 11:1577
   treatment 8:1078
   venous 8:1075
claustrophobia 11:1562–1563
cleft palate 2:207; 3:376, 401; 11:1483,
   1484, 1485; 12:1612–1613
   speech and 15:2030
clostridia, and gas gangrene 5:669

Clostridium spp.
  C. botulinum 2:261; 5:659
  C. tetani 2:166; 8:1030; 16:2197
clubfoot 2:207; 3:379; 12:1594
clumsiness, in children 3:414
cold, the common *see* common cold
cold sores 2:223; 3:382; 6:825; 9:1263;
  14:2008
  eczema and 3:382; 4:543
  sunlight and 14:1970
colic 3:356; 4:444, 445; 5:702
  biliary 5:668
color blindness 3:388–389; 5:606
coma 3:394–395; 5:611; 17:2321
  diabetic 1:26; 3:395; 4:473; 7:1006;
  17:2321
  hypoglycemic 4:473
  resembling death 2:270
comedones *see* blackheads
common cold 3:396; 7:938; 9:1170;
  10:1374
  antibiotics ineffective against 1:99
  deafness with 4:453
  leading to pneumonia 12:1624
  symptoms 2:282
    runny nose or nasal congestion
    10:1371; 13:1825, *1826*
    treatment 2:157, 282; 10:1374
    herbal remedies 6:812
  vaccination useless against 7:936
  vitamin A deficiency and 17:2373
compulsions 10:1387
concussion 2:266, 267; 6:762; 17:2318,
  2321
conduct disorder 2:152
confabulation 12:1722
congenital disorders 3:401–402
  bone 2:259
  cleft palate 2:207; 3:376, 401;
    11:1483, 1484, *1485*; 12:1612–1613
  clubfoot 2:207; 3:379; 12:1594
  congenital cataracts 2:207, 219;
    3:326
  congenital cysts 4:446
  congenital deafness 4:455
  genetic *see* genetic diseases and
    disorders
  Gilbert's syndrome 7:989
  heart defects and blue babies
    2:242–*243*; 3:401, 402; 6:788
  hip dislocation 3:402; 4:499;
    6:829–830; 10:1434; 15:2048;
    16:*2254*
  hydrocephalus 7:879
  of the kidney 17:2325
  pyloric stenosis 15:2067
  tests for 3:401; 11:1518
  tracheoesophageal fistula 5:644
  of the uterus 17:2327, 2328–2329
    in vitro fertilization and 7:971
  see also birth defects; Down
    syndrome; spina bifida
conjunctivitis 3:403; 5:*588*, 607
constipation 3:385, 404–405; 5:596,
  619, 624
  in babies 1:69
  before menstruating 9:1201
  causing anal fissures 1:102
  in children 1:69
  during pregnancy 3:404; 8:1045;
    12:1662, 1675
  flatulence and 5:645
  hemorrhoids and 6:807
  spurious diarrhea and 7:925
  treatment 3:405; 15:2152
    enemas 4:572
    laxatives 3:404, 405; 8:1045–1046
    suppositories 15:*2132*, 2133

contagious diseases 7:935
contusions *see* bruises
conversion disorder 7:906–907
convulsions 3:413
  febrile 3:413; 5:583, 585, 641
  see also epilepsy, seizures
copper bracelets 13:1819
coprolalia 16:2244
copropraxia 16:2244
corns 3:417–418; 12:1627
  differ from verrucas 17:2362
coronary arteries and thrombosis
  1:118; 3:419–421; 6:783–784
  coronary artery surgery 3:420–421;
    10:1403
  coronary disease 6:789
    prevention 3:421
    risk factors 3:421
  coronary thrombosis 3:419–420;
    6:783–784; 16:2215–2216, 2217
  see also angina; atherosclerosis;
    heart attack; thrombosis
coronaviruses 3:396
  SARS and 13:1863, 1864
Corynebacterium diphtheriae 4:497;
  14:*2013*
coughing 3:348, 426; 13:1751
  blood (hemoptysis) 3:371, 426;
    11:1560
  causing purpura 13:1755
  croup 3:426
  food "going down the wrong way"
    5:592; 8:1036
  needing medical attention 3:348,
    426
  phlegm 11:*1560*
  smoker's cough 3:371, 426; 5:603;
    8:1036
  treatment 3:426; 9:1177
    cough syrup 3:426, 427
    expectorants 3:426; 5:603
  whooping cough 3:426;
    17:2412–2413
cowpox, and smallpox vaccination
  7:911; 14:*1986*, 1988; 17:2331
Coxiella burnetti 13:1762
crabs (pubic lice) 8:1066
cradle cap 14:1972–1973
cramp 4:437; 5:599
  anaerobic exercise and 1:50
  during pregnancy 4:437; 12:1662
  heat cramp (stoker's cramp; miner's
    cramp) 6:796; 11:1544
  night cramps 4:437; 13:1764, 1861
  treatment 4:437; 13:1861
    quinine 13:1764, 1765
  see also stitch
crepitus 10:1437
cretinism 16:2226
Creutzfeldt-Jakob disease (CJD) 2:231;
  4:438–439; 12:1709
Crohn's disease 4:442–443
  fistulas and 5:644
cross-eye 10:1407; 10:1407
croup (laryngotracheobronchitis)
  2:282; 3:426; 8:1037, 1038, 1039;
  17:2414
Cryptococcus infection 10:1409
cryptosporidiosis 12:1704
Cushing's syndrome 1:46; 12:1601;
  15:2152
cuts *see* abrasions and cuts;
  lacerations
cyanide poisoning 12:1631
cyanosis 2:242; 3:295, 371;
  11:1464
  emphysema and 4:564
cyclothymia 10:1358

cyst 4:446–447
  bone 4:447
  breast 2:277; 4:446, 447; 9:1159
  congenital 4:446
  Dandy-Walker 7:879
  eruption 16:2178
  eyelid (meibomian cyst) 4:447;
    15:2112
  joint 4:447
  liver (hydatid) 4:446, 447
  ovarian 4:446, 447, *568*, 569; 6:733;
    11:1459; 16:2195
  polycystic kidney disease 2:207;
    4:447; 8:*1018*; 17:2325
  polycystic ovary syndrome 1:32
  skin
    dermoid 4:*446–447*
    sebaceous 4:446, 447; 6:726;
      14:*1900*; 15:*2147*, *2148*
  testicular 4:447; 16:2191, 2193–2194
cysticercosis 11:1498
cystic fibrosis 2:192; 4:448; 5:678, 684;
  11:1487
  detection 3:367
  pigeon chest and 12:1592
  treatment 4:448; 11:1581
    gene therapy 5:680
cystitis 2:217, 218; 3:409; 4:449–450;
  7:886; 17:2324
  treatment 4:450; 6:857
cystocele (bladder prolapse) 7:925;
  12:1686, *1687*
cytomegalovirus 5:587

dandruff 4:451–452
  sties and 15:2112
  see also dermatitis, seborrheic
Dandy-Walker cysts 7:879
deafness 4:453–456; 5:692; 10:1307
  causes 4:455–456
    earwax 4:453, 537; 15:2156–2157
    loud noises 4:453, 455, 456; 6:777;
      10:1363, 1365–1366
    measles 6:777
    Ménière's disease 2:168; 4:455;
      9:1194
    otosclerosis 4:453, 456; 12:1696,
      1700
  mutism and 10:1307–1308
  as plane takes off 4:454
  treatments 4:455, 456
    cochlear implants 2:191; 6:780
    hearing aids 6:779–780; 9:1194
    prosthetic earbones 12:1696,
      1699, 1700
death 4:457–458
  biological clocks and 2:187
  brain death 2:265, 269–270; 3:394;
    4:503, 504; 10:1356
    organ donation and 4:503, 504;
      16:2264
  causes 4:457; 10:1399; 12:1682
    cancer 8:*1125*; 10:1399; 14:*1998*,
      1999
    drowning 4:521
  mind still functions after 9:1226
  out-of-body experiences 9:1229
decompression sickness (the bends)
  2:178
deep vein thrombosis *see* thrombosis,
  deep vein
dehydration 13:1862
delirium tremens (the "DTs") 1:61
delusions 12:1719, 1720–1721
dementia 2:267; 4:459; 5:692, 693;
  10:1347; 12:1719
  alcohol and 7:897
  hydrocephalus and 7:880

  see also Alzheimer's disease;
    Creutzfeldt-Jakob disease
demyelination 9:1280–1281
dengue fever 16:2282
depression 4:464–466; 9:1208, 1209,
  1247; 12:1713
  in adolescence 1:44, 45
  dysthymia 10:1353
  in the elderly 14:1911
  fatigue and 5:618, 619; 8:1056
  hair loss following 6:735
  manic *see* bipolar disorder
  postpartum *see* postpartum
    depression and psychosis
  sleeplessness and 7:957, 958;
    8:1056–1057
  suicide and 15:*2123*, 2124
  treatment 4:466; 12:1712
    drugs 4:464, 466; 12:1710;
      13:1737–1738
    electroconvulsive therapy 4:466;
      9:1209; 10:1354
    occupational therapy 10:1397
    psychotherapy 13:1735
    unpleasant taste sensations and
      16:2171
  see also seasonal affective disorder
dermatitis 4:467–468; 7:946; 13:1782;
  14:1974
  ammoniacal 4:481, 482
  atopic *see* eczema
  contact 1:71, 73; 4:467, 468; 6:747;
    14:*1974*
  industrial 14:1974
  perioral 7:948
  rubber 14:*2009*
  seborrheic 1:32; 4:468, 482, 483;
    7:988, 989; 13:*1783*
    sties and 15:2112, 2113
    see also dandruff
  solar (photodermatitis) 4:468
dhobie itch 13:1838
diabetes 3:323; 4:471–473; 5:703; 9:1215;
  11:1487; 15:2121
  acidosis 1:27
  boils 2:255, 256
  breath smells 6:740, 741; 7:1006
  diabetes insipidus 4:471;
    8:1018–1020; 16:2210
  diabetes mellitus 4:471
  diabetic coma 1:26, 27; 3:395; 4:473;
    7:1006
  dietary sugar restricted 15:2120
  drowsiness and 4:523
  during pregnancy 7:960
  excessive urine secretion 16:2209
  eye changes 2:219; 3:327; 4:472;
    5:609
    treatment 8:1040, 1041
  fatigue and 5:619
  foot problems 3:418; 5:669
  gum diseases and 6:731; 13:*1760*
  hypoglycemia 4:471; 7:896, 960
  itches 7:987
  juvenile 4:472
  kidney damage and 8:1017
  noninsulin-dependent (maturity-
    onset diabetes; type II diabetes)
    4:472; 10:1367–1368
  pregnancy and 15:2082
  thirst and 15:2152; 16:2209, 2210
  thrush (Candida) and 10:1368;
    16:2219, 2220; 17:2437
  treatment
    herbalism 6:813
    insulin 4:472–473; 7:960
    pancreas transplants 16:2264
    weight and 10:1384

neurasthenia 10:1352–1353
  see also chronic fatigue syndrome
neuritis 10:1377
  optic 2:222
neurofibrillary tangle 1:83
neurofibromatosis (Von
    Recklinghausen's disease) 6:727;
    14:1891
neuroma, acoustic 16:2228
neuronitis, vestibular 10:1347
neuropathy 10:1347
  peripheral 8:1049
  X-linked bulbospinal 9:1259
neuroses 9:1207, 1208, 1227;
    10:1357–1358; 11:1540; 12:1713
  nervous breakdown and 10:1340
nevi 2:208, 209
  blue 9:1243
  compound 8:1091; 9:1243
  congenital melanocytic 9:1182
  dysplastic 8:1091
  giant melanocytic 9:1182
  intradermal 8:1091
  junctional 8:1091
  strawberry 12:1613
  see also moles
night blindness 10:1362; 17:2373, 2374
nocturia 2:218
noninsulin-dependent diabetes
    (maturity-onset diabetes; type II
    diabetes) 4:472; 10:1367–1368
nonspecific urethritis (NSU)
    14:1931–1933
nosebleeds 4:568; 6:803; 10:1371
  treating 10:1374
nuclear disasters
  radiation sickness 13:1771
  see also Chernobyl disaster
numbness 10:1376–1378
  see also pins and needles
nystagmus 2:219

obesity 4:492; 5:655; 6:846;
    10:1383–1386
  atherosclerosis and 3:372
  body mass index (BMI) and 17:2400
  brown fat theory and 9:1171
  diabetes and 10:1368
  a form of malnutrition 8:1127, 1128;
    10:1382
  glands and 1:46; 4:566; 10:1383
  Pickwickian syndrome 7:898
  reflux esophagitis and 6:787
  a symptom of Cushing's syndrome
    15:2152
  varicose veins and 17:2344–2345
  yoga and 17:2444
obsessions 7:894; 10:1387
obsessive-compulsive disorder 3:398;
    10:1342, 1358, 1387–1388
Onchocerca 11:1500, 1501
oncoviruses 3:314; 8:1126
onycholysis 6:747
oophoritis 9:1284
ophthalmia neonatorum 5:705
Opisthrocus viverina 17:2421
opportunistic infection 10:1409
oppositional defiant disorder 2:152
orchitis 9:1284; 16:2193
organic brain syndromes 12:1722
osteoarthritis 1:123, 123; 3:325; 5:691;
    10:1435–1438; 11:1581; 14:1968
  cause 1:123, 126
  causing lower back pain 8:1095
  cysts and 4:447
  dislocation and 4:498
  of the elbow 4:547
  of the hands 6:746; 14:1968

of the knee, hydrotherapy and 7:883
  stiffness and 10:1436, 1437;
    15:2077–2078
  symptoms 1:123, 126
  treatment 1:126
osteoid bumps 13:1836
osteomalacia 2:259; 13:1835, 1836;
    17:2381
osteomyelitis 2:258, 260
osteophytes 2:161
osteoporosis 2:258, 260; 3:310, 311;
    5:693; 6:854, 855; 9:1199;
    11:1450–1451; 14:1968
  backache and 2:161, 163
  causing limping 8:1078
  fractures and 2:161; 3:310; 5:660;
    6:828; 8:1078
  HRT and 2:260; 6:855, 856; 9:1199;
    11:1450, 1451
  immobilization 2:260
otitis 11:1452–1453
  otitis externa 4:452, 456; 7:988;
    11:1452–1452
  otitis interna 11:1453
  otitis media (middle ear infection)
    4:453, 456; 6:758; 11:1453;
    13:1826; 16:2213
    chronic 11:1453
    mastoiditis after 9:1160, 1161;
      16:2171
    perforated eardrum and 15:2156
    sore throat and 11:1555; 14:2011
    tonsillitis and 16:2236
    vertigo and 17:2366
otosclerosis 4:453, 456; 6:777; 12:1696,
    1700; 16:2228

pain 11:1474–1477
  analysis in the spinal cord
    16:2240–2241
  chronic 11:1474, 1477
  endorphins and 1:38; 11:1477, 1481
  function of 11:1474–1475, 1480
  the gate theory and 1:38
  hypnosis and 7:891
  radiation of 15:2149
  religious initiates and 11:1476
  tolerance to 2:188; 11:1474
  types 11:1476–1477
    from the nervous system
      11:1476–1477
    internal pain 11:1476
    phantom pain 1:127; 10:1344;
      11:1477
    referred pain 1:38; 11:1476; 15:2149;
      16:2212
    skin pain 11:1476
palilalia 1:108
palpitations 4:550; 6:789, 790
  treatment 2:157
palsy
  pseudobulbar 9:1258, 1259
  see also Bell's palsy; cerebral palsy
pancreatitis 9:1283; 11:1486
panic attacks, treatment 2:182; 5:630
panic disorder 10:1358
papilledema 10:1411
papillomatosis 16:2213
papules 13:1783
paralysis 8:1069; 11:1490–1493; 15:2150
  of cerebral palsy 3:336
  Guillain-Barré syndrome and 6:729
  hyperkalemic 9:1292
  hypokalemic 9:1292
  hysterical 11:1492
  spastic 10:1347
  treatment
    bionics and 2:191

physical therapy 11:1579–1580
  splints 8:1048–1049
paralytic ileus 11:1534
paraphimosis 11:1531
paraphrenia, late 14:1911
paraplegia 3:336; 11:1494–1497; 15:2043
parasites 11:1498–1502
  bedbugs 2:174, 175
  causing blindness 2:220
  causing malaria 8:1121
  cysts and 4:447
  fleas 2:211; 5:646–647
  lice 2:211; 7:885; 8:1064–1066
    typhus and 8:1066; 16:2299,
      2300, 2301
  mites, and scabies 13:1865, 1866
  worm see worms
paratyphoid see typhoid and
  paratyphoid
Parkinson's disease 2:267; 9:1266;
    10:1347; 11:1506–1507, 1581
  speech and 15:2032
  tremor 11:1506; 16:2274, 2275
paronychia see whitlow
pathogens 11:1508–1510
pathomimicry see Munchausen
  syndrome
Patterson Brown-Kelly syndrome
  16:2211
pediculoses 8:1065
pellagra 17:2376
pelvic inflammatory disease (PID)
    1:131; 2:161; 7:943; 11:1520–1521;
    14:1933
  from gonorrhea 5:706
pemphigoid 2:223, 224
pemphigusis 2:224
Pendred's syndrome 16:2226
penicillin-resistant Streptococcus
  pneumoniae (PRSP) 1:98
pericarditis
  pain 3:348
  tuberculous 16:2289
peridontal disease see pyorrhea and
  gingivitis
peritonitis 1:111; 4:501; 9:1189; 11:1532,
    1533–1535
pernicious anemia 1:88, 89, 90; 11:1514,
    1536–1537; 17:2376
  vitiligo and 17:2388
persistent generalized
  lymphadenopathy (PGL) 1:57
persistent vegetative state 2:270;
    3:394
Perthes' disease 6:830; 8:1076; 11:1546
petechiae 13:1755
Peyronie's disease 14:1929
phantom pregnancy 11:1548–1549
pharyngeal web 16:2211
pharyngitis 11:1556, 1557; 14:2011;
    16:2212
phenylketonuria (PKU) 3:401; 5:581,
    654, 684; 11:1558–1559
phimosis 3:374; 11:1531
phlebitis 16:2218; 17:2345
phlegm (sputum) 3:348, 426; 11:1560;
    13:1757
  examination 13:1752
  expectorants and 5:603
  tests 15:2025
phobias 9:1209; 10:1358; 11:1561–1563
  treatment 9:1209; 11:1563; 12:1710
    flotation therapy 5:649
  see also agoraphobia
photodermatitis 4:468
photosensitivity 11:1564–1565; 15:2126,
    2129
Pickwickian syndrome 7:898

picornaviruses 17:2371
pigeon chest 3:347; 12:1590–1592
pigeon toes 5:625, 628; 8:1076;
    12:1593–1594
piles 6:807
  see also hemorrhoids
pimples see acne and pimples
pins and needles 3:372; 10:1343, 1377;
    12:1595–1597; 16:2242
  with multiple sclerosis 9:1281
pinworms see threadworms
Pityrosporum ovale 4:451
PKU see phenylketonuria
placenta previa 3:341; 9:1277; 12:1605
plague 12:1606–1607
  a biological weapon 2:185, 186;
    12:1606
plaque 4:460, 461; 6:730, 731;
    12:1608–1610
  gum diseases and 6:730, 731;
    13:1759–1760
  testing for 4:461
Plaquenil 8:1105
plaques
  atheromatous see atheroma
  in the brain 1:83
Plasmodium spp., and malaria 8:1121;
    11:1500, 1501; 12:1704
pleurisy 2:281, 282; 3:426; 9:1189;
    12:1618–1620; 13:1751, 1752
  pain 3:348
  pneumonia and 12:1625
  treatment 12:1620; 15:2151
PMS see premenstrual syndrome
Pneumococcus spp. 2:166
pneumoconiosis 2:282; 4:564; 12:1621;
    13:1752
  treatment 2:282; 13:1752
Pneumocystis carinii pneumonia
  12:1625
Pneumocystis jiroveci 10:1409
pneumonia 2:282; 3:347, 348; 7:937,
    938, 940; 8:1103, 1104;
    12:1622–1625; 13:1752
  aspiration pneumonia 12:1624, 1625,
    1631
  bronchopneumonia 8:1104; 12:1623,
    1624–1625
  a complication of other diseases
    12:1625
    chicken pox 3:350
    influenza 7:950
    measles 9:1165
  double 12:1622
  lobar 8:1104; 12:1622, 1623, 1624, 1625
  pneumonic plague 12:1607
  prevention 12:1624
  secondary drowning 4:522
  treatment 2:282; 8:1103; 12:1624,
    1625; 13:1752
  see also Legionnaire's disease
pneumonitis 6:853
pneumothorax 13:1751, 1752
poisoning 12:1629–1632
  carbon monoxide 1:59; 3:395;
    12:1630, 1637–1638; 17:2320
  dementia and 4:459
  food see food poisoning
  headaches and 6:758
  lead 3:413; 4:573; 5:583;
    8:1048–1050; 10:1394, 1395;
    12:1630, 1638; 13:1746
    treatment 3:345; 8:1049
  methanol 10:1411
  toxic metals 2:230
    chelation therapy and 3:345, 346
    see also lead poisoning; mercury
    poisoning

poisoning (cont'd)
treatment 4:556; 12:1632
use of emetics 4:562
unconsciousness and 17:2321
see also irritants
poison ivy, oak, or sumac 2:211
poliomyelitis (polio) 6:728;
12:1633–1635; 16:2285
limping and 8:1077
paralysis and 11:1492, 1493; 12:1635
post-polio syndrome and 9:1259;
12:1635
scoliosis 14:1891
treatment and outlook 12:1634–1635
vaccination 7:911, 912; 12:1633, 1635;
13:1763; 16:2285; 17:2332
polyarthritis, symmetrical 13:1821
polydactyly (extra fingers) 2:257;
10:1305; 12:1613
polymorphic light eruption 11:1564,
1565
polymyalgia rheumatica 9:1292
polyneuritis 6:728
polyps 6:727; 12:1642–1643
cervical 3:339; 5:642; 6:733; 11:1488;
17:2327
in the intestines 12:1642
colon 3:386, 387; 12:1642, 1643
nasal 10:1372, 1375; 12:1642, 1643
in the rectum 13:1787
in the uterus 5:642; 12:1642, 1643;
17:2327, 2329
polysplenia 6:805
porphyria 11:1565; 14:1958
"porter's neck" 1:122
Portuguese man-of-war stings 2:210,
211
port-wine stains 2:208, 209
postnasal drip 11:1557
postpartum depression and psychosis
4:465; 8:1062; 9:1247; 10:1322;
12:1648–1651
post-polio syndrome 9:1259;
12:1635
post-traumatic stress disorder (PTSD)
10:1358; 12:1652–1655; 15:2102
complex 12:1653
postural syncope 2:214, 215
postviral fatigue syndrome see
chronic fatigue syndrome
preeclampsia (preeclamptic toxemia;
PET; proteinuric hypertension)
3:322; 7:931; 8:1106; 12:1659–1660;
17:2399
premature babies 2:204, 279; 7:933;
10:1338; 11:1516, 1517;
12:1666–1669
giving oxygen to 11:1464, 1466
premenstrual syndrome (PMS) 6:859;
8:1056; 9:1201, 1202; 12:1671–1674
headaches 6:758
treatment 12:1674
light therapy 14:1898
presbyacusis 4:455
presbyopia 5:608
priapism 12:1700; 14:1928; 16:2196
prickly heat 6:795; 11:1545; 12:1685;
15:2130
prions 4:439; 11:1509
proctalgia fugax 1:102
professional patient syndrome see
Munchausen syndrome
prolactinomas 12:1598, 1600–1601
prolapse 11:1526; 12:1686–1688
bladder (cystocele) 7:925; 12:1686,
1687
cord 12:1687–1688
invertebral disk see slipped disk

mitral valve 17:2341, 2342
rectal 1:103; 12:1686, 1687, 1688
uterine (womb) 2:161; 6:733; 7:904,
905; 12:1686–1687, 1688; 17:2327,
2335
vaginal wall 17:2335
Propiobacterium acnes 1:31, 32, 34
prostatitis 5:690; 9:1284; 12:1690–1691
Proteus spp.
P. mirabilis 2:166
P. vulgaris 2:166
Proteus syndrome 2:209
protozoal infections 7:936; 11:1510;
12:1703–1704
PRSP (penicillin-resistant
Streptococcus pneumoniae) 1:98
pruritus
of pregnancy 7:988
pruritus ani 1:103
pruritus vulvae 17:2393, 2394
see also itches
pseudobulbar palsy 9:1258, 1259
pseudocyesis see phantom pregnancy
pseudohypoparathyroidism 11:1505
Pseudomonas aeruginosa 13:1758
psittacosis 12:1624, 1705
psoriasis 4:469; 6:739; 7:989;
12:1706–1708
tattooing and 16:2173
types 12:1706, 1708
psychogenic disorders 12:1712–1713
psychoses 9:1207; 11:1540–1541; 12:1713,
1719–1722
antisclerotic 14:1911
nervous breakdown 10:1340
paranoid 12:1720
amphetamines and 1:87
postpartum psychosis 12:1649, 1651
senile 14:1911
treatment 12:1722; 14:1905
see also bipolar disorder;
schizophrenia
psychosomatic problems 9:1206, 1209;
12:1714, 1723–1725
back pain 2:161
self-healing 5:614
stress and 5:616
ptomaine poisoning 5:658
PTSD see post-traumatic stress
disorder
ptyalism 13:1854
pulled muscles 9:1292, 1294;
13:1747–1748; 15:2054
treatment 13:1747, 1748
pulmonary disorders 13:1749–1752
asbestosis 1:136; 12:1639; 13:1751
bronchiectasis 6:741; 12:1623–1624;
13:1750, 1751
cancer see cancer, lung
chronic obstructive pulmonary
disease (COPD) 3:370–371
oxygen therapy for 11:1465, 1467
edema 2:283; 3:348; 4:545; 17:2407,
2408
fibrosing alveolitis 13:1751, 1752
pneumoconiosis 2:282; 4:564;
12:1621; 13:1752
pulmonary embolism 13:1751, 1752;
16:2215
tuberculosis 16:2287–2289, 2290
see also asthma; bronchitis;
coughing; emphysema; pleurisy;
pneumonia
punch-drunk 2:266
punctures see wounds, puncture
purpura 2:228; 3:318; 13:1755–1756
Henoch-Schönlein 13:1755, 1756
senile 13:1756

pus 2:225; 13:1757–1758
in abscesses 1:21; 13:1757
anchovy-sauce (chocolate-sauce)
13:1757
in boils 2:255, 256
in wounds 1:19
pyelonephritis 17:2325
pyorrhea and gingivitis 13:1759–1761
gingivitis 6:731; 9:1263; 13:1759–1761
acute ulcerative 6:731
necrotizing ulcerative 13:1760
halitosis 6:740
pyorrhea (peridontal disease) 4:461;
6:731, 759; 12:1610; 13:1759–1761

Q fever 13:1762
quadriplegia 3:336; 15:2043
quinsy 14:2012–2013; 16:2236–2237

rabies 13:1766–1769
incubation period 7:927; 13:1766,
1767–1768
vaccination 13:1766, 1769; 16:2270,
2280
radiation 8:1060; 11:1510
a cause of cancer 8:1126; 13:1772
a cause of leukemia 8:1061
environmental 4:574; 12:1641
mutations 3:330
UV 11:1469, 1470
working with 10:1395
see also Chernobyl disaster;
radiation sickness
radiation sickness 13:1770–1771
Ramsay Hunt's syndrome 14:1939
rashes 13:1782–1784
allergy 13:1782; 14:1969
to tattoo pigments 16:2172, 2173
chicken pox 2:223, 224; 3:349;
13:1782, 1783, 1784
confluent 13:1783
drug-induced 13:1784
gold 13:1821
herpes 6:825; 13:1784
hives 6:831; 13:1783
hookworm infection and 6:852–853
lupus
discoid lupus erythematosus
8:1105, 1106, 1107
systemic lupus erythematosus
8:1105, 1107
macular 13:1783
maculopapular 13:1783
measles 9:1163, 1164; 13:1782, 1783,
1784
papular 13:1783
penicillin allergy 1:99, 100
photosensitive 11:1564, 1565; 15:2126
prickly heat 12:1685; 15:2130
purpuric 13:1755, 1756
pustular 13:1783
Rocky Mountain spotted fever
13:1845
rubella (German measles) 13:1784,
1849
scabies 13:1865, 1866
scarlet fever 13:1784; 14:1878, 1879
sex flush 5:590
shingles 14:1938, 1939
smallpox 14:1987, 1988
syphilis 13:1784; 14:1932, 1933;
15:2154, 2155
typhoid and paratyphoid 13:1784;
16:2297
typhus 16:2300
vesicular 13:1783
see also dermatitis; diaper rash;
eczema

Raynaud's syndrome 5:669; 6:747;
8:1105; 10:1378
biofeedback and 2:183, 184
scleroderma and 14:1888, 1889
reactive arthritis 13:1785–1786
genitourinary (urogenital) 13:1786
rectocele 12:1686
reflux, gastroesophageal 6:786–787;
17:2313
halitosis and 6:740
Reiter's syndrome 13:1786; 17:2312
repetitive strain injury (RSI) 10:1396;
11:1475; 13:1803–1804
respiratory distress syndrome 12:1667,
1668–1669
retained products of conception (RPC)
17:2338
retinal artery occlusion 2:222; 10:1411
retinal vein thrombosis 2:222
retinitis pigmentosa 2:222; 13:1811, 1812
retinopathy
diabetic 5:609; 13:1811, 1812
hypertensive 13:1812
retroviruses 5:680
Reye's syndrome 5:641; 10:1369;
11:1478, 1479; 13:1813–1814
rheumatic fever 6:788; 13:1817–1818,
1819; 15:2097
heart valves and 13:1817; 15:2067;
16:2215, 2216; 17:2341
symptoms 13:1818
Saint Vitus' dance 13:1818, 1851
rheumatism 11:1581; 13:1819
rheumatoid arthritis 1:126; 3:323;
7:1002, 1003; 11:1581; 13:1820–1824
in adults 1:122–123
in children 1:123
in the hands 6:746; 13:1820, 1821,
1823, 1824
monitored using thermography
16:2207, 2208
stiffness and 8:1027; 15:2077
treatment 13:1823–1824;
15:2072–2073
rheumatoid nodules 13:1821
rhinitis 11:1560; 13:1825–1826; 14:2002,
2003
season allergic see hay fever
vasomotor 14:2003
rhinoviruses 17:2372
rickets 2:260; 3:311; 11:1526;
13:1835–1836; 17:2381
rickettsia
Rocky Mountain spotted fever and
13:1844, 1845
typhus and 7:937, 938; 16:2300, 2301
rickety rosary 13:1836
rigors 5:640
ringworm 7:938, 939; 10:1315;
13:1837–1838; 14:1974
see also athlete's foot
risus sardonicus 16:2198
rituals 7:894
river blindness 11:1500, 1501; 16:2282,
2283, 2284; 17:2419
Rocky Mountain spotted fever
13:1844–1845
rosacea 1:34; 7:875
roseola infantum 5:588
roundworms (nematodes) 11:1498;
17:2419–2420
see also Ascaris
RSI see repetitive strain injury
rubella (German measles)
13:1849–1850
arthritis and 1:124
during pregnancy 13:1849, 1850
birth defects and 2:207; 3:326,

336, 402; 7:910; 13:1850
rash 13:1784, 1849
subclinical infection 7:935
vaccination 2:206; 6:748; 7:910, 912;
13:1739, 1849, 1850
avoiding pregnancy after
13:1849

SAD see seasonal affective disorder
Saint Vitus' dance 13:1818, 1851
salmonella 2:166; 13:1855–1857
encephalitis and 11:1513
food poisoning and 5:657, 659;
7:928; 13:1855, 1856–1857
paratyphoid and 13:1855, 1857;
16:2296
typhoid and 13:1855, 1857;
16:2295
Salmonella paratyphi 16:2296
Salmonella typhi 16:2295, 2296
salmon patches 2:208, 209
salpingitis 3:400; 6:733; 7:943;
13:1858–1860
salpingoophoritis 7:943
sarcoma 3:312; 16:2291
fibroids and 5:642; 17:2327
Kaposi's 1:56
osteogenic 2:260; 14:1966
SARS (severe acute respiratory
syndrome) 7:938, 962; 13:1763,
1863–1864
scabies 3:349; 11:1516; 13:1865–1866
scalded skin syndrome 15:2062
scalding 13:1867–1868
treatment 3:304; 13:1867, 1868
see also burns
scalp disorders see hair and scalp
disorders
scarlet fever (scarlatina) 14:1878–1879
rash 13:1784; 14:1878, 1879
scars 6:765; 14:1880–1881, 1971, 1972;
17:2422, 2423, 2424
acne 1:31; 14:1880
appendix-removal 1:109
discharge from 5:644
chicken pox 3:349; 13:1782, 1783
how to prevent 14:1881
keloid 7:1005; 14:1880, 1881
numbness in and around 10:1376
plastic surgery and 12:1617
surgical, healing 15:2136
schistosomiasis (bilharzia) 11:1499,
1501; 16:2281, 2284; 17:2420, 2421
schizophrenia 9:1208, 1209, 1247, 1278;
12:1720; 14:1882–1884; 15:2150
cause 12:1722
hypochondria and 7:895
nervous breakdown and 10:1342
paranoid 10:1342
treatment 9:1209; 12:1710; 13:1737
sciatica 2:161–163; 8:1078, 1094, 1095;
10:1349; 14:1885–1887, 1983
diagnosis 10:1355
sclerodactyly 14:1888
scleroderma (systemic sclerosis)
14:1888–1889; 15:2148
scoliosis 8:1078; 11:1448; 14:1890–1891
scotoma 10:1411
scratches 1:19
scurvy 2:260; 10:1379; 14:1896–1897;
17:2378
hemorrhaging and 6:804
sea sickness see motion sickness
seasonal affective disorder (SAD)
9:1186; 10:1353; 14:1898–1899;
17:2380
seborrhea see dermatitis, seborrheic
seborrheic tendency 4:451

seizures 2:215
epileptic see epilepsy, seizures
senility 14:1908–1911
sensitization 14:1912–1913
sepsis 14:1914–1915
puerperal 17:2338–2339
septic shock 4:441; 14:1915, 1943
septicemia 2:236; 14:1914
severe combined immune deficiency
(SCID) 5:677
sexual dysfunction 14:1928–1929
female
failure to achieve orgasm
10:1424; 14:1929
lack of libido and sex difficulties
after childbirth 8:1062; 14:1921,
1928
male
impotence 1:130; 5:590;
7:919–920; 11:1531; 14:1924
Peyronie's disease 14:1929
premature ejaculation 5:589,
590; 14:1924, 1928
priapism 12:1700; 14:1928; 16:2196
sexually transmitted diseases (STDs)
1:22, 45; 7:943; 11:1530;
14:1930–1935
casual sex and 14:1931
chlamydial infection 14:1931–1933,
1935; 16:2192; 17:2338
genital herpes 3:337, 341; 6:825;
11:1531; 14:1932, 1933, 2009
genital warts 11:1530; 14:1933, 1935;
17:2393, 2395, 2396–2397
treatment 17:2397
kidney disease and 8:1018
pregnancy and 12:1675; 14:1932,
1933, 1935
prevention 14:1934–1935
pubic lice 8:1066
salpingitis and 13:1858
thrush as 14:1934
trichomoniasis as 16:2278–2279
vaginal discharge and 14:1933–1934
vulval inflammation and 17:2393
where to go for help 14:1935
see also AIDS; gonorrhea; syphilis
shaking see tremor
shellfish
allergy to 15:2145
poisoning 8:1086
shell shock 10:1358; 12:1653; 15:2102
see also post-traumatic stress
disorder
Shigella 2:166; 4:533, 573
shingles 2:224; 6:825; 10:1349;
14:1938–1939
back pain and 2:161, 163
chicken pox and 3:349, 350; 6:825;
14:1938
lesions and rash 2:223; 7:935;
10:1349; 14:1938, 1939
shock 4:555; 14:1943–1947
after bites or stings 2:212
anaphylactic 14:1945
cardiogenic 14:1944, 1945, 1947
causing loss of voice 10:1334
coma and 3:395
effects of 14:1946
from bleeding 6:806
internal 8:805; 14:1945
from burns or scalds 3:304, 305;
6:806; 13:1867, 1868; 14:1943, 1944
hypovolemic 14:1944–1945
neurogenic 14:1945
psychological 14:1943, 1944
septic (endotoxic) 4:441; 14:1915,
1943, 1945, 1946

surgical 4:540; 12:1646
symptoms 14:1946
treatment 14:1946–1947
unconsciousness and 17:2320–2321
wounds and 1:20
shock lung 14:1943, 1946
short sight see myopia
Siamese twins 14:1950–1951
sick building syndrome 14:1952–1953
sickle-cell anemia 1:89, 90;
14:1954–1955
malaria and 16:2201
sickle-cell trait 14:1954
silicosis 10:1395; 14:1961
sinusitis 6:741; 9:1269; 10:1375; 13:1826;
14:1962–1963
headaches and 6:758, 759; 15:2150
sixth disease 5:588
Sjogren's syndrome 8:1149; 9:1149
SLE see lupus
sleep apnea 16:2236
sleeping sickness 12:1704;
16:2281–2282
sleep and sleep problems
14:1976–1980
problems
depression and 7:957, 958;
8:1056–1057
myoclonic jerks 16:2293, 2294
narcolepsy 7:897, 899; 15:2083
nightmares 4:511, 512; 14:1978
PTSD and 12:1653
sleeplessness see insomnia
sleepwalking 14:1981
sleep 5:620; 14:1976–1977
amount necessary 14:1978
in babies and children 1:85; 3:354;
14:1976, 1977, 1980
brain activity 14:1977
deprivation 14:1978
"early birds" and "night owls"
2:187, 188; 14:1976
hallucinations when waking or
falling asleep 12:1721
induced by alcohol 6:752
mind active during 9:1226
rapid eye movement (REM) 4:511,
512; 7:957; 13:1781; 14:1978–1980
versus unconsciousness 17:2319
wet dreams 5:589; 14:1906
slipped disk 2:160, 161–163; 3:325;
14:1968, 1982–1985
fibrositis and 5:643
paralysis and 11:1491–1493
reoccurrence 2:163
sciatica and 2:161–163; 10:1349;
14:1885–1887, 1983
scoliosis and 14:1890
treatment 11:1446; 14:1982, 1983–1985
traction 16:2255
smallpox 9:1217; 14:1986–1988
a biological weapon 2:185, 186
vaccination 7:910, 911, 912
smoking
heart attacks and 6:783; 16:2214
vision and 3:388
snakebites 2:212; 14:2000–2001;
16:2280
sneezing 10:1373; 11:1524;
14:2002–2003
with hay fever 6:757
snoring 1:41; 14:2004–2005
solvents, dangers of working with
10:1393, 1395
somatoform disorders 10:1358
sores 14:2008–2009
canker (aphthous ulcers) 17:2311
chrome 14:2009

decubitus ulcers see bedsores
genital 14:2009
industrial 14:2009
mouth, from solvent abuse 14:2007
treatment 14:2008, 2009
tropical 14:2009
see also blisters; cold sores; ulcers
sore throat 11:1555, 1557; 14:2010–2013
laryngitis 7:946; 8:1038, 1039;
10:1335; 14:2011, 2013; 16:2212;
17:2389
acute 8:1036, 1037–1039
chronic 8:1036, 1037, 1039
peritonsillar abscesses (quinsies)
14:2012–2013
pharyngitis 11:1556, 1557; 14:2011
streptococcal throat (strep throat)
11:1555, 1556, 1557; 14:2010;
15:2097; 16:2212
treatment 14:2010, 2013; 16:2213
see also tonsillitis
spastic colon 15:2022–2023
spasticity 2:149; 3:335, 336
speech difficulties and 10:1308
see also cerebral palsy
spina bifida 2:206, 207; 3:401, 402;
4:574; 5:684; 10:1351;
15:2037–2039, 2041–2043
chance of having another child
with 7:878; 15:2038
detection 3:367; 17:2316
hydrocephalus and 7:879
inherited 5:682; 15:2037
leg braces 10:1432
prevention, folic acid supplements
and 2:206; 3:401; 5:638, 682;
10:1351; 15:2037, 2039; 17:2377
treatment 3:402; 15:2039
plastic surgery 12:1614
types 15:2037–2039
meningocele 10:1351; 15:2037,
2039
meningomyelocele 7:879; 15:2039
see also birth defects
spirochetes 2:165; 11:1510; 17:2402
splinters 15:2047
spondylolisthesis 14:1968
sports injury 15:2050–2051, 2052–2055
bursitis 3:308
carpal tunnel syndrome 3:323
cramp 4:437
dislocations 15:2055
first aid 1:50
fractures 15:2050–2051, 2054
hamstring injuries 6:743–744
muscle stiffness 15:2054
muscle strain 15:2054
osteoarthritis and 10:1435
prevention 8:1027
pulled muscles 13:1747; 15:2054
sprains 15:2055
torn knee cartilage 3:325; 10:1434;
15:2055
torn muscles 9:1290, 1292
to tendons 15:2054
treatment 15:2051
cold and hot 6:797, 799
see also dislocation; fractures;
pulled muscles; sprains; tennis
elbow
spots before the eyes 2:219
sprains 8:1072; 15:2056–2057
ankles 6:764; 15:2057, 2145
splints used for 15:2048
sports injuries 15:2055
treatment 15:2051, 2056, 2057
sputum see phlegm
squint 2:219; 4:505; 5:609

2531

stammering and stuttering 1:107;
  15:2032, **2058–2061**
staphylococcus 2:164; 5:*670*; 11:1510;
  15:2062
  abscesses and 13:*1758*
  food poisoning and 5:657, 659;
    7:928; 15:2062
  pneumonia and 12:1623
  in skin lesions 2:255; 5:657; 7:918
  Staphylococcus aureus 1:34; 2:166;
    15:*2062*; 16:*2247*
    methicillin-resistant (MRSA) 1:98;
      11:1508; 15:2062
  toxic shock syndrome and 16:*2247*,
    2248
steatorrhea 5:624
stenosis 15:2067
  aortic 15:2067; 17:2341
  coronary artery 15:2067
  laryngeal 15:2067
  mitral 15:2067
  pulmonary 15:2067
  pyloric 1:67; 15:2067
  spinal 8:1078
sterility *see* infertility
stiffness **15:2076–2079**
  arthritis and 10:1436, 1437;
    15:2077–2078
  muscle 15:2054, 2076–2077
  treatment 15:2076, *2078, 2079*
stillbirth **15:2080–2082**
Still's disease 1:123
stings *see* bites and stings
stitch 1:49; **15:2086–2087**
stomatitis 9:1263
  aphthous (viral) 9:1263; 17:*2311*
stork marks 2:208, 209
strain 15:2098
  see also tension
strains
  eyestain 9:1233
  ligament 8:*1072*
  pulled or strained muscles 6:799;
    9:1292, 1294; 13:*1747–1748*; 15:*2051,*
    2054
strangulation **15:2094–2096**
strawberry marks 2:208, *209*
strawberry tongue 14:*1879*
streptococcus 2:164; 5:*670*; 11:1510;
  14:*1914*; **15:2097**
  glomerulonephritis and 8:1020
  impetigo and 7:918
  rheumatic fever and 13:1817, *1818*
  scarlet fever and 14:*1878–1879*
  streptococcal throat (strep throat)
    and 11:*1557*; 14:*2010*; 15:*2097*;
    16:*2212*
  Streptococcus fecalis 15:2097
  Streptococcus mutans 15:2097
  Streptococcus pneumoniae 15:2097
    penicillin-resistant (PRSP) 1:98
  Streptococcus pyogenes 2:166;
    14:*1878–1879*; 15:2097
  Streptococcus viridans 15:2097
stress **15:2098–2102**, 2103
  acne and 1:32
  the blood-brain barrier and
    2:230
  blood pressure and 2:237
  cancer and 3:314
  family relationships and 5:616–617
  the heart and 7:997
  post-traumatic stress disorder (PTSD)
    10:1358; 12:**1652–1655**; 15:2102
  psychosomatic symptoms and
    5:616; 12:1723, 1724
  ulcers and 4:530; 15:2102
  see also anxiety; tension

stretch marks 9:*1276*; 12:1661, 1662,
  1679; 15:**2105–2106**
stroke 2:265, 267; 5:691–692; 6:803;
  10:*1347*; 15:**2107–2111**; 16:2217–2218
  assessment, MRI scans 2:*269*
  associated with heart attacks
    15:2108
  brain scars after 14:*1881*
  causes 2:267; 15:2107–2108; 16:2217
    cerebral infarction (blood vessel
      blockage) 1:121; 15:2107–*2108,*
      2109; 16:2217
    hemorrhage 15:2108, *2109*
    high blood pressure and 15:2107,
      2108
  fits and 5:583
  limping and 8:1078
  loss of second languages and 1:107
  paralysis and 11:1490, 1493
    affecting sense of touch 16:2239
  patients at home 15:2110, *2111*
  prevention 15:2107, 2108, 2110–2111;
    16:2261, 2262
  risk 15:2108–2109
  the sense of touch and 16:2239,
    2242
  sight and 2:222; 5:606–607; 10:1411
  smart drugs 14:1989
  speech and 1:107; 10:1307; 15:2030,
    2033, 2107, 2110
  transient ischemic attacks and
    15:2109, 2111; 16:2261, *2262*
  treatment 1:108; 4:557; 5:692;
    15:2109–2110
    exercises 15:*2111*
    hydrotherapy 7:881
    occupational therapy 10:1397
    physical therapy 11:1580; 15:*2107*,
      2110
    rehabilitation 13:1796, *1797*
    surgery 15:2107
stuttering see stammering and
  stuttering
sty 2:256; 4:447; 6:799; 15:**2112–2113**
sudden infant death syndrome (SIDS)
  15:**2116–2117**
suffocation **15:2118–2119**
  babies 1:135
  first aid 15:*2119*
summer flu *see* gastroenteritis
sunburn 3:303; 11:*1470*; 15:**2126–2129**
  blisters 2:223; 15:2127, 2128
  in children 15:2128, 2129
  prevention 11:*1470*; 15:2128–2129
  rash and itching from 6:831
  treatment 15:2128; 16:*2272*
sunstroke (heatstroke) 6:796; 11:1545;
  15:**2130–2131**
swayback (lordosis) 13:1848
swellings **15:2145–2148**
  see also edema; elephantiasis
swimmer's itch 11:*1509*
Sydenham's chorea see Saint Vitus'
  dance
symptoms 4:474–475; 15:**2149–2152**
syncope *see* fainting
syndactyly 12:1613, *1614*
synovitis 9:1189
syphilis 4:459; 6:803; 7:938; 11:1531;
  14:1931; 15:**2153–2155**
  congenital 14:1931
  diagnosis 15:2153, 2154, 2155
  latent 15:2154
  neuralgia with 10:1349
  pregnancy and 12:1675; 14:1931, 1932;
    15:2154, 2155
  primary sore or ulcer 15:2153–2154,
    2155

rash 13:1784; 14:*1932, 1933*; 15:2154,
  2155
  spinal cord affected by 15:2042
  tongue or lip ulcers and 17:2311
  treatment 15:2155
  ulcers or sores in the groin
    15:2153–2154; 17:2314, 2334
systemic lupus erythematosus see
  lupus
systemic sclerosis *see* scleroderma

tachycardia 13:1754
Taenia saginata 17:*2420–2421*
Taenia solium 17:*2421*
talipes equinovarus *see* clubfoot
tapeworms 11:1498, *1500*, 1501; 17:2419,
  2420–2421
tarsal tunnel syndrome 3:322
tartar (calculus) 12:1609; 13:*1761*
Tay-Sachs disease 16:*2174*
  detection 3:367; 16:*2174*
TB *see* tuberculosis
tendonitis 6:799
tenesmus, rectal 3:383; 13:1788
tennis elbow 1:124; 4:547; 6:799;
  14:*1968*; 16:*2187*
tenosynovitis 5:629; 8:1105; 16:2185,
  2186; 17:*2430*
tension 16:**2188–2190**
  headaches and 6:758, 759; 9:1230
  necessity of 13:1801–1802; 16:2188
  treatment
    massage 8:1142; 9:1142
    mind-body therapy 9:1230
    relaxation 13:1800–1801
  see also stress
tetanus 1:20; 2:236; 7:*937*, 938;
  16:**2197–2198**, 2285; 17:2426
  vaccinations 1:17; 2:206; 7:910, 911,
    912; 8:1030; 16:2197, 2198, 2285;
    17:2424, 2426
tetany 3:311; 11:1504
  hyperventilation 6:745; 11:1504
tetralogy of Fallot 2:243
thalassemia 1:88, 89, 90;
  16:**2200–2201**
  detection 3:367
threadworms (pinworms) 1:103; 7:988;
  11:1498, 1501; 17:2419, 2420
thrombophlebitis 16:2214, 2215, 2218
thrombosis 1:119, 120; 16:**2214–2218**
  arterial 16:2217
  in the brain, and stroke 15:2107;
    16:2217–2218
  cerebral 16:2217–2218, 2262
  coronary 3:419–420; 6:783–784;
    16:2215–2216, 2217
    see also heart attack
  deep vein 2:223; 10:1417;
    15:2146–2147; 16:2218; 17:2345
  edema and 4:544
  in the heart's atria or ventricles
    16:2215–2216
  obesity and 10:1385
  the Pill and 10:1417; 16:2214
  prevention, warfarin 16:2214, 2216
  venous 16:2217
thrush (Candida; candidiasis) 7:987;
  16:**2219–2220**; 17:2337, 2436
  chronic mucocutaneous candidiasis
    16:2220; 17:2437, 2438
  genital 10:1368; 14:*1934*; 16:2220
  in the mouth 9:1263; 16:2219, 2220;
    17:*2436*, 2437
  of the nails 16:2220; 17:2437,
    2438
  people at risk from 16:2219, 2220
    diabetics 10:1368; 16:2219, 2220

on the skin 16:2220
  diaper rash and 4:481–482
  feet 16:2220; 17:*2436*
  systemic infections 17:2437,
    2438
  treatment 16:2220
  vaginal discharge and 6:733;
    16:2220; 17:2334, 2336
  see also yeast infections
thymomas 16:2222
thyroiditis 5:704; 16:2224, 2226
thyrotoxicosis (overactive thyroid;
  hyperthyroidism) 5:*704*; 6:857;
  10:1332; 11:1450, 1503; 15:2150;
  16:2223–2224, 2226
  Graves' disease 5:704; 16:**2225–2226**
  heat production and 16:2182
  treatment 13:1774; 15:2150; 16:2223,
    2224
  tremor and 16:2275
TIA *see* transient ischemic attack
ticks 2:211
  Lyme disease and 8:*1108*; 16:*2199*
  Q fever and 13:1762
  Rocky Mountain spotted fever and
    13:*1844–1845*
tics *see* twitches and tics
Tietze's disease 13:1831
tinea pedis *see* athlete's foot
tinnitus 10:1365; 16:**2227–2228**
  unilateral 2:227
toeing in *see* pigeon toes
togaviruses 17:2372
tongue-tied 16:2232
tonsillitis 2:281, 282; 8:1112; 14:2010,
  2011–2012; 16:2212, **2235**,
  2236–2237
  swollen lymph nodes and 8:1109
tophi (chalk stones) 5:*708*
total allergy syndrome 16:2238
Tourette's syndrome 2:152;
  16:**2243–2244**, 2293, 2294
toxemia 2:236
  preeclamptic (PET) 7:931
toxic confusional state 15:2150
toxic shock syndrome 16:**2247–2248**
Toxocara canis 2:220
toxocariasis 11:1500
Toxoplasma gondi 2:220
trachoma 2:220; 3:416; 16:2282
transient ischemic attack (TIA)
  16:**2261–2262**
  strokes and 15:2109, 2111; 16:2261,
    2262
translocation 5:676–677
tremor 16:**2274–2275**
  benign essential 16:2274, 2275
  intention 16:2275
  of Parkinson's disease 11:*1506*;
    16:2274
  physiological 16:2274, 2275
  red nucleus 16:2275
trench mouth 13:1760
Treponema pallidum 2:166; 14:*1932*;
  15:2155
Trichinella 11:1499; 16:2276
trichinosis 16:**2276–2277**
trichlorethylene 10:1393
Trichomonas vaginalis 16:2278, *2279*;
  17:*2325, 2336*, 2337–2338
trichomoniasis 12:1703; 14:1934;
  16:**2278–2279**; 17:*2325*, 2337–2338
  as a urinary tract infection 17:*2325*
trophoblastic disease 17:2327
tropical diseases 16:**2280–2285**
  see also under names of individual
    diseases
Trychophyton fungus 13:*1837, 1838*

trypanosomiasis 12:1704
  African *see* sleeping sickness
tuberculosis (TB) 2:282; 7:927, 938,
    940; 13:1752; 16:2285, **2287–2290**
  abdominal 16:2288, 2290
  arthritis following 1:124
  diagnosis 16:*2289*
  fatigue and 5:619
  meningitis following 9:1195
  miliary 16:2288
  open 16:2289
  pigeon chest and 12:1592
  pleurisy and 12:1619
  prevention 16:2290
    vaccination 7:912; 13:1763;
      16:2285, 2287, 2290; 17:2330
  silicosis and 14:1961
  of the spine 2:161
  treatment 2:282; 7:982; 9:1194;
    13:1750, 1752; 16:2288, 2290
    surgery 16:2287
tularemia, a biological weapon 2:185,
    186
tumors 16:**2291–2292**
  benign 3:312, 313; 8:1124, 1125; 16:2291
    see also fibroids; polyps
  malignant 8:*1124–1126*; 16:2291, *2292*
    see also cancer
  mixed 9:1254
  pressing on the spinal cord 15:2043
  treatment 16:2292
tunnel vision 2:*219*; 13:1812
Turner's syndrome 10:1305
twins, Siamese 14:*1950–1951*
twitches and tics 16:**2293–2294**
  tics 9:1266; 16:2293, *2294*
    Tourette's syndrome and 16:2243,
      2293, 2294
  twitches 16:2293–*2294*
typhoid and paratyphoid
    16:**2295–2298**
  paratyphoid 13:1855; 16:2295, 2296,
    2298
  rash 13:1784; 16:2297
  typhoid 4:485, 533; 5:623; 7:*937*, 938;
    13:1855–1856; 16:2285,
    2295–2298
    carriers 16:2296, 2297
    gallstones and 16:2295
    prevention 16:2298
    in the small intestine 16:*2295*,
      2297
    treatment 16:2297–2298
    vaccination 7:955; 16:2285
typhus 4:573; 7:*937*, 938; 16:2295,
    2299–2301
  epidemic 16:2299, 2300, *2301*
  murine (endemic typhus) 16:2299,
    2300
  scrub 16:*2300–2301*

ulcers 14:2008; 17:**2310–2314**
  cancer/malignancy and 3:312; 8:1124
  colon-wall 3:387
  decubitus *see* bedsores
  diabetic foot, treatment 2:190
  duodenal (intestinal) 4:495, 530, *531*
    bleeding from 6:803–804; 8:1042
    body weight and 15:2090
    excess salivation and 13:1854
    kissing ulcers 17:2313
    pain 17:2313
    perforated 11:1534, 1535; 17:2313
    treatment 2:157, 158; 4:531; 8:1042;
      15:2138; 17:*2340*
    see also ulcers, peptic
  in the groin 17:2310, 2314, 2334
  leg 1:17; 17:*2310*, 2312–2313, 2343

mouth 9:1260, 1263; 14:2008;
    16:2234; 17:2310–2311
  general disease and 17:2311–2312
  treatment 17:2312
  treatment in AIDS patients
    16:2204
oesophageal 17:2313
peptic 7:930; 17:2313–2314
  stress and 4:530; 15:2102
  surgery for 17:2312
  see also ulcers, duodenal; ulcers,
    stomach
skin
  from chromium 10:1392
  rodent ulcers 14:1975; 17:2314
  sepsis and 14:*1915*
stomach (gastric) 1:11; 4:495; 5:581;
    15:*2088*, 2089–2090; 17:*2313*, 2314
  aspirin and 1:122; 11:1479
  asymptomatic 17:2312
  biopsy 3:192
  bleeding from 6:803–804;
    8:1042; 14:1945
  body weight and 15:2090
  causes 15:2089; 17:2313
  gastritis and 5:671
  gastroscopy and 4:570, 571;
    8:1042
  stomach or arm pain and 14:1948
  treatment 2:157, 158; 5:581; 8:1042;
    15:2090
  see also ulcers, peptic
see also sores
unconsciousness 17:**2318–2321**
  after a blow to the head 17:*2318*,
    2320, 2321
  coma and 3:394–395; 17:2321
  common causes of 17:2321
  dealing with an emergency
    4:555–556
  memory loss and 9:1190
  see also blackouts; fainting
undulant fever *see* brucellosis
unipolar disorder 9:1247
uremia 15:2150; 17:2322
urethral syndrome 4:449
urethritis 11:1531; 17:2323, 2325
  nonspecific 14:*1931–1933*
urticaria *see* hives
uveitis 17:2311–2312

vaccinia *see* cowpox
vaginal discharge 6:733; 17:2333, 2334,
    2335, **2336–2339**
  after childbirth 17:2338–2339
  after miscarriage 17:2338
  bloodstained 3:338; 5:642; 17:2339
  caused by cancer 17:2339
  caused by chlamydia 17:2338
  caused by gonorrhea 17:2334, 2338
  during pregnancy 12:1662
  from retained material 17:2335,
    2336, 2338
  Gardnerella vaginalis infection
    17:2336, 2338
  normal 17:2334, 2336
    during sexual arousal and
      intercourse 17:*2334*
  Pap tests and 11:1489
  of STDs 14:*1933–1934*
  thrush (Candida; candidiasis) 6:733;
    16:2220; 17:2334, 2336
  trichomoniasis 14:1934; 16:2278,
    2279; 17:*2336*, 2337–2338
vaginismus 7:919, 965; 14:1924–1925;
    17:2334
vaginitis 17:2336
  atrophic 4:496; 9:1202; 17:2334, 2335

of trichomoniasis 16:2278, 2279;
    17:2336
vancomycin-resistant enterococci
    (VRE) 1:98
varicella *see* chicken pox
varicocele 7:943–944; 16:2194
varicose veins 16:*2216*, 2218;
    17:**2343–2346**
  during pregnancy 5:637; 12:1662,
    1675–1676; 17:2344
  edema and 4:544
  hemorrhoids and 6:807
  obesity and 17:2344–2345
  the Pill and 10:1414
  in the scrotum (varicocele)
    7:943–944; 16:2194
  swollen ankles and 15:2146–2147
  thrombophlebitis and 16:2218
  thrombosis and 16:*2216*
  treatment 17:2343, *2345–2346*
  ulcers and 17:2312, 2343
  varicose eczema 7:987; 17:2345
  venular flares and 17:2344
variola virus 14:1986, *1987*, 1988
vascular disease, peripheral 1:120
ventricular fibrillation 17:2359–2360
ventricular septal defect 2:242, *243*;
    3:402
venular flares 17:2344
verruca (plantar wart) 3:418; 5:625;
    7:886; 12:1627; 17:**2361–2363**, 2395
  treatment 17:2361, 2362–*2363*
vertigo 4:502; 17:**2364–2366**
  Ménière's disease and 9:*1194*
  positional 17:2365, 2366
  see also dizziness
vibration white finger 10:1394, 1395,
    1396
  see also Raynaud's syndrome
vibrio 2:164
Vibrio cholerae 3:365
Vincent's organisms 13:1760
viral hemorrhagic fevers 2:186
viruses 7:935, 936; 11:1510;
    17:**2369–2372**
  causing cancer 3:314; 7:935
  causing fever 5:641
  coma and 3:395
  damaging effects 7:939
  encephalitis and 3:395
  infection by 7:927
    incubation period 7:927, 928
    lymphocytes and 8:1113
    prevention 17:2372
  reproduction 7:*939*; 17:*2370*
  treatments 17:2369, 2372
    antibiotics ineffective 11:1528;
      17:2369
vitiligo 9:*1181*; 17:**2388**
vocal nodes 6:832; 8:*1037*
volvulus neonatorum 15:2094
vomiting 10:1330; 15:2088–2089;
    17:**2390–2391**
  in babies 1:69
    projectile 1:67, 69
  blood 4:495; 17:2391
  bulimia and 1:*95*, 96; 10:1384; 17:2391
  in children 1:69
  "coffee grounds" material 4:495;
    17:2391
  emetics and 4:562
  food poisoning and 4:531;
    5:657–658
  with a hangover 6:752
  induction, not recommended when
    corrosives are swallowed 7:*981*
  with morning sickness 9:1248, 1249;
    17:2391

motion sickness 9:1253–1254;
    10:1330, 1331; 17:*2390*, 2391
  psychogenic 10:1331
  treatment 7:1004; 17:2390, 2391
  unpleasant foods and 11:1484
  see also nausea
von Economo's disease 8:1057
Von Recklinghausen's disease *see*
    neurofibromatosis
von Willebrand's disease 17:*2392*
vulvitis 17:*2394*
vulvovaginitis 5:705; 17:2437

warts 6:726; 14:*1975*; 17:**2395–2397**
  adult 17:*2396*, 2397
  filiform 17:2396
  genital 11:1530; 14:1933, 1935;
    17:*2393*, 2395, 2396–2397
    treatment 17:2397
  plantar *see* verruca
  seborrheic 14:*1975*
  tattooing and 16:2173
  treatment 17:2397
  wartlike growths in the throat
    17:2395
wasp stings 2:210, 212
water brash 7:930
waxy flexibility 14:1882
weakness 15:2150
Weil's disease 17:**2402**
welts 13:1783
Wernicke's encephalopathy 12:1722
West Nile virus 17:**2406**
wet lung (shock lung) 14:1943, 1946
wheezing 17:**2407–2408**
whiplash injury 10:1334, *1335*;
    13:1747–1748; 17:**2409–2410**
whipworms 17:*2420*
whiteheads 1:31
whitlow (paronychia) 6:747; 10:1314;
    17:**2411**, 2438
whooping cough 3:426; 17:**2412–2415**
  treatment 17:2413–2414
  vaccination 7:911, 912; 11:1516;
    17:2412, *2413*, 2414–2415
Wilm's tumor 17:**2325**
Wilson's disease 9:1235; 16:2249, 2250
worms 17:**2419–2421**
  appendicitis and 1:110
  in the feces 5:623
    tests for 15:2025
  filarial 17:2419
    elephantiasis and 4:554; 8:1112;
      16:2283
  flukes
    liver fluke 8:1088–1089; 11:*1500*,
      1501; 17:2420, *2421*
    see also schistosomiasis
  from undercooked or raw food
    17:2419, *2421*
  hookworms 2:241; 6:852–853;
    11:1499, *1500*, 1501; 17:2419–*2420*
  malnutrition and 16:2282
  roundworms (nematodes) 11:*1498*;
    17:*2419–2420*
    see also Ascaris
  tapeworms 11:1498, *1500*, 1501;
    17:2419, *2420–2421*
  threadworms (pinworms) 1:103;
    7:988; 11:1498, 1501; 17:2419, 2420
  trichinosis and 16:*2276–2277*
  whipworms 17:*2420*
wounds 17:**2422–2426**
  foreign bodies in 17:2426
  gunshot 17:2422
    treatment 17:2425
  healing 6:765; 14:1971–1972;
    17:2423

wounds *(cont'd)*
zinc and **16**:2250
see also scars
infections **17**:2425–2426
tetanus and **16**:2197; **17**:2424, 2426
needing medical attention **1**:19
puncture **1**:*19*, 20; **17**:2423, 2425
splinters **15**:2047
treatment **17**:*2424–2425*
cleaning **1**:*18*
dressings **1**:17, *18*; **4**:*513–515*
see also abrasions and cuts; bruises; lacerations
Wucheria bancrofti **4**:554; **17**:2420

xanthelasma **3**:366

yeast infections **7**:938; **17**:2436–2438
causes **17**:2436–2437
see also thrush
dandruff and **4**:451
diaper rash and **4**:481–482
oral **9**:1263; **11**:1484; **17**:*2436*, 2438
treatment **17**:2438
vaginal **7**:937; **17**:2436, 2438
during pregnancy **5**:634
yellow fever **2**:186; **16**:2285; **17**:2439
vaccination **16**:2272, 2285; **17**:2439
Yersinia pestis **12**:1607
"**yuppie syndrome**" **3**:369

TREATMENTS AND CURES

abrasion, chemical *see* dermabrasion
accidents
occupational hazards **10**:*1391–1396*
see also emergencies
acetaminophen (Tylenol; Tempra) **1**:137, 138; **11**:1479, 1482
damage to the kidneys **8**:1020
liver damage and **8**:1084, 1087; **11**:1479
overdose **11**:1479; **12**:1629, 1631; **15**:2093
acetyl-L-carnitine (ALC) **14**:1989
aciclovir (Zovirax) **3**:382; **14**:1939
Acticoat7 **3**:301
Activase **4**:557
acupressure **1**:35–36; **3**:359; **8**:*1144*; **9**:*1144*
acupuncture **1**:37–39, 77, 80; **3**:359, *360*; **6**:837, *838*; **10**:1328; **11**:1474
the pulse and **13**:1753
to treat pain **1**:38; **11**:1478
withdrawal from drugs and **17**:*2416*
adenoidectomy **1**:41; **16**:2212
alendronate **11**:1451; **16**:2259
Alexander technique **1**:65–66, 78–79; **6**:837, *838*
allografts **5**:709, 710
aloe **10**:1329
alternative medicine **1**:75–81
Alexander technique **1**:65–66, 78–79; **6**:837, *838*
anthroposophical medicine **1**:79
aromatherapy **1**:79, 114–117; **6**:837
ayurvedic medicine **1**:75, 79, 80
Bach flower remedies **1**:79
chiropractic **1**:77–78; **3**:362–364; **6**:*836*; **11**:1446
color therapy **3**:390–391
crystal therapy **1**:80
cupping **1**:80, 81; **6**:835
flotation therapy **5**:648–650
herbal medicine *see* herbs and herbalism
homeopathy **1**:78; **6**:837, 842–845; **10**:1326

hypnotherapy **1**:79; **6**:837; **12**:*1712*; **13**:*1735*, 1736
iridology **1**:80–81; **7**:975–976
kinesiology **1**:81; **6**:836
meditation **1**:75, 80; **9**:1178–1179; **11**:*1477*; **13**:1802; **15**:*2104*
transcendental **9**:1178; **15**:2104
mud therapy **9**:1270–1273
naturopathy **1**:81; **10**:1326–1329
osteopathy **1**:78; **2**:161; **3**:362; **6**:837; **11**:1446–1449
qigong (chi kung) **1**:81; **3**:358, 360–361
reflexology **1**:78, 80; **6**:837; **8**:*1143*; **9**:*1143*; **13**:1793–1794
reiki **1**:81
shiatsu **1**:80; **6**:776; **8**:*1144*; **14**:1936–1937
see also acupuncture; faith healing; holistic medicine; massage
amantadine **7**:927, 950
aminoglycosides **1**:100
aminophylline **15**:2085
ampicillin **1**:99
amylobarbital **2**:170
analgesics *see* aspirin and analgesics
anesthesiologists **1**:91; **15**:*2137*
anesthetics **1**:91–93; **15**:2135
aftereffects **1**:93
dental uses **1**:92–93
epidural **1**:92, 93
for cesarean births **3**:*342*
for labor **1**:93; **2**:201, 285; **8**:1093; **15**:*2041*
general **1**:*91–92*, 93; **10**:1405–1406; **15**:2135
recovery from **12**:1645
local *see* local anesthetics
premedication **1**:91, 93; **12**:1670; **14**:1902
regional **15**:2135
spinal **1**:92, 93; **15**:2134, 2135
see also anesthetics, epidural
angioplasty
balloon **3**:346, 421; **9**:*1170–1171*, 1172
cerebral **4**:557
antacids **6**:787; **7**:930
anthroposophical medicine **1**:79
antianxiety drugs *see* tranquilizers
antibiotics **1**:99–100; **2**:165; **7**:940; **9**:1174
ineffective against viruses **11**:1528; **17**:2369
side effects **1**:100; **14**:1959; **17**:2364
see also penicillin; tetracycline
anticoagulants, side effects **14**:1959
anticonvulsants **5**:585
antidepressants **4**:464, 466; **13**:1737–1738; **14**:1903–1904; **15**:2084
side effects **14**:1958, 1959
antihistamines **1**:72, 74; **6**:756, 831
rashes and **13**:1784
sedative **7**:893
side effects **7**:893; **14**:1956, 1959
antipsychotic drugs **12**:1720, 1722; **13**:1737; **14**:1905
side effects **14**:1959
antiretroviral agents **17**:2372
antiseptics
garlic **6**:*814*
Lister and **15**:2135, *2137*
antivenin **14**:2000, *2001*
antiviral drugs **17**:2369
see also aciclovir
anxiolytic drugs *see* tranquilizers
appliances, orthodontic **10**:*1426*, *1428–1429*; **16**:2175, *2177*

aromatherapy **1**:79, 114–117; **6**:837
arthrodesis **1**:126
arthroplasty, hip **2**:189
artificial insemination **1**:129, 130; **15**:2141
by donor (AID) **1**:129, 130; **7**:942, 945
by husband (AIH) **7**:945
artificial limbs **1**:127–128; **8**:1076; **10**:*1344*; **12**:*1696–1699*
arms **1**:127, *128*; **12**:*1696*, *1697*, *1698*
bionic **2**:191
legs **1**:127; **12**:*1696–1698*
physical therapy and **11**:1580
see also bionics; prostheses
artificial methods of conception **1**:129–131
in vitro fertilization (IVF) **1**:129, 131; **7**:971–974; **11**:1520
artificial respiration (kiss of life; mouth-to-mouth resuscitation) **1**:132–135; **3**:*321*; **4**:522, 555; **13**:*1809*
for a baby or child **1**:*134*
cardiopulmonary resuscitation (CPR) **1**:134, 135; **3**:320, *321*; **13**:1807, 1808, *1809*, 1810
art therapy **3**:390
aspirin and analgesics **1**:137–138
analgesics (painkillers) **1**:*137–138*; **11**:1478–1480, 1481–1482
see also acetaminophen; codeine; ibuprofen; morphine
aspirin **1**:137, *138*; **11**:1478–1479, 1482, 1554
allergy **10**:1370
damage to the esophagus **6**:787
damage to the kidneys **8**:1020
dangerous to suck **16**:2235
deafness and **1**:122; **4**:455
dosage **1**:137; **11**:1460
gargle **14**:2013; **16**:2213
gastric ulcers and **1**:122; **11**:1479
heart attacks and **6**:785; **11**:1478
interaction with warfarin **14**:*1957–1958*
overdose **4**:562; **11**:1460; **12**:1629
Reye's syndrome and **5**:641; **11**:1478, 1479; **13**:*1813–1814*
side effects **14**:1959
stomach irritation **7**:1002
stroke prevention **15**:2111; **16**:*2261*, 2262
treatment for arthritis **1**:122
treatment for stiffness **15**:2079
see also painkillers
assertiveness training **15**:2104
assisted living programs **6**:841
atropine
as a medication **7**:1004; **12**:1670
allergy to **12**:1670
autogenic training **2**:183
autografts **5**:709, 710
aversion therapy **2**:176, 177; **7**:969
emetics and **4**:562
Awareness Through Movement (ATM) **5**:*630*, 631, 632
ayurvedic medicine **1**:75, 79, 80
azathioprine **4**:443
AZT **2**:230

Bach flower remedies **1**:79
bandages *see* dressings and bandages
barbiturates **2**:170; **4**:527; **7**:892–893; **14**:1903, 1904
abuse **4**:525, 526
overdose **2**:170; **3**:395
withdrawal **5**:583; **17**:2417, 2418
behavior therapy **2**:176–177; **10**:1358; **11**:1482, 1541; **12**:*1712*, 1714–1715; **13**:*1734–1736*

bentonite **9**:1273
benzodiazepines **7**:892, 893; **14**:1903, 1904, 1905, 1978; **16**:2256–2257, *2258*
see also chlordiazepoxide; diazepam; nitrazepam
benzoyl peroxide **1**:33
beta-blockers **2**:158
effect on blood pressure **2**:239
side effects **14**:1959
in asthmatics **3**:419
sedative action **14**:1904
as tranquilizers **16**:2257
treatment for angina **3**:420
bicalutamide (Casodex) **12**:1694–1695
bicarbonate of soda **7**:929
bill of rights, a patient's **7**:873
bioenergetics **9**:*1222*; **13**:1735
biomedical engineering **2**:189–190
see also kidney dialysis; pacemaker; prostheses
bionics **2**:191
birth, cesarean **2**:204–205; **3**:340–342; **7**:931, 932
bisacodyl, suppositories **15**:2133
blepharoplasty **17**:2427
blood donors **2**:231–232; **6**:810; **7**:977, 990; **12**:1611
blood transfusions **2**:240–241; **6**:806; **7**:970
before transplant surgery **16**:2265
blood groups and **2**:234, *240*, *241*
rh factor **2**:233; **13**:1815
exchange transfusions **2**:240; **7**:992
malaria and **11**:1500
plasma **12**:1611; **13**:1867
body wraps, marine algae **6**:776
bone marrow *see* marrow
borage **6**:*814*
botox injections **17**:2428
BR-16A **14**:1989
braces **15**:2048
dental
invisible **10**:*1428*
sports injuries and **15**:2050
brachytherapy **10**:1400; **12**:*1693*
brain surgery **2**:271; **8**:1092; **10**:1354, *1355*, 1356; **15**:*2134*
psychosurgery **12**:1715
bridges, dental **4**:*463*
bromides **14**:1903
bromocriptine **12**:1601
Brompton cocktail **6**:861
bronchodilators, as drugs **1**:74, 139, 141; **7**:953, 953–954
Broselow tape **4**:560
bupivacaine **1**:92; **8**:1092
burn center **3**:301–302
buspirone (BuSpar) **16**:2257–2258
bypass surgery **3**:346, 420–421; **10**:*1402*, 1403; **17**:2357
see also open-heart surgery

calamine lotion **7**:987
calcitonin **3**:311
cannulas **17**:2357
nasal **11**:1464
Captopril **9**:*1170–1171*
cardiac massage **1**:*134*, 135; **3**:320–321; **4**:555
cardiac monitors **13**:*1807*, 1808
cardiopulmonary resuscitation *see* CPR
cascara **8**:1046
Casodex (bicalutamide) **12**:1694–1695
castor oil **8**:1045–1046
casts
plaster **10**:*1430*; **11**:1580; **15**:*2048*

limping after removal 8:1076
physical therapy after removal 8:1076
cayenne (chili pepper) 6:812–813
cephalosporins 1:100
cesarean birth 2:204–205; 3:340–342; 7:931, 932
preeclampsia and 12:1659
chelation therapy 3:345–346
chemical dependency units 4:528
chemosurgery 3:424
chemotherapy 3:314, 316–317; 10:1400; 13:1775
for leukemia 8:1061
resistance to 3:312
side effects 3:317; 8:1145; 9:1145
Chinese medicine 3:358–361
cupping 6:835
dietary therapy 3:358, 361
herbal medicine 1:80; 3:359–360
qigong exercises 1:81; 3:358, 360–361
see also acupressure; acupuncture
chiropractic 1:77–78; 3:362–364; 6:836; 11:1446
chives 6:813
chloral hydrate 7:892, 893
chloramphenicol 16:2295, 2297
chlordiazepoxide (Librium) 14:1903, 1904; 16:2257
chlorofluoroquine 8:1123
chlorpromazine (Largactil) 11:1565; 13:1738; 15:2126; 16:2256
cholecystectomy (gallbladder removal) 2:179, 180; 5:667; 6:764; 9:1236
cimetidine 11:1486
cinchona bark 13:1765
ciprofloxacin 16:2295, 2297–2298
Clinical Risk Index for Babies (CRIB) 10:1338
clonidine 2:152; 6:824; 16:2259
cloning 3:377–378
humans 3:378; 9:1166
clotrimazole 16:2220
codeine 1:137, 138; 9:1250; 10:1319; 11:1479–1480
cognitive enhancers see smart drugs
cognitive reappraisal 15:2104
cognitive therapies 13:1734–1736
cold therapy 11:1579
collars, cervical 10:1334, 1430
colonic irrigation (colonic hydrotherapy; colonic lavage) 3:384–385
color therapy 3:390–391
colostomy 3:392–393; 5:644; 13:1787, 1788
complementary medicine and therapies 1:76; 16:2206
see also alternative medicine
compresses
cold 15:2056
hot 13:1757
for sties 15:2113
see also poultices
conception
artificial methods of 1:129–131
in vitro fertilization (IVF) 1:129, 131; 7:971–974; 11:1520
conditioning, operant 2:177
contact lenses 3:403, 406; 10:1417
astigmatism and 1:142
convalescence 3:412
cordotomy 11:1481
corticosteroids 1:74
injections 13:1804
the skin and 12:1706
cortisone 1:74

cough syrup 3:426, 427
see also expectorants
counseling 3:428–430; 12:1712; 13:1733, 1735
drug counseling 4:528–529
genetic 5:683, 684, 686; 6:749
for blood relatives 7:921, 922
CPR (cardiopulmonary resuscitation) 1:134, 135; 3:320, 321; 13:1807, 1808, 1809, 1810
cranioplasty (skull replacement) 10:1354, 1355, 1356
crash teams 13:1807–1808, 1810
creative therapies 13:1735
CRIB (Clinical Risk Index for Babies) 10:1338
cricothyroidotomy 16:2251, 2252
critical care unit (CCU) 4:440–441
see also intensive care unit
crowns, dental 4:462, 463
crystal therapy 1:80
cupping 1:80, 81; 6:835
cyclosporine 7:913; 8:1022, 1024; 16:2265
adverse effects 7:914
Cylert 2:152

D & C see dilatation and curettage
D & E (dilatation and evacuation) 1:16
Dacron 5:709, 711
dance therapy 9:1230, 1231–1233
danthron, suppositories 15:2133
decongestants, nasal drops 1:40
deep heat lotions 6:797
defibrillators 13:1807, 1808; 17:2360
Demerol 1:137
dental care 4:460–461; 6:740
anesthetics 1:92–93; 8:1092; 10:1378
avoiding plaque 4:461; 12:1610
during pregnancy 12:1676
fluoride 4:461; 5:651–652; 12:1636; 16:2176
gums and gum diseases 4:461, 462; 6:730–731
heart murmurs and 9:1287
orthodontics 10:1425–1429; 16:2175, 2177
while wearing orthodontic appliances 10:1425, 1426
dentures, crowns, and bridges 4:462–463
dentures 4:462–463; 8:1149; 9:1149; 13:1760
dermabrasion (chemical abrasion) 1:31; 3:424; 17:2428
for tattoo removal 16:2172, 2173
Dermagraft 2:190
desensitization 1:74; 6:757; 14:1912
systematic 2:177; 3:398
desferrioxamine 15:2093
Desipramine 2:152
Detoxamin 3:346
Dexedrine 2:152
dextromethorphan 10:1319
dialysis, kidney see kidney dialysis
diathermy, shortwave 11:1579
diazepam (Valium) 7:893; 14:1903, 1904; 16:2257
dichloralphenazone 7:893
diet pills 1:85; 4:493, 524
digitalis 14:1957, 1958
digoxin 14:1957, 1958; 15:2083
dilatation and curettage (D & C) 4:496; 5:642; 9:1202; 17:2329
dilatation and evacuation (D & E) 1:16
dilaudid 1:137
dill water 6:813
dimercaprol 3:346

dimethylaminoethanol (DMAE) 14:1989
diphenhydramine 7:893
dipyramidol 16:2262
disodium cromoglycate 1:74; 7:954; 14:2003
dispensers 11:1551
diuretics 4:500
for high blood pressure 2:239
for premenstrual syndrome 12:1674
side effects 14:1959
DMPS chelation 3:345, 346
DMSA chelation 3:345, 346
doctors
choosing 6:766
emergency-room 4:561
finding 6:766
Dolly (sheep) 3:377
donors 4:503–504; 6:791; 16:2264–2265
blood 2:231–232; 6:810; 7:977, 990; 12:1611
bone marrow 8:1139, 1140; 9:1139, 1140
kidney 8:1017, 1022, 1023–1024
doxapram 15:2085
doxycycline 6:787
dressings and bandages 4:513–520; 17:2425
bandages 1:17; 4:516–520
allergies to 4:513, 516
when not to bandage 4:520
dressings 1:17; 4:513–515, 516
drug compliance 11:1552
drug counseling 4:528–529
drugs
acetylation 14:1958–1959
affecting the autonomic nervous system 2:156
allergies to 9:1174; 14:1959
penicillin 1:70, 99, 100; 11:1527, 1528, 1529; 14:1959; 16:2199
antacid 4:531
anticonvulsants 5:585
antidepressant see antidepressants
anti-inflammatory 4:468
antiviral 17:2369
see also aciclovir
the blood-brain barrier and 2:229–230
central nervous stimulant (CNS) 13:1737
delivered via transdermal patches 16:2259–2260
dispensing 11:1553
dosage 14:1957–1958
first-pass metabolism 16:2260
health risks associated with 13:1840
hypnotic 7:892–893, 959
see also sedatives; sleeping pills
immunosuppressive see immunosuppressive drugs
interaction with other drugs 14:1957–1958
manufacture 11:1550–1553, 1554
names of medications 11:1550, 1551
new
development 11:1552, 1554
medical research and 9:1170–1172
side effects and 14:1956
nonsteroidal anti-inflammatory (NSAIDs) 6:787; 10:1369–1370; 11:1482
see also aspirin and analgesics
overdose 11:1460–1462
acetaminophen 11:1479; 12:1629
amphetamine 1:87
aspirin 4:562; 11:1460; 12:1629

barbiturate 2:170; 3:395
coma and 3:395
suicide and 15:2124
teenage "suicidal gestures" 12:1630
tranquilizers 16:2256, 2257
treatment 2:170; 6:824; 11:1462, 1479; 15:2091–2093
photosensitizing 11:1565; 15:2126
psychotropic 13:1737–1738
smart 14:1989
taken as suppositories 15:2132–2133
testing 11:1552, 1554
see also antibiotics; medicines; pharmacy; side effects

ECT see electroconvulsive therapy
EDTA 3:345–346
effleurage 8:1142–1143; 9:1142–1143
electric shock therapy see electroconvulsive therapy
electroconvulsive therapy (ECT; electric shock therapy; electrotherapy) 4:466; 9:1209; 10:1354; 11:1578, 1579; 12:1712, 1715; 14:1884
electrolysis 4:553
electromyographs (EMGs) 2:181, 183
electrosurgery 12:1628
electrotherapy see electroconvulsive therapy
emergencies 4:555–556
emergency department 4:440, 557–561; 11:1456
see also trauma center
emergency medical technicians (EMTs) 4:561
emetics 4:562; 15:2092–2093
endotracheal tubes 13:1805
enemas 3:384; 4:572
barium 4:478, 572; 15:2096
ephedra 6:813
ephedrines 4:493; 6:813
epidural injections 1:92
for cesarean births 3:342
for labor 1:93; 2:201, 285; 8:1093; 15:2041
episiotomy 2:203, 285; 5:586; 8:1030; 10:1322, 1324
Epley maneuver 17:2366
Epsom salts 8:1046
ergotamines 9:1224
esophageal obturator airway 13:1808–1810
Estraderm 16:2260
ethyl chloride 13:1747
evacuation of retained products of conception (ERPC) 17:2338
existential therapy 13:1735
expectorants 3:426; 5:603
see also cough syrup
eye pads 4:515

face-lifts (rhytidectomy) 3:424, 425; 12:1612; 17:2428
face-and-neck lift 12:1615
scars 14:1880
face masks 9:1270, 1272
faith healing 5:613–614; 12:1603
fasting 10:1327
fecal softeners 8:1046
Feldenkrais method 5:629–632
fennel 6:812; 10:1329
Fentanyl 12:1670; 16:2259, 2260
fertility drugs 7:972, 974
multiple births and 7:942; 9:1274, 1275
FES (functional electrical stimulation) 2:191

feverfew 9:1222
first aid 10:1393
  after a traffic or other accident
    4:556
  bites and stings 2:210, 211; 4:556
  bleeding/hemorrhaging (external)
    6:804; 16:2246; 17:2422
  burns 3:304; 4:556; 10:1393
    chemical 10:1393
  chemicals in the eye 10:1393
  choking 1:132, 135; 16:2212, 2252
  common emergencies and their
    treatment 4:556
  convulsions 3:413
  CPR (cardiopulmonary
    resuscitation) 1:134, 135; 3:320,
    321; 13:1807, 1808, 1809, 1810
  drowning 4:521, 522, 556
  elbow injuries 4:546
  electric shock 4:549, 556; 10:1393
  fevers 5:641
  foreign body in the eye 5:606;
    10:1393, 1406; 15:2047
  fractures 4:556; 5:663; 10:1393
  frostbite 5:666
  gas inhalation 4:556; 10:1393
  heart attack 6:784
  the home medicine chest
    9:1175–1177
  lacerations 8:1031
  minor injuries 1:18
  multiple injuries 17:2426
  nosebleeds 10:1374
  poisoning 4:556
  rabies 13:1769
  requirements for overseas travel
    16:2272
  shock 14:1947
  sports injuries 1:50
  sprained ankle 15:2057
  sties 15:2111, 2113
  suffocation 15:2119
  for suspected drug overdose 6:824;
    11:1462
  tongue, swallowing the 15:2118;
    16:2232
  vomiting 17:2390, 2391
  see also dressings and bandages
flotation therapy 5:648–650
flucloxacillin 11:1528
fluconazole 16:2220
fluoxetine see Prozac
functional electrical stimulation (FES)
    2:191
Functional Integration 5:631–632

gamma rays, radiotherapy and
    13:1773–1774, 1775
gargling, for a sore throat 14:2010,
    2013; 16:2213
garlic 6:814, 815; 10:1329
gastrectomy, partial 17:2314
gastric lavage see stomach pump
gastroenterostomy 17:2314
gene therapy 5:677, 679
  cancer treatment 10:1400
  germ-line 5:679
  somatic 5:679–680
Gestalt therapy 5:695–696; 13:1735
ginger 10:1329
gingivectomy 13:1759, 1761
gingko biloba 14:1989
glasses 5:604; 10:1412, 1413
glycerol, suppositories 15:2132, 2133
glyceryl trinitrate 16:2259
goat's rue 6:813
"golden hour" 4:560
gold injections 13:1820, 1821, 1823

grafting 5:709–711
  blood vessels 5:711; 10:1403
  bone 5:709, 711; 10:1430, 1432
  cartilage 5:711
  corneal 3:416; 4:504; 5:710, 711;
    10:1407
    passing on rabies 13:1766
  graft-versus-host (GVH) disease
    and 5:677
  hair 5:709; 6:739
  heart valves 5:711
  rejection and 5:710
  skin 5:709, 710–711; 9:1221; 12:1612,
    1615–1616
    after burns 3:302, 304
  tendons 5:711
  see also bypass surgery; transplants
Granuflex 4:515
grommets 4:456
group therapy 5:713–714; 13:1736

haptics 16:2180
healing 6:764–765
health care system 6:766–767
  home care 6:839–841
  managed care 8:1133–1134
  see also hospice care; hospitals
health spas 3:412; 6:774–776
hearing aids 6:779–780; 9:1194
heart transplants 4:504; 6:791–794;
    10:1422; 16:2263, 2264, 2266
    repeated 16:2263
heat treatment 6:797–799
  for abscesses 6:797, 799; 13:1757
  for stiffness 15:2076, 2079
Heimlich maneuver 1:132; 15:2119
Hellerwork 13:1846, 1847, 1848
hemodialysis 8:1014–1015
heparin 8:1015
herbs and herbalism 1:78; 6:812–815,
    837
  Chinese herbal medicine 1:80;
    3:359–360
  fragrant herbs 14:1991, 1993, 1994
  for migraines 9:1222
  naturopathy and 10:1327, 1329
holistic medicine 6:835–838; 17:2403,
    2404
  herbalism and 6:815
  homeopathy and 6:843–844
  see also alternative medicine
home care 6:839–841
homeopathy 1:78; 6:837, 842–845;
    10:1326
hormone replacement therapy (HRT)
    2:260; 4:566; 5:594; 6:733,
    854–856
  osteoporosis and 2:260; 6:855, 856;
    9:1199; 11:1450, 1451
  the risk of breast cancer and 6:856;
    7:875
  skin patches 16:2259, 2260
hospice care 6:841, 860–861; 7:872,
    959
hospitals 6:767; 7:870–873
  children in 7:870, 871; 11:1516–1517,
    1518
  coronary care units 6:785
  crash teams 13:1807–1808, 1810
  day 11:1457
  emergency department 4:440,
    557–561; 11:1456
    see also trauma center
  occupational therapists 10:1398
  operating room 10:1404–1406
  outpatients 11:1454–1457
  patients as part of studies in
    9:1170

  see also hospice care; intensive care
    unit
human potential therapies 13:1734
Humulin 5:679
hydergine 14:1989
hydrocortisone 4:467, 468
  for eczema 4:543
  for joint pain and stiffness 15:2078,
    2079
  suppositories 15:2133
hydroquinone 8:1090, 1091
hydrotherapy 6:799; 7:881–883;
    10:1328; 11:1579; 13:1795; 16:2206
hydroxychloroquine 8:1107
hyoscine 9:1255
hypnosis 7:890–891; 9:1229
hypnotherapy 1:79; 6:837; 12:1712;
    13:1735, 1736
hypnotic drugs 7:892–893, 959
  see also sedatives; sleeping pills
hysterectomy 7:903–905, 906; 10:1421
  abortion and 1:16
  cystitis and 4:450
  endometriosis and 4:568, 569; 7:905
  fibroids and 5:642; 7:905
  Pap smears after 11:1488
  sex life after 6:732
  for sterilization 7:905; 15:2069, 2071

ibuprofen 1:138; 6:787; 10:1369
ice therapy 13:1804; 15:2051
imidazopyridine derivatives 7:893
Imipramine 2:152; 13:1738
immunosuppressive drugs 7:913–914
  after transplant surgery 6:794;
    7:913, 914; 8:1022, 1024, 1139;
    9:1139
  to treat autoimmune disorders
    7:914; 8:1113
immunotherapy 10:1400
incubators 10:1337; 11:1517; 12:1667, 1668
indomethacin 1:138
induction of labor 2:201; 7:931–934;
    10:1322
  in the case of stillbirth 15:2082
inhalants 7:953–954
inhalers 7:954; 13:1750
injections 7:955–956
insight-oriented therapy 10:1358
integrative therapies 1:76
Integra TM 3:301
intensive care unit 7:961–962; 12:1646
  neonatal 7:962; 10:1336–1338;
    11:1516; 12:1667, 1669
  physical therapy in 11:1581
  respirators 13:1806
  thermistors 16:2184
  see also critical care unit
intensivists 4:441
interferon 7:927
  cancer and 3:312
intracytoplasmic sperm
    injection/transfer (ICSI/T) 1:130,
    131; 7:974
intravenous infusions (IVs) 7:970;
    12:1646
in vitro fertilization (IVF) 1:129, 131;
    7:971–974; 11:1520
iodine 10:1334
  radioactive (radioiodine) 13:1774;
    16:2223
iontophoresis 4:470
ipecac syrup 4:562
iproniazid 13:1738
iridology 1:80–81; 7:975–976
iron lungs 13:1805
irradiation (body), whole-body, and
    bone marrow transplants 3:317

irradiation (food) 7:979
isometrics 5:602, 664; 7:984–986
IVF see in vitro fertilization

joints, replacement 7:998–999

kaolin 7:1004
  kaolin and morphine 7:1004; 9:1250,
    1251
  kaolin and pectin 7:1004; 9:1177
kidney dialysis 2:190; 5:598;
    8:1014–1016, 1020; 17:2322
  treatment for poisoning 12:1632
kidney transplants 4:503, 504;
    8:1022–1024; 16:2263, 2264–2266
  ultrasound and 17:2315
kinesiology 1:81; 6:836
kiss of life see artificial respiration

LAAM (L-alpha acetyl methadol) 6:824
labor, induced see induction of labor
lactulose 8:1046
L-alpha acetyl methadol (LAAM) 6:824
laminectomy 14:1886, 1984, 1985
Largactil see chlorpromazine
laryngectomy 17:2389
lasers 8:1040–1042
  acne treatment 1:34
  argon 8:1041
  carbon dioxide (laser knife) 8:1042
  eye treatment
    the cornea and see LASIK surgery
    diabetic 8:1040, 1041, 1042
    the retina and 2:221; 8:1041, 1042
  tattoo removal 16:2173
LASIK surgery 8:1043–1044
laughter therapy 9:1232, 1233
lavage, gastric see stomach pump
laxatives 3:404, 405; 4:572; 5:598;
    8:1045–1046
  abuse 8:1045
laying on of hands 5:613, 614
L-dopa 11:1506, 1507
lemon balm 10:1329
Librium (chlordiazepoxide) 14:1903,
    1904; 16:2257
lidocaine 1:92; 8:1092
life, prolonging, ethics of 9:1166–1167
life-support systems 2:266
  coma and 3:395
  turned off 3:394; 5:595; 9:1167
    organ donation and 4:503
ligatures 15:2137
light therapy (phototherapy)
  for jaundice 7:991; 11:1581; 12:1669
  for seasonal affective disorder
    14:1898, 1899
lignocaine 15:2078
linear accelerators 8:1115
linopirdine 14:1989
lipectomy 3:424, 425
liposuction 3:424, 425; 8:1079–1080;
    12:1615
lithium 4:466; 12:1720; 13:1738
  lithium carbonate 2:199
lithotripsy 8:1020, 1021
lobotomy, prefontal 12:1715
local anesthetics 1:92; 8:1092–1093;
    10:1378; 15:2135
  for fingers 10:1378
  topical 8:1092
lozenges, throat 14:2010, 2013
lumpectomy 8:1098–1099, 1147, 1172;
    11:1513
  see also mastectomy

macrolides 1:100
magnesium sulfate 8:1046

ma-huang **14**:1989
malathion **8**:1065
malaxone **1**:138
managed care **8**:1133–1134
manipulation **8**:1135–1136; **11**:1578–1579
  chiropractic **3**:364
  see also massage; physical therapy
marjoram **6**:*815*
marrow and transplants **2**:258;
    8:1139–1140
  marrow
    diseases **8**:1139–1140; **13**:1755
    and red blood cells **2**:*226*, 227
    samples taken **8**:*1061*; **11**:1514,
      1536
    stem cells **15**:2065
    transplants (grafting) **3**:317; **4**:*504*;
      5:711; **8**:1139, *1140*
massage **1**:79–80; **8**:1141–1144
  aromatherapy **1**:115, 117;
    14:*1936*
  around joints **3**:363
  cardiac **1**:*134*, 135; **3**:320–321; **4**:555
  Chinese (tui na) **3**:360, 361
  facial **1**:*35*; **8**:1141; **9**:1141; **14**:*1936*
  foot **5**:625; **8**:1141, *1143*; **9**:1141, *1143*
  neck **10**:*1334*
  osteopathy and **11**:1447, *1448*
  for pulled muscles **13**:1747
  reflexology **1**:*78*, 80; **6**:837; **8**:*1143*;
    13:1793–1794
  rolfing **13**:1846, 1847, *1848*
  scalp **6**:*739*
  self-massage **9**:1233
  shiatsu **1**:80; **6**:776; **8**:*1144*;
    14:*1936*–1937
  to relieve stiffness **15**:2078, *2079*
  to treat sprains **15**:2056
  see also acupressure; manipulation
mastectomy **8**:1112, **1145**–1148, 1172
  breast implants following **8**:*1145*;
    10:1421; **12**:1614, 1698
  external prostheses following
    12:1698, *1699*
  see also lumpectomy
mastoidectomy **9**:1161
mastoplexy **3**:424
mechanical percutaneous myocardial
    revascularization (MPMR)
    10:1403
medicines **9**:1173–1177
  cough
    cough syrup **3**:426, **427**
    expectorants **3**:426; **5**:**603**
  cure-all **11**:1552
  homeopathic **6**:843–844
  names of medications **11**:1550, 1551
  overdose **11**:1460–1462
  over-the-counter **11**:1460
  reactions to medications **11**:1550
  reducing risk of poisoning from
    12:1629
  see also drugs; pharmacy
Medline **9**:1168, 1169
melatonin, medication **7**:994; **9**:1186,
    1187
menthol **13**:1825
meperidine hydrochloride **10**:1319, 1320
metamorphic technique **13**:1794
methadone **6**:824; **10**:1320; **17**:2418
methicillin **1**:98
methyldopa **15**:2045
methyl prednisolone **7**:914
metronidazole (Flagyl) **16**:2279;
    17:2337–2338
microscopes, operating **9**:*1218*, 1219
microsurgery **5**:709; **9**:1218–1221;
    10:1434; **15**:2139

mifepristone **1**:14
mind-body therapy **9**:1230–1233
minimally-invasive
    (keyhole/laparoscopic) surgery
    6:764; **9**:1236–1237; **15**:*2138*, 2139
  telesurgery and **16**:2180
minoxidil (Rogaine) **2**:169; **14**:1969
Mogadon (nitrazepam) **16**:2257
monoamine oxidase inhibitors
    (MAOIs) **4**:466
morphine **1**:138; **6**:*822*, 861;
    9:1250–1251; **10**:1319; **11**:1480
  kaolin and morphine **7**:1004; **9**:1250,
    1251
  side effects **14**:1959
  withdrawal **6**:823; **17**:2417–2418
moxibustion **1**:*39*; **3**:359
mucolytics **5**:603
mud therapy **9**:1270–1273
myomectomy **5**:642

naloxone **6**:824
naproxen **11**:1479
nasal drops, decongestant **1**:40
nasal spray or drops **13**:1825; **14**:2002
nasogastric tubes **15**:2134
natural healing **5**:614
naturopathy **1**:81; **10**:1326–1329
neonatal intensive care unit **7**:962;
    10:1336–1338; **11**:1516; **12**:1667,
    1669
nephrectomy **10**:1339
nerve block procedures **8**:*1093*
nettle **6**:*814*
nitrazepam (Mogadon) **16**:2257
nitroglycerine, skin patches **16**:2260
nitroimidazoles **1**:100
nonsteroidal anti-inflammatory drugs
    (NSAIDs) **6**:787; **10**:1369–1370;
    11:1482
  interactions with other drugs
    10:1370
  see also aspirin and analgesics
novocaine **15**:2078
NSAIDS see nonsteroidal anti-
    inflammatory drugs
nuclear cell transfer **3**:377, 378
nuclear medicine **2**:190
nurses **7**:871
  emergency **4**:561
  home-care **6**:840
  postoperative care by **12**:1644–1645
  psychiatric **12**:1712
nursing
  barrier **7**:*982*, 983
  reverse barrier **7**:*982*, 983

occupational therapy **6**:839;
    10:1397–1398; **12**:1715; **13**:1796,
    1797–1798
  see also physical therapy
oils, essential *see* aromatherapy
open-heart surgery **10**:1401–1403
  see also bypass surgery
operating room **10**:1404–1406
operations *see* surgery
opiates **1**:137–138
opioids **10**:1320; **11**:1481–1482
orchiopexy **16**:2192
organ removal **10**:1421–1422
orlistat **10**:1385
osteopathy **1**:*78*; **2**:161; **3**:362; **6**:837;
    11:1446–1449
  cranial **11**:*1447*, 1449
osteotomy **10**:1438; **12**:1594
outpatients **11**:1454–1457
oxygen chambers, hyperbaric **3**:302;
    11:1465, *1467*

oxygen cylinders **11**:1467
oxygen masks **11**:*1463*, 1464, *1466*
oxygen tents **11**:1467
oxygen therapy **11**:1464–1465,
    1466–1467
oxytetracycline **15**:2126

pacemaker **11**:1472–1473
  artificial **2**:*190*; **3**:*421*; **11**:*1472*–1473
    failure **11**:1472
    replacing **6**:788
  natural (sinoatrial node) **6**:*782*;
    9:1267; **11**:1472
painkillers **1**:*137–138*; **11**:1478–1480,
    1481–1482
  see also acetaminophen; aspirin
    analgesics; codeine; ibuprofen;
    morphine and
pain management **11**:1481–1482
  acupuncture **1**:38; **11**:1478
  cold therapy **11**:1579
  electrical stimulation **11**:1481, 1579
    transcutaneous electrical nerve
      stimulation (TENS) **11**:1482, 1579
  flotation therapy **5**:649
  in hospices **6**:861
  pain clinics **11**:1482
  painkillers (analgesics) **1**:*137–138*;
    11:1478–1480, *1481–1482*
    see also acetaminophen; aspirin
      and analgesics; codeine;
      ibuprofen; morphine
  skin patches **16**:2260
  surgery **11**:1481
  ultrasound **11**:1579, *1580*
  wax treatment **11**:1579
palatoplasty **14**:*2005*
palliative care **7**:961
papaverine **10**:1319
paraffin, liquid **8**:1046
paramedics **4**:561
penicillamine **13**:1823
penicillin **1**:*99*, 100; **10**:1304;
    11:1527–1529
  allergy to **1**:70, 99, 100; **11**:1527, 1528,
    1529; **14**:1959; **16**:2199
  semi-synthetic **11**:1528
  sensitization to **14**:1912
pentobarbital **7**:893
pentothal (thiopental) **2**:170
peppermint **6**:812, *813*; **10**:1329
"pep pills" **1**:86
pessaries, ring **12**:1686
petrissage **8**:*1142*, 1143; **9**:*1142*, 1143
pharmaceutical companies
    11:1550–1553
pharmacists **11**:1551, *1552*
pharmacology **11**:1551, 1554
pharmacy **11**:1550–1554
  see also drugs; medicines
Phenacetin **1**:137; **8**:1020
phenobarbital **2**:170; **7**:893
phenothiazines **14**:1903
phenylbutazone **1**:138
photocoagulation **8**:1041
phototherapy *see* light therapy
physical therapy **11**:1578–1581;
    13:1797–1798; **16**:2205, 2206
  after surgery **13**:1795
  hydrotherapy **6**:799; **7**:881–883;
    10:1328; **11**:1579; **13**:1795; **16**:2206
  for stroke victims **11**:1580; **15**:2107,
    2110
  see also manipulation; occupational
    therapy
physician assistants (PAs) **4**:561
Pinel, Philippe **12**:*1722*
pin and plate operation **10**:*1431*, 1433

piracetam **14**:1989
placebo effect **12**:1602–1603
  ethical use of placebos **9**:1167
  tonics and **15**:2083; **16**:2231
plants
  as medicines **1**:114
    see also herbs and herbalism
  a source of starch **15**:2063
plasma exchange **6**:729
plasmapheresis **12**:1611
plaster casts *see* casts, plaster
plastic and reconstructive surgery
    12:1612–1617
PMS Escape **12**:*1674*
podophyllum **17**:2397
polymerase chain reaction (PCR)
    3:377–378
postoperative care **12**:1644–1647
postural drainage **3**:295; **11**:1580–1581
potassium chloride **6**:787
poultices
  bread and starch **15**:2063
  see also compresses, hot
practolol **14**:1956, *1957*
prednisolone **7**:914
prednisone **4**:442
premedication **1**:*91*, 93; **12**:1670; **14**:1902
prenatal care **12**:1665, 1675–1679, 1680
  dangers of smoking **5**:638; **10**:1361;
    12:1604, 1665
  dental care **12**:1676
  diet **2**:206; **3**:402; **4**:491; **8**:1127, 1128;
    10:1379; **12**:1662, 1665, 1675, 1678
    to avoid listeriosis **8**:1083
  exercise **5**:601, 634; **12**:1665
  exercises(s) **11**:1570; **12**:1665, *1677*,
    1678–1679
  nipples **12**:1675
  obstetricians and **10**:1389–1390
  posture **12**:1656, *1677*, 1678
  prenatal clinics **6**:769, 770
  routine checkups and tests **6**:749;
    12:*1659*, 1660, 1663–1664, 1676
  to avoid preeclampsia **12**:1660
  vitamin or mineral supplements
    5:638; **12**:1675
    folic acid **2**:206; **3**:401; **5**:638, 682;
      10:1351; **15**:2037, 2039; **17**:2377
    iron **12**:1675
  weight gain **12**:1665
prescribers **11**:1551
prescriptions **11**:1552, *1553*, 1554
primal therapies **13**:1735
promethazine **7**:893
prostheses **12**:1696–1700
  breast
    external **8**:1145, 1146, *1148*; **9**:1145,
      1146, *1148*; **12**:1698, *1699*, 1700
    internal (implants) **8**:*1145*; **9**:*1145*;
      10:1421; **12**:1614, 1615, *1616*, 1698,
      1700
  earbones **12**:1696, *1699*, 1700
  joint replacement **7**:998–999;
    12:1698–1699
    hips **1**:122; **2**:189; **6**:829, 830;
      7:998, *999*, 1000; **10**:*1438*;
      12:1696, 1699
    knees **7**:998, *999*; **10**:1430
  male genitalia **12**:1700
  see also artificial limbs
protein C, activated **14**:1915
proton pump inhibitors **4**:531; **6**:787
Prozac **4**:466; **13**:1737, 1738; **16**:2258
psychic healing **5**:614
psychoanalysts **12**:1712
psychoanalytic therapies **13**:1735
psychodrama **12**:1715; **13**:1735
psycho-oncology **10**:1399

psychosurgery 12:1715
psychosynthesis 13:1735
psychotherapy 3:428; 9:1228; 11:1541;
    12:1712, 1714; 13:1733–1736; 16:2206
    formal 12:1714
    Gestalt therapy 5:695–696; 13:1735
    insight-directed 12:1714
    the subconscious and 15:2114, 2115
    supportive-expressive 4:529
    to treat phobias 11:1563
    see also behavior therapy; hypnosis
psychotropic drugs 13:1737–1738
Pudenz-Heyer shunt 7:880
Putti-Platt operation 4:498
pyloroplasty 17:2314
pyridostigmine 10:1313

quinalbarbital 2:170
quinidine 13:1765
quinine 4:437; 8:1123; 13:1764–1765
    deafness and 4:455, 502
quinolones 1:100

radiation therapy see radiotherapy
radiopharmaceuticals 2:190
    radioiodine 13:1774; 16:2223
radiotherapy 3:314, 315–316; 10:1400;
    13:1772–1776; 17:2435
    for lymphoma 8:1115
    in outpatients departments 11:1457
    as palliative treatment 13:1776
    postsurgery treatment using
        13:1776
    radioactive implants 3:316; 10:1400;
        12:1693; 13:1774
    side effects 13:1770–1771, 1776
ranitidine 6:786
rebirthing 13:1735
recovery position 1:134
recovery rooms 12:1644–1645
reflexology 1:78, 80; 6:837; 8:1143;
    13:1793–1794
rehabilitation 13:1795–1799
reiki 1:81
renodialysis machines 8:1014–1015,
    1016
reserpine 2:198
respirators 13:1805–1806
restricted environmental stimulation
    therapy (REST) 5:648
resuscitation 13:1807–1810
    after drowning 4:521, 522
    cardiopulmonary (CPR) 1:134, 135;
        3:320, 321; 13:1807, 1808, 1809,
        1810
    mouth-to-mouth see artificial
        respiration
retinoids 1:33
retinoscopes 10:1413
rhinoplasty (changing shape of the
    nose) 3:424, 425; 12:1613
rhytidectomy 3:424
rhytidectomy see face-lifts
RICE (mnemonic) 1:50; 15:2051
rifampin 1:99
rights, patient's bill of 7:873
ring pads 4:519
Ritalin 2:152; 13:1738
Rogaine (minoxidil) 2:169; 14:1969
rolfing 8:1144; 9:1144; 13:1846–1848
rosemary 10:1329

salazopyrin 3:383
salicylic acid 6:813; 17:2362–2363
salt gargle 16:2213
scalpels 15:2137–2138
sclerotherapy 3:424
scopolamine 12:1670

secobarbital 7:893
sedatives 14:1902–1905
    causing drowsiness 7:892
    dangerous mixed with alcohol
        7:892
    premedication 1:91, 93; 12:1670;
        14:1902
    see also antidepressants;
        antipsychotic drugs; sleeping
        pills
selective serotonin reuptake inhibitors
    see SSRIs
self-healing 5:614
self-massage 9:1233
senna 5:598; 8:1045–1046
sensate focusing 14:1925
sensitization, covert 2:177
sex therapy 16:2206
sheep
    cloning 3:377
    transgenic 5:681
shiatsu 1:80; 6:776; 8:1144;
    14:1936–1937
Shirodkar operation 3:338
sibutramine 10:1385
side effects 11:1554; 14:1956–1959
    of antibiotics 1:100; 14:1959; 17:2364
sign language 10:1307, 1308
sildenafil (Viagara) 7:963; 14:1928
skin patch see transdermal patch
sleeping pills 5:620; 7:958, 959;
    14:1980
    children and 7:892
    dangerous on long flights 7:993
    dangerous mixed with alcohol
        7:892
    disadvantages 7:892, 957; 14:1978
    drowsiness and 4:523; 8:1057
    overdose, treatment 11:1462
    postoperative 3:412
    used for anxiety 1:104
slings 4:516, 519
smart drugs 14:1989
smelling salts 5:601
sodium bicarbonate 5:645
sodium cromoglycate 4:543; 6:757
sound therapy 9:1231
spas 9:1272
special-care baby unit see neonatal
    intensive care unit
speculum 6:734; 11:1488–1489; 15:2027
speech therapy 10:1309; 13:1798;
    15:2032–2033; 16:2206
    for aphasia 1:107, 108; 15:2110
spinal fusion 7:1002
spiritual healing 5:614
Spitz-Holter shunt 7:880
splints 15:2048–2049
    inflatable 15:2048
    joint, for rheumatoid arthritis
        13:1822
sports medicine 15:2052–2055
    biofeedback 2:181
springs, thermal 9:1272–1273
SSRIs (selective serotonin reuptake
    inhibitors) 4:466; 13:1738
    see also Prozac
statin drugs 8:1119
steam cabinets 6:776
Stelazine (trifluorperazine) 16:2256
sterilization (microbial), for surgery
    10:1404–1405; 15:2135–2136
sterilization (reproductive)
    15:2068–2071; 16:2286
    failure 16:2286
        ectopic pregnancy and 15:2068,
            2069, 2070; 16:2286
    hysterectomy 7:905; 15:2069, 2071

involving the fallopian tubes
    15:2069, 2070, 2071; 16:2286
involving the ovaries 15:2069, 2071;
    16:2286
laparoscopic 8:1034; 15:2071
the menopause and 15:2070;
    16:2286
reversal 15:2068; 16:2286
    assessment 8:1034
steroids 1:48; 15:2072–2073
    for asthma 7:953, 954; 15:2072
    for dermatitis 4:468
    for eczema 4:543
    immunosuppressive 7:914
    side effects 14:1956–1957, 1959;
        15:2073
    structure 15:2073
stethoscope 4:474, 475; 15:2074–2075
stitches see sutures
stomach pump 4:562; 15:2091–2093
stone therapy 6:798
streptomycin
    balance and 9:1194
    deafness and 4:455
stress management 15:2103–2104;
    17:2405
    biofeedback 2:181–183
    meditation 1:75
    rolfing and 13:1846
    visualization 9:1231
sulfasalazine 4:443
sulfonamides 1:100
suppositories 15:2132–2133
surgeons 15:2139–2140
    training 15:2134
surgery 15:2134–2140
    brain see brain surgery
    bypass 3:346, 420–421; 10:1402,
        1403; 17:2357
    for cancer 3:315
    "clean" and "dirty" 15:2135
    cosmetic 3:424–425; 12:1612, 1615
        for moles 9:1243
    dressings used after 4:515
    effects of 12:1646–1647
    hemorrhaging after 6:806
    instruments used in 15:2136,
        2137–2139
    laparotomy 8:1035
    LASIK 8:1043–1044
    microsurgery 5:709; 9:1218–1221;
        10:1434; 15:2139
    minimally-invasive
        (keyhole/laparoscopic) 6:764;
        9:1236–1237; 15:2138, 2139
        telesurgery and 16:2180
    open-heart 10:1401–1403
    operating rooms and 10:1404–1406
    operating tables 10:1406
    plastic and reconstructive
        12:1612–1617
    postoperative care 12:1644–1647
    respirators used during
        13:1805–1806
    risks 15:2136
    side effects 13:1840
    sterilization during 10:1404–1405
    telesurgery 16:2180
    tourniquets used in 16:2246
    under hypothermic conditions 7:900
    viewing rooms 10:1406
    see also transplants
sutures (stitches) 8:1031; 12:1647;
    15:2136–2137, 2138, 2144; 17:2425
    abdominal, bursting 15:2138, 2144
    absorbable (dissolving) 15:2144;
        17:2422, 2425
    internal 15:2144; 17:2422

nonabsorbable 17:2425
    removal 15:2144
    a stitched cut healing 6:765
    sweep 7:932
swimming 7:881; 8:1094, 1095; 11:1573
    eczema and 4:542
    otitis and 11:1452, 1453
synovectomy 1:126; 13:1824
syringing 4:454, 456, 537, 538;
    15:2156–2157

tacrolimus 7:913, 914; 8:1024
taurine 14:1989
tea 14:1902, 1905; 16:2256
    herbal 6:815; 11:1480
Telehomecare 6:839
Tempra see acetaminophen
TENS (transcutaneous electrical nerve
    stimulation) 11:1482, 1579
tetracyclines 1:100; 4:468; 16:2199
    side effects 11:1565; 14:1957; 16:2178,
        2199, 2272
    taken during pregnancy 1:99;
        16:2178, 2199
tetrahydrobiopterin 11:1559
thalidomide 8:1119; 16:2202–2204
    taken during pregnancy 2:206;
        3:402; 6:749; 9:1170; 11:1550;
        16:2202–2204
    victims using prostheses 12:1698
therapeutic communities (TCs) 4:528
therapy 16:2205–2206
    complementary therapies 16:2206
        see also alternative medicine
    group therapy 5:713–714; 13:1736
    mind-body therapy 9:1230–1233
        see also physical therapy;
        psychotherapy; speech therapy
thiopental (pentothal) 2:170
thyroidectomy 16:2225
tissue engineering 2:190
tissue expanders 16:2266
tonics 3:412; 15:2083, 2084; 16:2229,
    2231
tonsillectomy 8:1113; 14:2012–2013;
    16:2235, 2236, 2237
toothpaste, fluoride 5:651, 652
tourniquet 1:17; 16:2245–2246; 17:2422
toxicologists 11:1551
tracheal tubes 13:1808
tracheostomy 7:946; 8:1037; 13:1805;
    16:2251–2252; 17:2389
tracheotomy 10:1333; 16:2251
traction 16:2253–2255
    for fractures 10:1431–1432, 1433;
        16:2253, 2254, 2255
    intermittent 16:2253
tranexamic acid 17:2392
tranquilizers 14:1903, 1904, 1980;
    16:2256–2258
    alternatives to 16:2256, 2257, 2258
    side effects 16:2272
    see also sedatives
transactional analysis 13:1735
transcutaneous electrical nerve
    stimulation (TENS) 11:1482, 1579
transdermal patch 16:2259–2260
Transderm Nitro 16:2260
transpersonal therapy 13:1735
transplants 16:2263–2266
    artificial 16:2265
    from animals 4:503
    heart 4:504; 6:791–794; 10:1422;
        16:2263, 2264, 2266
    kidney see kidney transplants
    liver 4:504; 8:1084; 16:2263, 2265,
        2266
    living donor 16:2264–2265

lung 4:504; 13:1750
marrow see marrow transplants
pancreas 16:2264
postoperative care 16:2266
rejection 16:2265
    suppression of 6:794; 7:913, 914;
        8:1022, 1139; 9:1139; 15:2072,
        2073; 16:2265
    umbilical cord blood 5:676, 677
    see also donors; grafting
transurethral resection of the prostate
    (TURP) 12:1693
trauma center 16:2267–2269
    see also emergency department
triazolam 7:893
tricyclic drugs 4:466
trifluorperazine (Stelazine) 16:2256
trimeprazine 7:893
tubal ligation 16:2286
TURP (transurethral resection of the
    prostate) 12:1693
twelve-step facilitation (TSF)
    programs 4:529
Tylenol see acetaminophen

Vacuflex 13:1794
vagotomy 2:158; 17:2314, 2340
Valium (diazepam) 7:893; 14:1903,
    1904; 16:2257
venlafaxine 4:466
Viagara 7:963; 14:1928
viruses, used in gene therapy
    5:679–680
visualization 9:1231
voice synthesizers 3:335

water pills 4:544
wax treatments 6:799; 11:1579
wheelchairs 11:1495, 1497
willow bark 6:813
withdrawal symptoms 17:2416–2418
    fits 5:583
    from alcohol abuse 1:61; 6:742;
        17:2417, 2418
    heroin or morphine 6:823; 17:2416,
        2417–2418
workstations 11:1493

xenografts (animal tissue grafts)
    5:709, 710

yoga 1:80; 5:602; 11:1477; 17:2440–2445
    during pregnancy 12:1679; 17:2444
    relaxation and 13:1802; 17:2440,
        2444
yttrium 5:698

Zantac 6:786
zinc pyrithione 6:739
zolpidem 7:893
Zovirax (acyclovir) 3:382; 14:1939

PREVENTION AND DIAGNOSIS OF DISEASE

accident prevention 1:23–25
    drowning 4:522
    electric shock 4:549
adipometers 11:1577
aerobics 1:49–52; 7:995–997; 11:1573,
    1575; 17:2401
    aerobic capacity test 11:1575
amniocentesis 1:84; 2:207; 3:367;
    4:506, 508; 5:677, 686; 12:1664,
    1676
    miscarriage after 1:84; 3:368

sex of the baby and 5:638; 12:1675
    spina bifida and 15:2038
amnioscopy 4:571
Amsler grid 8:1119
angiography 4:478; 10:1356
    cardiac 6:790
    carotid angiogram 17:2357, 2431,
        2434
    fluorescein 8:1119
antioxidants 1:101; 7:946; 9:1187;
    10:1328, 1382; 17:2379, 2384, 2387
arteriograms 1:118
    cerebral 2:265, 266
arthrograms 17:2432
arthroscopy 1:125; 4:571; 10:1432, 1434
aseptic techniques 15:2135–2136
audiometers 6:778
auriscopes 15:2157
autoanalyzers 15:2025
autopsies 11:1511, 1512, 1514, 15:2080

Babinski's sign 6:763
barium liquids 2:171–172; 4:443, 475,
    478; 17:2433, 2434
    enemas 4:478, 572; 15:2096
BCG vaccine 7:912; 16:2287, 2290
beta-carotene 1:101
BioChips 3:334
biofeedback techniques 2:181–184;
    5:648, 650; 9:1232, 1266; 11:1482
biopsy 2:192–193; 4:570; 8:1029;
    15:2025–2026
    heart muscle 6:794
    for malignancy 6:726
        breast 8:1132
        skin 9:1184
body plethysmography 3:371
bone marrow puncture 8:1061
bracelets, medical alert 16:2270
bronchoscopy 4:571; 8:1100, 1104;
    13:1752

calcium 3:310–311; 9:1234, 1235; 10:1381
    bones and 2:259; 13:1835
    during pregnancy 3:310, 311; 12:1678
    parathyroid glands and
        11:1503–1505
callisthenics 5:602
caloric testing 9:1194
carbohydrates
    dietary 4:487–488; 10:1380;
        15:2063–2064, 2120, 2121
    breakdown 5:702, 703; 9:1215;
        15:2063
    during pregnancy 12:1678
    processed in the liver 8:1086
    see also starch; sugars
carbolic acid 15:2135
catheterization 17:2357
    cardiac 6:788; 9:1289; 10:1401;
        17:2342
CAT scans see CT scans
central venous pressure (CVP) 14:1945,
    1947
checkups 4:474; 6:766; 12:1680, 1684
    for children 11:1518–1519
    see also physical examination
chi kung see qigong
chorionic villus sampling (CVS) 2:207;
    3:367–368
    Huntington's disease and 7:877
    sex of the baby and 5:638
chromium 9:1235; 16:2250
cobalt, in high doses 16:2249, 2250
cod liver oil 13:1835
colonoscopy 3:386–387; 4:501, 570, 571;
    12:1643
colposcopes 11:1489

computerized (axial) tomography see
    CT scans
computerized ultrasound fetal
    cardiotocography (CTG) 3:340
copper 9:1235; 16:2249, 2250
    poisoning 9:1235; 16:2249, 2250
cryotherapy 4:470; 12:1627; 17:2363
CT scans (CAT scans) 2:266; 3:394;
    4:477, 478; 10:1355; 17:2434–2435
    dyes used in 13:1869
cystoscopy 4:570, 571; 9:1236
    used in prostate surgery 12:1693
cystourethrography, micturating
    (MCU) 17:2324
cytology 11:1513

dermatology 4:469–470
diagnosis 4:474–476
    see also specimens
diagnostic imaging 2:190; 4:477–480
    potential risks 4:480
    see also CT scans; Doppler scans;
        MRI; PET scanning; radionuclide
        scanning; thermal imaging;
        ultrasound; X rays
diet 4:487–491; 17:2404
    acidic 9:1263
    calcium in 3:310–311; 10:1381; 11:1451;
        12:1678
    Chinese 3:358, 361
    cholesterol and 1:120; 3:366;
        5:621–622
    during convalescence 3:412
    during pregnancy 2:206; 3:402;
        4:491; 8:1127, 1128; 10:1379;
        12:1662, 1665, 1675, 1678
    elimination diets 1:73–74
    fats 4:489; 5:621–622; 8:1086;
        9:1215; 10:1380; 12:1682
        cholesterol and 1:120; 3:366
        digestion 2:180; 5:621
        during pregnancy 12:1678
        malabsorption 5:624
    feces and 5:624
    fish 2:266
    gluten-free 3:329
    health foods 6:772–773
    high-fiber 5:645; 8:1045; 10:1382
        for irritable bowel syndrome
            7:980
    importance of antioxidants 1:101;
        10:1328
    iron in 1:89
    macrobiotics 8:1116–1118; 17:2353
    naturopathic 10:1326, 1327, 1328
    for patients on dialysis 8:1014
    of PKU-affected children 11:1559
    proteins 4:488–489; 6:772, 773;
        10:1380; 12:1701
        during pregnancy 12:1678
    reducing see dieting
    roughage 1:102; 3:404; 4:490
    special diets 4:491
    sugar-free 7:896
    to avoid coronary disease 3:421
    tooth care and 4:461
    unhealthy 6:769–770
    while breast-feeding 4:485
    see also carbohydrates; minerals;
        nutrition; vegetarianism;
        vitamins
dieting 4:488, 492–493; 6:768; 10:1385
    basal metabolic rate and 2:173
    constipation and 3:404, 405
    diet clubs and 10:1386
    diet pills 1:85; 4:493, 524
    eating disorders and 1:94, 95, 96
    in health spas 6:774

ketone production during 7:1006
    using diuretics 4:500
    yoga and 17:2441
disclosing agents, dental 4:461;
    12:1608, 1609
Doppler scans 4:479
douching 14:1935
    vaginal 5:689
DTaP vaccines 17:2415
DTP vaccines 4:497; 17:2413, 2414, 2415
dyes, Evan's Blue 11:1503

echocardiography 17:2317
electrocardiograms (ECGs) 4:475,
    550–551, 559; 6:790; 17:2341
    fetal 10:1390
electroencephalograms (EEGs) 2:263,
    266; 4:552; 10:1356; 14:1892
    biofeedback and 2:183, 184
    epilepsy and 4:552; 5:584
    unconsciousness and 3:394–395;
        17:2319
electromyography (EMG) 10:1356
endoscopy 4:570–571; 11:1455
    amnioscopy 4:571
    arthroscopy 1:125; 4:571; 10:1432, 1434
        and biopsy 2:193
    bronchoscopy 4:571; 8:1100, 1104;
        13:1752
    colonoscopy 3:386–387; 4:501, 570,
        571; 12:1643
    for Crohn's disease 4:443
    cystoscopy 4:570, 571; 9:1236
        used in prostate surgery 12:1693
    of the duodenum 4:531
    gastroscopy 4:570, 571
    laparoscopy 4:568, 569, 570, 571;
        8:1033–1034; 9:1236; 11:1459,
        1520; 15:2138
        infertility investigation 7:945;
            8:1033–1034
    sigmoidoscopy 4:501, 570; 14:1960
    telesurgery and 16:2180
epidemiology 9:1172
essential (medical term) 4:474
examinations, medical 4:474
    see also internal examination;
        physical examination
exercise testing 4:551

fiber, dietary see roughage
fitness, physical see physical fitness
flavonoids 1:101; 10:1382
floss, dental 4:461; 6:731; 12:1610
fluids, not to be given to accident
    victims 4:555
fluoride 4:461; 5:651–652; 9:1235;
    10:1381, 12:1636; 16:2176
folic acid see vitamin B, folic acid
Food and Drug Administration (FDA)
    5:655; 13:1745; 14:1956
    smart drugs and 14:1989
freeze-fixing, biopsy samples
    2:193
fructose 15:2121
fruit and vegetables, antioxidants in
    1:101

gas dilution 3:371
gastroscopy 4:570, 571
    gastroscopic laser coagulation
        8:1042
genetic engineering 5:678–681
geriatric medicine 5:691–694
    physical therapy and 11:1581
Guthrie test 3:401
gynecology 6:732–734
    laparoscopy used in 8:1034

hammers, rubber (patellar) 4:475
health education 6:768–771;
    12:1682–1684
    see also medical information
        highway
health foods 6:772–773
heel-prick test, PKU 11:1559
hematology 11:1513–1514
histopathology 11:1512–1513; 15:2026
Holter machines 6:790
humidifiers 7:876
hygiene 2:165, 166; 7:884–888; 11:1544
    in the bathroom 5:671; 7:888
    body odor and 2:249
    food and in the kitchen 2:166; 5:671;
        7:884, 886–887
    foot 5:625, 627; 11:1543
    vaginal 17:2334
        vaginal douching and 5:689
    washing your hands 5:657; 7:884
hysterosalpingography 7:945; 13:1860

idiopathic (medical term) 4:474
imaging, diagnostic see diagnostic
    imaging
immunization 2:166; 7:910–912
    schedule for children 11:1519
    sudden infant death syndrome and
        15:2117
    WHO scheme 16:2283
    see also vaccination
immunohematology 8:1029
immunology 8:1029; 11:1514
inoculation see immunization;
    vaccination
interdental cleaners 4:461
internal examination 1:14; 6:732, 734;
    7:966–967; 15:2027
Internet
    Internet2 16:2179
    medical information highway
        9:1168–1169; 16:2180
intravenous pyelograms (IVPs) 4:475;
    8:1020
iodine 9:1235; 16:2250
    deficiency 5:704; 10:1334
iron 7:977–978; 9:1234–1235; 16:2250
    blood donors and 7:977
    deficiency 1:88–89, 90; 7:977; 8:1128
        detection 7:978
    dietary 7:977, 978; 10:1381
        during pregnancy 12:1678
    excess 6:800; 7:978
    hemochromatosis and 6:800
    loss 7:977–978
    supplements 6:787; 12:1675
        black feces and 5:623; 7:977
        children accidentally swallowing
            4:555; 7:977; 9:1234
        overdose 9:1234; 11:1460; 15:2093
    vitamin E absorption and 17:2382
Ishihara cards 3:388
isolation 7:982–983
    see also quarantine
isotope scans see radioisotope scans

jogging 5:599; 7:995–997

keratometers 3:328
Koplik's spots 9:1163, 1164

laboratory tests 8:1028–1029
    see also pathology
laparoscopy 4:568, 569, 570, 571;
    8:1033–1034; 9:1236; 11:1459, 1520;
    15:2138
    infertility investigation 7:945;
        8:1033–1034

laparotomy 8:1035
lepromin test 6:755
lifting 2:163; 12:1688; 14:1985
lumbar puncture 2:266; 4:475, 565;
    8:1097; 9:1196
    myelography and 10:1355
lymphangiograms 8:1112, 1114

magnesium 9:1235
magnetic resonance imaging see MRI
mammography 2:192; 3:312;
    8:1129–1132; 14:1895; 16:2292;
    17:2432
manganese 9:1235; 16:2250
medical alert bracelets 16:2270
medical information highway
    9:1168–1169; 16:2180
    see also health education
medical research 9:1170–1172
meditation 1:75, 80; 9:1178–1179;
    11:1477; 13:1802; 15:2104
    transcendental 9:1178; 15:2104
Medline 9:1168, 1169
microbiology 8:1029; 9:1216–1217;
    11:1514
micturating cystourethrography
    (MCU) 17:2324
"mind mirrors" 2:183
minerals 4:490; 9:1234–1235; 10:1381
    see also trace elements
MMR vaccination 2:206; 7:911, 912
molecular biology 9:1240–1241
MRI (magnetic resonance imaging)
    4:478, 479; 13:1869, 1870
    of the brain 2:190, 230, 266, 269;
        6:758; 10:1356
    of the breasts 8:1132
    of carpal tunnel syndrome 3:322
myelography 10:1355
    myelograms 2:163; 14:1885, 1886,
        1887, 1984

neurology and neurosurgery
    10:1354–1356
    physical therapy and 11:1579–1580
neurosurgery see neurology and
    neurosurgery
nuclear medicine 2:190
nutrition 10:1379–1382
    see also diet; health foods

obstetrics 10:1389–1390
    physical therapy and 11:1580
oncology 10:1399–1400
    integrative 10:1399
ophthalmology 10:1407–1408
ophthalmoscopes 4:475, 476; 5:604;
    10:1408
optometrist 10:1412–1413
    tests for color blindness 3:388
orthermography 16:2207
orthodontics 10:1425–1429; 16:2175,
    2177
    interceptive 10:1427
orthopantomography 17:2434
orthopedics 10:1430–1434
    physical therapy and 11:1580
otoscopes 4:475, 476; 6:779

Pap smear (cervical smear) 3:313, 314,
    337, 338; 6:734; 7:966, 967; 8:1126;
    11:1488–1489, 1513; 14:1894
    after sterilization 15:2071
    during pregnancy 12:1676
paternity testing 2:233
pathology 11:1508, 1511–1514
    chemical 11:1514
    forensic 11:1513

see also biopsy; laboratory tests;
    microbiology
peak flow meters 13:1752
pediatric medicine 10:1389;
    11:1515–1519
    physical therapy and 11:1580
Pel-Ebstein fever pattern 1:114
percussion 4:475
PET scanning 2:190; 4:480; 10:1355;
    11:1547; 13:1869, 1870
phosphorus 9:1235
photoic stimulation 5:583, 585
physical examination 11:1566,
    1566–1569
    for children 11:1518–1519, 1568
    see also checkups
physical fitness 11:1570–1573, 1574, 1575
    aerobics and 1:50; 11:1573
    jogging and 7:997
    pulse rate and 1:50; 11:1572, 1574
physical fitness testing 11:1574–1577
plethysmography, body 3:371
pleural rub 12:1620
podiatry 12:1626–1628
polysomnographic (PSG) studies 7:958
positron emission tomography see
    PET scanning
potassium 9:1234, 1235
    paralysis and 9:1292
    supplements 4:544, 545
    overdose 9:1234
preimplantation genetic diagnosis
    (PGD) 5:677
preservatives, food 5:656
preventive medicine 12:1680–1684
prick test, for allergies 14:1913
primary (medical term) 4:474
psychiatry 12:1709–1715, 1716; 13:1734
psychology 12:1716–1718; 13:1734
psychoneuroimmunology 15:2102
public health 12:1680–1681;
    13:1743–1746
pulmonary function tests (PFTs) 3:371
pyelograms, intravenous (IVPs) 4:475

qigong (chi kung) 1:81; 3:358, 360–361
quarantine 13:1763
    see also isolation

radioisotope scans 2:268; 3:315;
    10:1354, 1355
radionuclide scanning 4:477, 480
    PET scannning 4:480
    SPECT 4:480
RDAs (recommended daily amounts)
    5:656
    vitamins 5:655, 656
Reed-Sternberg cells 6:833
refracting heads 5:609
relaxation 9:1230, 1232; 13:1800–1802;
    15:2103, 2104; 17:2405
    biofeedback and 2:182–183
    flotation therapy and 5:648, 649,
        650
    tai chi and 16:2166
    yoga and 13:1802; 17:2440, 2444
research, medical 9:1170–1172
risk analysis 13:1839–1840
roughage 1:102; 3:404; 4:490
Rubin's test 7:945

safety see accident prevention
salt 9:1235; 13:1861–1862
    dietary 5:653; 11:1484; 13:1861
    edema and 4:544
    loss 13:1862
        cramp and 4:437; 11:1544
    salt water as an emetic 4:562

scans 13:1869–1870
    see also CT scans; diagnostic
        imaging; MRI; PET scanning;
        ultrasound
Schick test 4:497
Schilling test 11:1536
scratch test 1:72, 73; 13:1783
screening 14:1892–1895
    babies 14:1893
        eye tests 10:1407
        hearing tests 4:454
    cancer 3:314–315; 14:1892
    children 14:1893–1894
    prenatal 14:1893
        see also amniocentesis; chorionic
            villus sampling; ultrasound,
            during pregnancy
selenium 5:655; 16:2250
serology 4:475
sex education 1:45; 6:768, 769
sigmoidoscopy 4:501, 570; 14:1960
silicon 16:2250
single-photon-emission computerized
    tomography (SPECT) 4:480
smears, cervical see Pap smear
sodium 9:1234
specimens 15:2024–2026
    blood tests 2:225; 4:475; 8:1029;
        15:2024–2025
    sputum tests 15:2025
    stool samples 15:2025
    urine tests 4:475; 5:596; 8:1029;
        12:1676; 15:2024, 2025, 2026
        for ketones 7:1006
        in pregnancy 15:2024
        for protein 8:1018, 1020
    see also biopsy; Pap smear
SPECT (single-photon-emission
    computerized tomography)
    4:480
sphygmomanometer 2:183; 4:475, 476;
    11:1569; 15:2036–2039
spinal tap 15:2042
spirometry and spirometers 3:371;
    13:1752
staining, biopsy samples 2:193
starch 15:2063–2064, 2121
    broken down by amylase 11:1487;
        15:2063
stress testing, cardiac 4:551; 11:1574
sucrose 5:702; 15:2121
sugars 15:2120–2121
    diabetes and 4:471, 473; 15:2121
    dietary 5:702
        teeth and 15:2120, 2121
        white and brown 5:653
    levels in the body 4:488; 7:960;
        15:2121
    see also sucrose
sunscreen 11:1470; 15:2128–2129;
    17:2428
suntanning preparations 14:1970

tai chi 16:2165–2168
telemedicine 16:2179–2180
tensilon 10:1312, 1313
tests
    laboratory 8:1028–1029
    see also laboratory tests
thermal imaging 16:2207–2208
thermistors 16:2184
thermometers 4:475; 16:2181,
    2183–2184
theta-wave training 2:182
tissue typing 16:2263, 2265
TNM classification 8:1098–1099, 1132
tomography
    computerized (axial) see CT scans

positron emission *see* PET scanning
single-photon-emission computerized (SPECT) 4:480
X-ray 17:2434
toothbrushes 6:731; 12:1608
trace elements 16:2249–2250
harmful 16:2250
see also minerals
travel and health 16:2270–2273, 2284–2285
basic precautions 16:2282
travel sickness pills, overdose 4:562
triage 4:560; 16:2268
trichogram analysis 6:739
tuning forks 4:454

ultrasound 4:478–479; 13:1870; 14:*1893*; 17:2315–2317
breast scans using 8:1132
for cataract removal 3:*326*, 328
Doppler 4:479
during pregnancy 2:207, 285; 4:477, 479, 480; 12:1664, 1676; 13:1869, 1870; 14:1893, *1894*; 15:*2143*; 17:2315, 2316–2317
taken with a full bladder 17:2315
lithotripsy and 8:1020
treatment (providing heat) 6:797, 798; 11:1579, *1580*; 17:2315
for hemophiliacs 6:*801*
ultrasound-assisted lipoplasty (UAL) 8:1080
urography, intravenous (IVU or IVP) 17:2433

vaccinations 2:166; 7:940; 9:1216; **17:2330–2332**
attenuated vaccines 7:911; 17:2330
before traveling overseas 16:*2270*, 2271–2272
during pregnancy 2:206; 16:2284
encephalitis and 4:565
see also immunization
vaccines, genetically engineered 5:680–681
variolation 7:911
VDRL test 15:2154
vegans and veganism 17:2351, 2352, 2353, 2354
illnesses associated with 17:2355
vegetarianism 4:488, *489*; 10:*1379*; **17:2351–2356**
minerals and 9:1234
videoconferencing 16:*2179*
vitallographs 17:2408
vitamin A **17:2373–2374**
an antioxidant 1:101; 10:1328, 1382
deficiency 5:606; 8:1118, 1128; 17:2373, 2374
during pregnancy 12:1678
excess 17:2373, 2374, 2387
genetically altered rice and 5:675
night vision and 10:1362
vitamin B **17:2375–2377**
B1 (thiamin) 17:2377
daily requirements 17:2376
deficiency 8:1128; 12:1722; 17:2376
B2 (riboflavin) 17:2376, 2377
daily requirements 17:2376
deficiency 17:2376
B3 (niacin; nicotinic acid) 17:2377
daily requirements 17:2376
deficiency 8:1128
B6 (pyridoxine) 9:1201, 1249; 12:1674; 17:2375, 2376, 2377
deficiency 17:2376
B12 (cyano-cobalamin) 17:2376

deficiency 8:1118; 11:1536, *1537*; 15:2043; 17:2355, 2376
excess 17:2355
B13 (orotic acid) 17:2377
B17 (laetrile) 17:2377
biotin, deficiency 17:2376
deficiency 5:606; 7:897; 8:1118, 1128; 9:1214; 11:1536, *1537*; 17:2375, 2376
during pregnancy 12:1678
excess 17:2375
folic acid (folacin) 17:2376
supplements 2:206; 3:401; 5:638, 682; 10:1351; 15:2037, 2039; 17:2377
pantothenic acid 17:2376
sources 17:2377
supplements 17:2377
toxicity 17:2377
vitamin C **17:2378–2379**
an antioxidant 1:*101*; 10:1328, 1382; 17:2379
collagen formation and 14:1896–1897; 17:2378
common cold and 3:396
daily requirements 17:2379
deficiency 2:260; 3:298; 5:606; 6:804; 8:1128; 10:1379; 14:1896–1897; 17:2378
people at risk from 17:2379
during pregnancy 12:1678
foods containing 14:1896; 17:2378–2379
vitamin D 8:1118; **17:2380–2381**
calcium absorption and 3:*311*; 11:1504; 13:1836
daily requirements 17:2381
deficiency 2:260; 3:*311*; 5:691; 8:1128; 13:1835–1836; 17:2381
veganism and 17:2355
during pregnancy 12:1678
excess 17:2381, 2387
sunlight and 17:*2380*
supplements 2:272; 13:1836
types 17:2380
vitamin E 4:510; **17:2382–2384**
an antioxidant 1:*101*; 10:1328, 1382; 17:2384
daily requirements 17:2384
deficiency 17:2383
during pregnancy 12:1678
iron supplements and absorption of 17:2382
overdosage 17:2384
supplements 17:*2383*
dangerous for babies 17:2384
vitamin K 2:228; **17:2385–2386**
during pregnancy 12:1678
vitamins 4:489–490; 10:1381; **17:2387**
RDA 5:655, 656
supplements 8:1127
during pregnancy 5:638
for elderly people 5:691
fatigue and 5:619
fluorinated 5:651
see also under the names of each vitamin eg: vitamin A

warfarin 16:2214
interaction with aspirin 14:*1957*–1958
washing 7:885
hands 5:657; 7:884, *887*
compulsive 3:397, *398*
water
acid rain and 1:29
balance, hypothalamus and 7:898–899
daily requirement 8:1017
drinking water 4:573

fluoridation of 5:651, 652; 13:*1744*
lead in 8:1048–1049
mineral water 9:1234
pollution 4:574; 12:1636, *1638*, 1639–*1640*
public health and 13:1744
wellness 17:2403–2405
well-woman clinics 14:1895
whiff test 17:2338
World Health Organization (WHO) 13:1746

X rays 4:*478*; 13:1772–1773; **17:2431–2435**
angiography and 4:478; 10:1355
carotid angiograms 17:*2357*, 2431, *2434*
arthrograms 17:2432
barium liquids and 2:*171*–172; 4:*443*, 478; 17:2433
contrast 4:478
dental 17:*2434*
digital radiography 17:2433–2434
during pregnancy 12:1664–1665, 1676; 17:*2431*
endoscopy and 4:570
intravenous urography 17:2433
mammography 2:192; 3:*312*; 8:**1129–1132**; 16:*2292*; 17:2432
risks from 11:1510; 17:2435
"10 day rule" 5:682; 17:2435
cancer 3:312
during pregnancy 2:206, 285; 4:478; 5:682; 17:2431
leukemia 8:1059
mutations 10:1306
negligible for radiation sickness 13:1770
teleradiology and 16:2180
therapy, heat treatment unwise after 6:798
used in radiotherapy 13:1772–1774; 17:2432
see also arteriograms; CT scans; myelography

yin and yang 1:37; 3:358; 5:650; 8:1116
shiatsu and 14:1937
tai chi and 16:2165
yoga 1:80; 5:602; 11:1477; **17:2440–2445**
during pregnancy 12:*1679*; 17:2444
relaxation and 13:1802; 17:2440, *2444*

zinc 9:1235; 16:2249, 2250

HUMAN BEHAVIOR

abortion 1:**14–16**
after diagnostic tests 1:84; 3:368; 4:506
bleeding after 1:16
ethics 9:1166
failure 1:14
salpingitis after 13:1858
sterilization not recommended at the same time 15:2068
subsequent miscarriages and 9:1238
absentmindedness 4:459
abstinence 1:22, 45
periodic *see* rhythm method
see also virginity
acid rain 1:28–30; 12:1638–1639
Adler, Alfred 3:398
adolescence 1:**42–45**
abstinence education 1:22

acne 1:*31*; 14:1974
anxiety 1:105
blushing 2:244; 14:1974
duodenal ulcers 4:530
fainting in 3:372; 5:612
growing pains 5:715, 716
growth in 4:532; 5:*716*, 717, 718
homosexuality and 6:850
hysteria 7:*906*
mood swings 9:1206, *1245*, 1246
need for privacy during 13:1739
"suicidal gestures" 12:1630
sweating 14:1974
see also chat room
affect 9:1245
flattening of 9:1247
incongruity of 9:1247
lability of 9:1247
air pollution 1:**59–60**; 4:573–574; 12:*1636*, 1637–1639, *1641*
acid rain and 1:29–30; 12:1638–1639
indoor 4:573
ozone 11:1468; 12:1639
sulfur dioxide 12:1639
see also chlorofluorocarbons
alcohol 4:526; 11:1510
abuse in adolescence 1:45
abuse affects the nervous system 10:1343
on an empty stomach 7:*896*; 15:2088
arterial disease and 1:120
capillary dilation 3:318
a cause of jaundice 7:991
cold weather and 5:666
effect on the brain 7:897
effect on the liver 3:375; 7:991; 8:1084, *1086*, *1087*
gastritis and 5:670, 671
hepatitis and 6:810
intoxication 7:**968–969**
memory loss and 9:1190
metabolized 2:188; 7:968
mixing your drinks 6:752
personality and 9:1278; 11:1540
poisoning 12:1629
recommended consumption 17:2403
for relaxation 13:1800, *1801*; 14:*1903*, 1904
resistance to 7:968
as a sedative 14:1903, 1904; 16:2258
sex and 14:1922, 1923
temporary impotence 14:1928
snoring and 14:2004
taken with analgesics 1:137
taken with antibiotics 1:99
vertigo and 17:2366
vision under the influence of 4:505; 6:752
amphetamines 1:**85–87**; 4:527; 13:1737; 15:2083
abuse 4:*524*, 526, 527; 15:2084
causing schizophrenic symptoms 14:1882
used to lose weight 10:1385
withdrawal 17:2417
androgynous people 5:672
appetite 1:**112–113**
aspartame 5:654
awareness 5:696

baby blues 9:1247; 12:1649
benzene 1:59
bereavement *see* grief, bereavement
Bhopal disaster 4:574
biofuels 5:674

biological and chemical warfare 1:97;
2:185–186; 4:440
bioterrorism, emergency departments
and 4:557
birth control *see* contraception;
rhythm method
bisexuality 6:851; 14:1929
body language 2:245–248; 12:1712
body piercing 2:250–251
ears 2:250, *251*
keloid scars and 14:1880
infected 11:1515
breath holding 1:132; 2:278; 3:413;
17:2320

Cain complex 3:398
cannabis *see* marijuana
castration complex 3:397–398
cellular telephones 3:333–334
CFCs *see* chlorofluorocarbons
chat room 3:343–344
chemical warfare 2:186
child abuse 3:351–353; 5:660
whiplash injury 17:2409
see also incest; sexual abuse
child development 3:354–357;
11:1518–1519
speech 15:2028, 2030–2031
chlorofluorocarbons (CFCs) 1:60; 4:574;
11:*1468*, 1471; 12:1636
circumcision 3:374; 5:688; 14:1918
female 5:*687–688*
cocaine and crack 3:380–381; 4:526,
527; 6:770
withdrawal 17:2417, 2418
complexes and compulsions
3:397–398
compulsions 3:397, *398*; 9:1208,
1209; 12:1713
obsessive-compulsive disorder
3:398; 10:1342, 1358, 1387–1388
compulsions *see* complexes and
compulsions
condoms 3:407, *408*, 410;
14:1934–1935; 16:2273
contraception 3:407–411
after the menopause 6:732
before penetration 7:964
during breast-feeding 2:272; 3:407
the Pill *see* oral contraceptives
sterilization 15:2068–2071
male *see* vasectomy
vaginal douches ineffective for
17:2333
withdrawal method 5:589
see also rhythm method
cosmetics 3:422–423
cosmetic surgery 3:424–425; 12:1612,
1615
for moles 9:1243
crack *see* cocaine and crack
crying 4:444–445; 10:1373
babies 4:444, *445*; 6:758;
10:*1366*

daydreams 6:742
DDT 4:574; 13:1839
Depo-Provera 3:411
diaphragms (contraceptives)
3:408–410
fitted after giving birth 17:2334
disaccharides 15:2120, *2121*
divorce 5:615
douching (contraceptive method)
3:411
dreaming 4:511–512; 5:620; 9:1190,
1228; 13:1781; 14:1978–1979; 15:2114
wet dreams 5:589; 14:1906

driving
relaxation while 13:1800
while pregnant 5:638
while using cellular phones 3:333
see also road rage
drug abuse 4:524–527, 528; 6:770
in adolescence 1:43, 44, 45
amphetamines 4:524, 526, 527;
15:2084
barbiturates 4:525, 526
drug counseling 4:528–529
hallucinations and 6:742; 8:1096
health education and 6:770
treatment 13:1798–1799
see also alcohol; cocaine and crack;
ecstasy; heroin; LSD; marijuana;
overdoses; smoking
dry-cleaning fluid 4:526, *527*

eccentricity 9:1206
ecstasy 1:85, 87; 4:526, 527; 6:770;
13:*1737*
Electra complex 3:398
emotions 9:1245
the brain and 2:262, 264
emotional outbursts 7:*907*
hormones and 6:859
puberty and 13:1741, 1742
smell and 2:262; 14:*1993*
see also moods
environmental hazards 4:573–574
see also occupational hazards;
pollution
ethics, medical *see* medical ethics
etiquette, medical 9:1166
euthanasia 5:595; 9:1167; 15:2125
see also suicide, assisted
exercise 5:599–602; 9:1230;
17:2404–2405
aerobics 1:49–52; 7:995–997; 11:1573,
1575; 17:2401
aerobic capacity test 11:*1575*
anaerobic 1:50
body temperature and 16:2181
callisthenic 5:602
cramp and 4:437
during pregnancy 11:1570; 12:1665,
1677, 1678–*1679*
effect on muscles 5:599; 9:1290
effects of overtraining 1:50
facial exercises 17:2427
with a fever 5:640
foot 5:*628*
the heart and 6:781
isometric 5:602, 664; 7:984–986
isotonic 5:602
lack of 6:769; 11:1574
ligaments and 8:1069
menstrual cycle and 15:2052
for the pelvis 11:*1524*
perspiration and 11:*1544*
qigong 1:81; 3:358, 360–361
stitch following 15:*2086*, 2087
for stroke patients 15:*2111*
to avoid backache 2:*162*
to avoid coronary disease or heart
attacks 1:118; 3:419, 421
to improve posture 12:*1658*
types, benefits 11:*1572*, 1573
warm-ups before 15:*2055*, 2086
yoga 17:2440–2445
extroversion 11:*1540*, 1542
eye contact 2:245–246

face packs or masks 3:422
family planning
natural *see* rhythm method
see also contraception

family relationships 5:615–617
fear 2:156
female genital mutilation (FGM)
5:*687–688*
fertilizers, as pollutants 12:1640
flavor enhancers, food 5:656
fluorine 12:1636, 1639
food
additives 4:574; 5:653–654, 656
color 5:*653*, 654, 655
monosodium glutamate 5:653,
654; 9:*1244*
preservatives 5:654
allergies 1:73; 4:485, 487, 562; 5:657
causing angioneurotic edema
7:*947*; 15:2145
causing migraine 9:1224
diagnosis 1:73–74
fish 1:72
hives and 6:831
itches and 7:989
milk 1:72
monosodium glutamate 5:653
prostaglandin involvement
12:1689
soy 5:675
antioxidants in 1:*101*; 10:1328, 1382
appetite and 1:*112*
canned 2:*261*
causing diarrhea 4:*485*, 486
dreaming and 4:511
energy from 4:490–491; 5:655–656;
9:*1215*
glucose 5:702–703
genetically altered (GA) 5:674–675;
10:1420
gluten-free 3:329
hazards 4:574
health foods 6:772–773
high-fiber 5:*645*; 8:1045
for irritable bowel syndrome
7:*980*
hygiene 2:166; 5:671; 7:884, 886–887
intolerance, celiac disease 1:71–72;
3:329; 4:485
iron in 7:*977*, 978
irradiated 7:*979*
labeling 5:655–656
irradiated food 7:*979*
listeriosis from 8:1083
organic 10:1328, 1418–1420
pesticides in/on 4:574; 5:657, 659;
10:1418, 1420
public health and 13:*1743*, 1745
purine-rich, and gout 5:707
raw 10:1326
salty 11:1484
toddlers spitting out food 9:*1262*
types 4:487–490
unpasteurized 3:297
use in the body 9:*1215*
freon 12:1636
Freud, Sigmund 3:397–398; 4:511–512;
7:*923*; 12:1653, *1711*
theory of personality 12:1711

gender and health 5:672–673
sex changes 5:672, 673
transsexuals 5:672, 673; 16:2196
genetically altered (GA) food
5:674–675; 10:1420
gestures 2:*245*, 246–248
glue-sniffing 4:526, 527; 14:*2006*,
2007
glycerol monostearate (GMS) 5:654
grass *see* marijuana
grief 5:712
after miscarriage 9:*1239*

family relationships 5:615–617

bereavement 4:458, 464, 465; 5:712;
9:*1206*; 17:2446
hallucinations 6:742; 12:1719
shock and 14:*1943*, 1944

hangover 6:752–753
cures for 1:62
haptics 2:246
heroin 4:524, 525, 526, *527*; 6:822–824;
10:1319, 1320
withdrawal 6:823, 824; 10:1320;
17:2416, 2417–2418
homesickness 6:848–849
homosexuality 6:850–851
hyperhidrosis 2:249

inbreeding 7:921–922
incest 7:923–924
denial of 5:615
inferiority complexes 3:*397*, 398
infibulation 5:687
inhalants, drug-abuse *see* solvent
abuse
intelligence 2:262
heredity and 6:817–818
memory and 9:1193
intoxication 7:968–969
intrauterine devices (IUDs) 3:407,
410–*411*; 4:496; 7:972; 8:1033
ectopic pregnancy and 4:541
morning-after 3:411
periods and 9:1204, 1205
salpingitis and 13:1859
introversion 11:1540, 1542
isolation 7:982–983
IUDs *see* intrauterine devices

Jocasta complex 3:398
Jung, Carl 3:397; 12:*1711*; 15:2115

Klein, Melanie 12:1711
Kohler, Wolfgang 5:696
Kyoto Protocol 1:60

Lear complex 3:398
learning 2:264
lesbianism 6:850, 851
life expectancy 1:53; 4:*458*;
8:1067–1068; 12:1682
biological clock and life span 2:188
of men and women 1:55
obesity and 10:1385
life span
biological clock and 2:188
heredity and 6:818
living wills 5:595; 15:2125
longevity *see* life span
LSD 4:526, *527*; 8:1096; 10:1320
Lunelle 3:411

macrobiotics 8:1116–1118; 17:2353
makeup *see* cosmetics
marijuana (cannabis; grass; pot) 4:526,
527; 6:822; 8:1137–1138
medicinal usage 8:1138; 9:1138
masturbation 9:1162, 1210; 13:1742
medical ethics 9:1166–1167
brain death and harvesting of
organs 16:2264
embryonic stem cells and 15:2066
intensive care and 7:962
surrogacy and 15:2142–2143
medical etiquette 9:1166
menstrual regulation 1:15
mirroring 2:247–248
moisturizers 3:*423*
monosaccharides 15:2120, *2121*
Montreal Protocol 11:1471

moods 9:1245–1247
in adolescents 9:1206, *1245*, 1246
disorders 10:1358
see also emotions
mother complex 3:398

narcotics 10:1319–1320; 11:1481–1482
addiction to 7:1004; 10:1319, *1320*
see also heroin; opiates
natural childbirth 2:200; 10:1321–1325
natural family planning *see* rhythm
method
nicotine 10:1359–1361
poisoning 10:1361
skin patches 14:1995; 16:*2259*, 2260
nightmares 4:511, 512; 14:1978
nitrogen oxides 1:28, 59, 60
noise 10:1363–1366, 1395
deafness and 4:453, 455, 456; 6:777;
10:1363, 1365–1366
tinnitus and 16:2227, 2228
NuvaRing contraceptive rings 3:411

occupational hazards 10:1391–1396
pneumoconiosis 2:282; 4:564;
12:**1621**; 13:1752
silicosis 10:1395; 14:**1961**
see also environmental hazards
Oedipus complex 3:397–398; 7:923
oil spills, detergents and 12:1638
opiates 11:1482
abuse 4:525
see also opium
opium 9:*1250*, 1251; 10:1319; 11:1482
oral contraceptives (the Pill)
10:*1414*–1417; 11:1458; 17:2326
age and 15:2107
antibiotics and 1:99
bleeding between periods and
9:1204, 1205
checkups while taking 10:1416
children swallowing 11:1462
coming off the 10:1416, 1417
common problems and solutions
10:1417
compared to HRT 7:874
D & C operation and 4:496
diarrhea and 4:485
during adolescence 1:42
forgetting to take 9:1202
internal examination before going
on 7:966
previous hepatitis infection and
6:809
side effects 5:593; 9:1158; 10:*1415*,
1417
on the breasts 10:1417; 14:1956
circulatory disorders 10:1417;
16:2214
cystitis 4:450
ectopic pregnancy 10:1417
on libido 7:963; 10:1414;
14:1920–1921
migraines 9:1222; 10:1417
premenstrual tension 9:1201
risk of stroke 15:2107
on sebaceous glands 14:1900
skin darkening 8:1091
and skin pigmentation on the
face 8:1090, 1091
weight 10:1416; 17:2398
taken during pregnancy 10:1416
taking a break from 10:1414
tanning and 9:1180
to treat acne 1:31; 14:1900
to treat endometriosis 4:569
to treat premenstrual syndrome
12:1674

types 10:*1415*, 1416–1417
varicose veins and 10:1414
while taking other medication
10:1414
organic food 10:1328, **1418–1420**
Ortho Evra patches 3:411
overdoses 11:**1460–1462**
acetaminophen 11:1479; 12:1629
amphetamine 1:87
aspirin 4:562; 11:1460; 12:1629
barbiturate 2:170; 3:395
coma and 3:395
suicide and 15:2124
teenage "suicidal gestures" 12:1630
tranquilizers 16:2256, 2257
treatment 2:170; 11:1479; 15:*2091*,
2092
emetics 15:2092–2093
first aid for suspected drug
overdose 6:824; 11:1462
stomach pump 15:2091–*2093*
overeating 3:397
appetite and 1:112, 113
during the menstrual cycle 1:112
ozone layer 1:59; 11:*1468*–1471
depletion 4:574; 11:1468, *1469*; 12:1636

periodic abstinence *see* rhythm
method
Perls, Fritz and Laura 5:695
persecution complex 3:398
personality 5:682; 11:**1538–1542**
A-type and B-type, and stress
15:2101
disorders 9:1207
multiple personality 9:1207,
1278–1279; 11:1540
moods and 9:*1247*
problems 12:1713
pesticides 13:1839
in/on food 4:574; 5:657, 659; 10:1418,
1420
as pollutants 12:1640
piercing *see* body piercing
Pill, the *see* oral contraceptives
pollution 12:**1636–1641**
lead 8:*1050*; 12:1638
light 12:1641
noise 12:1641
radiation poisoning 12:1641
soil 12:*1640*–1641
visual 12:1641
water 4:574; 12:1636, *1638*,
1639–*1640*
see also acid rain; air pollution
polyaromatic hydrocarbons (PAHs)
1:59
polychlorinated biphenyls (PCBs) 4:574
polysaccharides 15:2120, *2121*
pot *see* marijuana
psychoticism scale 11:1541
purple hearts 1:87; 15:2083

rape 13:**1777–1780**; 14:1926, 1927
post-traumatic stress disorder and
12:1652, 1653
rhythm method 3:411; 13:**1827–1830**
road rage 13:**1841–1843**

sewage 4:574; 12:1636, 1639; 13:1744
sex 14:**1916–1925**
12 steps to sexual intimacy 2:246
frequency 14:1916
libido 8:*1062–1063*; 14:1920–1921,
1922
aging and 1:53
the Pill and 7:963; 10:1414;
14:1920–1921

pituitary gland and 12:1598
safe sex
while traveling 16:2273
see also contraception
sexual attraction 14:1917
sexual awareness 14:1917
sexual problems 14:1919–1925
dyspareunia (painful intercourse)
4:568; 7:965; 8:1034; 9:1269;
13:1860; 14:1924–1925, 1929
impotence 1:130; 5:590;
7:**919–920**; 11:1531; 14:1924
premature ejaculation 5:589,
590; 14:1924, 1928
sex therapy and 14:1925, *1929*
what is "normal" 14:*1922*
sex changes 5:672, 673
sexual abuse 14:**1926–1927**
of children 3:353; 14:*1926–1927*
see also child abuse; incest
sleep and sleep problems, sleep,
dreaming 4:511–512; 5:620;
9:1190, 1228; 13:1781;
14:1978–1979; 15:2114
sleepwalking 14:**1981**
smogs 1:59–60; 4:574; 12:*1636*, 1637
smoking 3:*315*; 6:768, 770–771; 8:1100;
11:1510; 14:**1995–1999**
addiction to 17:2416
artery disease and 1:101, 118; 5:669;
6:783
cancer and 2:279, *283*; 3:314; 8:1067,
1104, 1126; 13:1749; 14:1996,
1997–1998
chest problems and 13:1750
children starting 14:1997
chronic bronchitis and 2:279; 3:294,
426
chronic obstructive pulmonary
disease and 3:370
the circulation and 1:*120*
damage by free radicals and 1:101
drugs
cocaine 3:*380*
marijuana 4:526; 8:1137
during pregnancy 5:638; 10:1361;
12:1604, 1665; 14:1995; 15:2080
effect on the lungs 8:*1103*
emphysema and 2:279; 3:294, 296;
4:563–564
filters on cigarettes 14:1996
giving up 2:283; 14:1999
acupuncture and 1:37
the body recovering from 10:1359;
14:1996
constipation and 3:404
flotation therapy and 5:649
hypnosis and 7:890
nicotine gum 14:1995
nicotine patches 14:1995; 16:*2259*,
2260
weight and 10:1384
withdrawal symptoms 10:1361;
17:2417, 2418
halitosis and 6:740, 741
heart attacks and 6:783; 16:2214
hoarseness and 6:832
immediate effects 10:1359,
1360–1361
longevity and 1:53; 14:1998, 1999
nicotine and 10:1359–*1361*;
14:1995–1996
nicotine staining 6:740
phlegm and 11:1560
public health and 13:1744, *1746*
reducing the effects of 14:1995,
1996
reflux esophagitis and 6:787

secondary (passive) 10:*1360*;
13:1840; 14:1999
sense of smell and 14:1990
sense of taste and 16:2169
skin damage and 9:1185; 17:2428
smoker's cough 3:371, 426; 5:603;
8:1036
teeth and 4:460; 14:*1999*
the tongue and 16:2232
wheezing 17:2407
why people smoke 14:1995–1997
work-related diseases and 10:1392
snuff 9:1188
soil, pollution 12:*1640*–1641
solvent abuse 4:526, 527;
14:**2006–2007**
somnambulism *see* sleepwalking
speech 10:1334; 15:**2028–2031**; 17:2389
esophageal 8:1036; 17:2389
the mouth and 9:*1262–1263*; 16:2233
problems 15:2030, 2031
aphasia 1:107–108; 10:1308;
15:2030
in children 8:*1081–1082*; 15:2028,
2030, 2032, *2033*
lisping 8:*1081–1082*; 11:1483;
15:2060
mutism 10:1307–1309
stammering and stuttering 1:107;
15:2032, **2058–2061**
stroke and 1:107; 10:1307; 15:2030,
2033, 2107, *2110*
signals 2:248
speed (drug) 1:87
spermicides 3:*407–408*, 409
stimulants 15:**2083–2085**
sports and 1:85
see also amphetamines
suicide 4:464; 15:**2122–2125**
assisted 15:2125
see also euthanasia
in the elderly 6:839
pacts 15:2124
teenage "suicidal gestures" 12:1630
sulfur dioxide 1:28, 29, 60; 12:1638
surrogacy 15:**2141–2143**

tantrums *see* temper tantrums
tattooing 2:*236*; 6:*809*; 16:**2172–2173**
medical uses 16:2173
tattoo removal 8:*1040*, 1042; 12:1614;
16:2172, *2173*
telephones, cellular 3:**333–334**
temper tantrums 3:356, 413; 7:906
texturizers 5:654
toning lotions 3:*423*
touching 2:246
transsexuals 5:672, 673; 16:2196
transvestites 5:*673*

Union Carbide disaster 4:574

vaginal sponges 3:*410*, 411
vasectomy 16:2286; 17:**2347–2350**
reversal 9:1218, *1220*; 16:2191; 17:2347,
2348, 2349, 2350
virginity 17:**2367–2368**, 2368
hymen and 7:889; 17:2367, 2368
internal examination and 7:966
see also abstinence
volatile organic compounds (VOCs)
1:59

warfare, biological and chemical *see*
biological and chemical warfare

zest 17:**2446**

PEOPLE INDEX

Adler, Alfred 3:398
Aesculapius 3:362
Alexander, Frederick Matthias 1:65
Ali, Muhammed 11:1506
Allen, Woody 10:1358
Alzheimer, Alois 1:82
Amenhotep IV 7:924
Argyle, Michael 2:246
Aserinsky, Edward 13:1781
Asher, Richard 9:1285–1286
Atlas, Charles 7:984

Bach, Edward 1:79
Berry, Halle 14:1917
Bichat, Marie Francois Xavier 10:1399
Bijani, Ladan and Laleh 14:1951
Billroth, Albert 15:2097
Bogart, Humphrey 14:1997
Bond, Thomas 7:870
Bradford Hill, A. 14:1997–1998
Braille, Louis 2:221–222
Brosnan, Pierce 14:1917
Brown, Louise 7:971
Bunker, Chang and Eng 14:1950
Burkitt, Denis 5:587
Bush, George W. 15:2066

Cade, John 13:1738
Caesar, Julius 16:2175
Capone, Al 15:2153
Carson, Rachel 13:1839
Celsus, Aurelius Cornelius 7:947
Chace, Marian 9:1231–1232
Chang and Eng (Siamese twins) 14:1950
Chang San-Feng 16:2168
Charbib, Rhadouane 14:1964
Charcot, Jean-Martin 7:906; 12:1653, 1710
Chichester, Francis 11:1541
Churchill, H.V. 5:651–652
Clinton, Bill 8:1133, 1134, 1138
Cobain, Kurt 15:2122
Coisins, Norman 9:1233
Cook, Frederick 14:1898
Cormack, Allan 17:2434
Crawford, Cindy 6:726
Crick, Francis 9:1240–1241
Cullen, William 10:1357
Cuthbert, Betty 9:1281

Davies, Mary Sue 15:2146
De Niro, Robert 11:1539; 12:1691
Descartes, René 14:1899
Doll, Richard 14:1997–1998

Economo, Constantin von 8:1057
Edwards, Robert 7:971, 972
Elephant Man, the 2:209; 6:727
Epstein, Anthony 5:587
Eysenck, Hans 11:1539

Fabricius, Hieronymus 10:1399
Feldenkrais, Moshe 5:629, 631
Fitzgerald, William 13:1793
Fleming, Alexander 11:1527, 1528
Fliess, Wilhelm 2:195
Franklin, Benjamin 7:870
Franklin, Rosalind 9:1241
Freud, Sigmund 3:397–398; 7:923; 12:1653, 1710, 1711; 13:1733
    cocaine and 3:380–381
    dreams and 4:511–512
    neuroses and 10:1352, 1357

psychoneuroses and 10:1357
    theory of personality 12:1711
Friedman, Meyer 15:2101

Galen 7:947
Gattefosse, René-Maurice 1:115
Gehrig, Lou 9:1256
George VI, King 15:2061
Gilles de la Tourette, George 16:2243, 2294
Gingrich, Newt 8:1138

Hahnemann, Samuel 6:842, 844
Harvey, William 17:2358
Hawking, Stephen 9:1256, 1258, 1259
Heller, Joseph 13:1846, 1848
Hippocrates 6:812; 10:1326
Holmes, Thomas 15:2100–2101
Houdini, Harry 11:1535
Hounsfield, Godfrey 17:2434

Ibrahim, Mohamed and Ahmed 14:1951
Ivan, Saint 9:1273

James I, King 7:921
James, Leon 13:1843
Janet, Pierre 12:1710
Jenner, Edward 7:911; 14:1986, 1988; 17:2331
Jenny, Hans 9:1231
John Paul II, Pope 13:1828
Jonah 9:1279
Jung, Carl 3:397; 12:1711; 15:2115

Kardiner, Abram 12:1653
Kasparov, Garry 16:2189
Keller, Helen 10:1308
Keller, Herbert 16:2202
Kelley, David E. 16:2244
Kennedy, John F. 1:48
Kevorkian, Jack 5:595
Kiss (rock group) 5:673
Klein, Melanie 12:1711
Kleitman, Nathaniel 13:1781
Kofka, Kurt 5:696
Kohler, Wolfgang 5:696
Kraepelin, Emil 12:1710
Kramer, Peter 13:1738
Kunz, Wilhelm 16:2202
Kurelek, William 14:1883

Laban, Rudolph 9:1231
Laennec, Rene-Theophile-Hyacinthe 15:2074–2075
Laing, R.D. 14:1883
Landsteiner, Karl 2:233, 235
Leboyer, Charles 10:1323
Leszczynski, Darius 3:334
Lewis, Tracy and Peter 15:2069
Lind, James 14:1896
Lister, Joseph 15:2135, 2137

McBride, William 16:2203
Martin, Dean 17:2349
Mary Tudor, Queen 11:1548, 1549
Menuhin, Yehudi 17:2445
Merrick, Joseph 2:209
Mesmer, Franz 12:1710
Minot, George 11:1537
Moon, Chris 1:127
Munchausen, Karl Friedrich Hieronymus von 9:1285
Murphy, William 11:1537

Nachran, Abi Kusno 17:2423
Napoleon 16:2175

Nerenberg, Arnold 13:1842–1843
Nijinsky, Vaslav 14:1884

Olsen, Mary Kate and Ashley Olsen 9:1274

Palmer, Bartlett Joshua 3:362
Palmer, Daniel David 3:362
Papanicolaou, George Nicolas 3:338; 11:1488
Parkinson, James 11:1506
Pasteur, Louis 15:2135; 17:2369
Perls, Fritz 5:695
Perls, Fritz and Laura 5:695
Pinel, Philippe 12:1722
Pope, the 13:1828
Porter, Rodney 6:728
Purce, Jill 9:1231

Rahe, Richard 15:2100–2101
Raspe, Rudolf Eric 9:1285
Ravert, Stephanie, Kristelle and Natasha 9:1277
Reich, Wilhelm 9:1230
Reye, Ralph Douglas 13:1813
Rivers, W.H.R. 12:1653
Rolfe, Ida P. 13:1846, 1848
Röntgen, Wilhelm Conrad 13:1773; 17:2431
Roosevelt, Theodore 15:2059
Rosenman, Ray H. 15:2101

Sassoon, Siegfried 12:1653
Schwing, Hans 2:197
Seyle, Hans 15:2098–2099, 2101
Steptoe, Patrick 7:971, 972
Still, Andrew Taylor 3:362
Swoboda, Hermann 2:195
Sybil 9:1279

Te Kanawa, Kiri 11:1556
Teltscher, Alfred 2:195
Thompson, Daley 8:1071
Typhoid Mary 16:2296

Waldeyer, Wilhelm 10:1399
Walton sextuplets 9:1276
Wang Chung-yueh 16:2168
Wang Yang Lu-chu'an 16:2168
Watson, James 9:1240–1241
Wertheimer, Max 5:696
White, Eve 9:1278–1279
Whitehead, Mary Beth 15:2142
Whitehouse, Mary 9:1231–1232
Williams, Cleveland 17:2318
Williams, Venus 16:2187
Winfrey, Oprah 11:1539
Wong, David 13:1738

Young, King 9:1279

Comprehensive index

Page numbers in **bold** refer to main articles; those in *italics* refer to picture captions. Numbers preceding a colon indicate the volume number.

A

abdomen 1:**11–13**
  ascites 4:545; 11:1533
  infertility investigation 7:945;
    8:1033–1034
  knife wound to 11:1534
  laparoscopy 4:*568, 569, 570,*
    571; 8:**1033–1034;** 9:1236;
    11:1459, 1520; 15:*2138*
  laparotomy 8:1035
  ligaments 8:1069
  pain 1:*11–13;* 6:797; 11:1475,
    1520–1521, 1578; 15:2152
  swelling 15:2148
  tuberculosis 16:2290
  tumors 16:2291
abortion 1:**14–16**
  after diagnostic tests 1:84; 3:368;
    4:506
  bleeding after 1:16
  ethics 9:1166
  failure 1:14
  salpingitis after 13:1858
  spontaneous *see* miscarriage
  sterilization not recommended at
    the same time of 15:2068
  subsequent miscarriages and
    9:1238
abrasion, chemical *see* dermabrasion
  abrasions and cuts 1:**17–20;** 17:*2422,*
    2423
  healing 6:*765*
  treatment 1:18, 20; 17:2424
  see also lacerations
abruption, placental 15:2081
abscess 1:21; 5:641; 13:1758
  heat treatment 6:797, 799;
    13:*1757*
  meibomian 15:2113
  parapharyngeal 16:2237
  peritonsillar (quinsy) 14:2012–2013;
    16:2236–2237
  releasing the pus 13:*1757, 1758*
    drainage 5:644
  tooth 1:*21;* 13:1758
absentmindedness 4:459
abstinence 1:22, 45
  periodic *see* rhythm method
  see also virginity
Acanthamoeba polyphaga 12:1704
accident prevention 1:**23–25**
  drowning 4:522
  electric shock 4:549
accidents
  occupational hazards 10:**1391–1396**
  see also emergencies
acetabulum 11:1523
acetaminophen (Tylenol; Tempra) 1:*137,*
    138; 11:*1479,* 1482
  damage to the kidneys 8:1020
  liver damage and 8:1084, 1087;
    11:1479
  overdose 11:1479; 12:1629, 1631;
    15:2093
acetone 6:740; 7:1006

acetylcholine 2:158; 6:*857;* 9:1266
  Alzheimer's disease and 1:82, 83
  myasthenia gravis and 10:1313
acetyl-L-carnitine (ALC) 14:1989
achalasia, of the esophagus 6:787
achondroplasia 4:532; 7:922; 10:*1306*
aciclovir (Zovirax) 3:382; 14:1939
acid-base balance 1:**26–27**
acidosis
  metabolic 1:26–27
  respiratory 1:27
acid rain 1:**28–30;** 12:1638–1639
acini 11:1486–1487
acne and pimples 1:**31–34;** 2:255; 7:*885;*
    14:1974
  acne rosacea 14:1975
  menstrual cycle and 1:32; 14:1970
  scarring from 1:31; 14:1880
  treatment 1:32–*34,* 75
acrodermatitis enteropathica 16:2250
acromegaly 5:697, 698; 12:1601
ACTH *see* adrenocorticotropic
    hormone
Acticoat7 3:301
actinomycosis, pulmonary
    13:*1749*
Activase 4:557
acupressure 1:**35–36;** 3:359;
    8:1144
acupuncture 1:**37–39,** 77, *80;* 3:359,
    360; 6:837, *838;* 10:1328; 11:1474
  the pulse and 13:1753
  to treat pain 1:38; 11:1478
  withdrawal from drugs and
    17:2416
acute abdomen 15:2152
Adam's apple 10:1332, *1335;*
    16:*2213*
adaptation syndrome 15:2099
ADD (attention deficit disorder)
    2:152; 13:1738
addiction
  to hospital or polysurgical *see*
    Munchausen syndrome
  psychological 14:1905
  to drugs 11:1554; 12:1710;
    17:2416
    sedatives 14:1902, 1905
    tranquilizers 16:2256
  treatment, using flotation
    therapy 5:649
  see also alcoholism
Addison's disease 1:48; 2:237;
    6:747; 7:896; 9:*1181;* 13:1862;
    15:2150
  fatigue and 5:619
  treatment 15:2072
adenoidectomy 1:41; 16:2212
adenoids 1:**40–41;** 2:281; 10:1372,
    1375; 11:1557; 16:2212–2213
  snoring and 14:*2005*
adenomyosis 9:1204; 17:2327
adenosine deaminase (ADA)
    deficiency 5:679, 680, 681
adenosine triphosphate (ATP)
    5:703
adenosis, sclerosing *see* mastitis,
    chronic
adenoviruses, used in gene
    therapy 5:680
ADHD *see* attention deficit
    hyperactivity disorder

adhesions 11:1533, 1534
  stiffness and 15:2077
adipometers 11:*1577*
adipose tissue 8:1079–1080
Adler, Alfred 3:398
adolescence 1:**42–45**
  abstinence education 1:22
  acne 1:*31;* 14:1974
  anxiety 1:105
  blushing 2:244; 14:1974
  duodenal ulcers 4:530
  fainting in 3:372; 5:612
  growing pains 5:**715,** 716
  growth in 4:532; 5:**716,** 717, 718
  homosexuality and 6:850
  hysteria 7:*906*
  mood swings 9:1206, *1245,* 1246
  need for privacy during 13:1739
  stretch marks 15:2105
  "suicidal gestures" 12:1630
  sweating 14:1974
  see also chat room; puberty
adrenal glands 1:**46–48;** 9:1246
  overactive 6:858
  pituitary gland and 4:567; 12:1598
  underactive 6:858
adrenaline (epinephrine) 1:47; 4:*566;*
    12:1724
  in the brain 2:229
  effects 1:*48;* 9:1246; 15:2085,
    2099
    blushing 2:244
    as a bronchodilator 1:140
    dry mouth 9:1262
    fat breakdown 5:622
    glycogen breakdown
      15:2064
    on the heart 6:781
    high blood pressure 1:46
  too much 6:858
  used as a drug 1:47
adrenocorticotropic hormone
    (ACTH) 12:1599, 1601
adult respiratory distress syndrome
    (ARDS; shock lung; wet lung)
    14:1943, 1946
aerobics 1:**49–52;** 7:**995–997;**
    11:1573, 1575; 17:2401
  aerobic capacity test 11:*1575*
affect 9:1245
  flattening of 9:1247
  incongruity of 9:1247
  lability of 9:1247
afterbirth *see* placenta
agammaglobulinemia 7:909
age spots 8:1090
  see also liver spots
aging 1:**53–55**
  absentmindedness 4:459
  Alzheimer's disease 1:82
  antiaging treatment
    melatonin 9:1186, 1187
    serums 9:1273
  arthritis 5:691
    osteoarthritis 1:*135–138*
  balance and 2:167; 11:1581
  blackouts 5:691
  cataracts 3:326
  causes 1:53–54
  cells and 1:54–55; 3:330
  cystitis and 4:450
  deafness 4:455; 5:692–693

dementia 5:692, 693
  drowsiness 4:523
  eyesight and 5:608; 10:1412
  fibrositis 5:643
  free radicals and 1:101
  frostbite and 5:665–666
  geriatric medicine 5:**691–694**
    physical therapy and 11:1581
  glaucoma 2:221; 5:701
  height loss 1:53; 3:324
  hip fractures 6:828, 830, 855
  hypothermia 5:693–694;
    7:900, *901,* 902
  impairment of faculties
    14:1910
  incontinence 5:693
  libido 1:53
  lower-back pain 5:630
  macular degeneration 2:220,
    222; 8:1119; 13:1811, *1812*
  malnutrition 8:*1127*
  memory and 9:1190, *1192;*
    14:1908, 1909–1910
  osteoporosis 5:693; 6:855;
    11:*1450–1451*
  physical disabilities 6:751
  prostate enlargement 12:1691
  psychiatric disorders
    14:1910–1911
  retirement and 8:1067
  sense of taste 16:2169
  skin 14:*1970,* 1975
    age spots 8:1090
    liver spots 8:*1091*
    wrinkles 14:*1970;* 15:2127;
      17:**2427–2428**
  strokes 5:691–692
  suicide in the elderly 6:839
  tiredness 5:620; 16:2229
  weight gain 10:1384
  see also menopause; senility
agoraphobia 10:*1357, 1358;* 11:1561, 1562,
    1563
AIDS 1:45, **56–58;** 7:938
  after acquiring a tattoo 16:2172, 2173
  AIDS hotline 1:56
  an occupational hazard 10:1395
  the blood-brain barrier and
    2:229, 230
  incubation period 7:928
  mouth ulcers, treatment 16:2204
  pigeon droppings and 10:1409
  pneumonia and 12:1623
  prevention 1:58; 7:936
  statistics 14:1935
  testing 1:56, *58*
  thrush 16:2219
  transmission 1:57; 7:936
    donated blood and 1:56, 57; 2:240
  treatment 1:58
    visualization 9:1231
  tuberculosis and 16:2287
AIDS-related complex (ARC) 1:57
air pollution 1:**59–60;** 4:573–574;
    12:*1636,* 1637–1639, *1641*
  acid rain and 1:29–30;
    12:1638–1639
  indoor 4:573
  ozone 11:1468; 12:1639
  sulfur dioxide 12:1639
  see also chlorofluorocarbons
airsickness *see* motion sickness

albinism **5**:684, 686; **6**:735; **7**:*921*, 922; **9**:1181; **10**:*1304*, *1305*
alcohol **4**:526; **11**:1510
  abuse in adolescence **1**:45
  abuse affects the nervous system **10**:1343
  arterial disease and **1**:120
  capillary dilation **3**:318
  a cause of jaundice **7**:991
  cold weather and **5**:666
  effect on the brain **7**:897
  effect on the liver **3**:375; **7**:991; **8**:1084, *1086*, *1087*
    gastritis and **5**:670, 671
  on an empty stomach **7**:*896*; **15**:2088
  hepatitis and **6**:810
  intoxication **7**:**968–969**
  memory loss and **9**:1190
  metabolised **2**:188; **7**:968
  mixing your drinks **6**:752
  personality and **9**:1278; **11**:1540
  poisoning **12**:1629
  recommended consumption **17**:2403
  for relaxation **13**:1800, *1801*; **14**:*1903*, 1904
  resistance to **7**:968
  as a sedative **14**:1903, 1904; **16**:2258
  sex and **14**:1922, 1923
    temporary impotence **14**:1928
  snoring and **14**:2004
  taken with analgesics **1**:137
  taken with antibiotics **1**:99
  vertigo and **17**:2366
  vision under the influence of **4**:505; **6**:752
alcoholism **1**:**61–64**; **7**:969; **14**:1903, 1904
  appetite and **6**:753
  cirrhosis of the liver and **3**:375
  pregnancy, fetal alcohol syndrome and **5**:633
  treatment **2**:176
    aversion therapy **2**:176, 177; **7**:969
    flotation therapy **5**:649
    rehabilitation **13**:1796, 1798
    tremor and **16**:2275
  ulcers and **4**:531
  vision and **3**:388
  withdrawal symptoms **1**:61; **6**:742; **17**:2417, *2418*
  see also hangover
aldosterone **1**:47; **2**:238, *239*; **4**:566; **6**:858; **8**:1020
alendronate **11**:1451; **16**:2259
Alexander technique **1**:**65–66**, 78–79; **6**:837, *838*
alimentary canal **1**:11, **67–69**
  see also colon; digestive system; duodenum; stomach
alkalosis
  metabolic **1**:27
  respiratory **1**:26, 27
allergies **1**:**70–74**; **3**:396; **16**:2238
  acute colitis and **3**:383
  blood cells and **2**:227
  breast-feeding and **13**:1750
  causes of **1**:72–73
  causing anaphylactic shock **14**:1945
  causing asthma **1**:140
  causing rhinitis **13**:1826; **14**:2002
  causing swelling **15**:2145, 2147
  diagnosis **1**:72, 73–74; **14**:1913
  ear **1**:71

eye **1**:71, *74*
  conjunctivitis and **3**:403
nose **1**:41, 71
self-help **1**:74
skin
  causing eczema **1**:71, 73; **4**:467, 468, 487, 542, 543
  contact dermatitis **1**:71, 73; **4**:467, 468; **6**:747; **14**:*1974*
  from tattoos **16**:2172, 2173
  heat and **6**:795
  urticaria *see* hives
to animals **1**:72
to bandages **4**:513, 516
to drugs and medicines **7**:893; **9**:1174; **14**:1959; **16**:2270
to food **1**:71–72; **4**:485, 487, 562; **5**:657
  causing migraine **9**:1224
  fish **1**:72
  milk **1**:72
  monosodium glutamate **5**:653
  shellfish **15**:2145
  soy **5**:675
to metal **4**:467, 468
  chrome **4**:467
  nickel **2**:251; **4**:467; **14**:1969
to penicillin **1**:70, 99, 100; **11**:1527, 1528, 1529; **14**:1959; **16**:2199
to soap **7**:884
total allergy syndrome **16**:2238
to tattoo pigments **16**:2172, 2173
treatment **1**:74
vaccines **11**:*1551*
see also hay fever; sensitization
allografts **5**:709, 710
aloe **10**:1329
alopecia *see* baldness
alpha-1 antitrypsin **4**:563, 564; **5**:681
alpha-linoleic acid **10**:1382
alpha thalassemia **16**:2201
alternative medicine **1**:**75–81**
  Alexander technique **1**:**65–66**, 78–79; **6**:837, *838*
  anthroposophical medicine **1**:79
  aromatherapy **1**:79, **114–117**; **6**:837
  ayurvedic medicine **1**:75, 79, 80
  Bach flower remedies **1**:79
  chiropractic **1**:**77–78**; **3**:**362–364**; **6**:*836*; **11**:1446
  color therapy **3**:**390–391**
  crystal therapy **1**:80
  cupping **1**:80, 81; **6**:835
  flotation therapy **5**:**648–650**
  herbal medicine *see* herbs and herbalism
  homeopathy **1**:*78*; **6**:837, **842–845**; **10**:1326
  iridology **1**:**80–81**; **7**:**975–976**
  kinesiology **1**:81; **6**:836
  meditation **1**:75, 80; **9**:**1178–1179**; **11**:1477; **13**:1802; **15**:2104
    transcendental **9**:1178; **15**:2104
  mud therapy **9**:**1270–1273**
  naturopathy **1**:81; **10**:**1326–1329**
  osteopathy **1**:78; **2**:161; **3**:362; **6**:837; **11**:**1446–1449**
  qigong (chi kung) **1**:81; **3**:358, 360–361
  reflexology **1**:*78*, 80; **6**:837; **8**:*1143*; **13**:**1793–1794**
  reiki **1**:81
  shiatsu **1**:80; **6**:776; **8**:*1144*; **14**:**1936–1937**
  see also acupuncture; faith healing; holistic medicine; massage

alternative medicine, hypnotherapy **1**:79; **6**:837; **12**:1712; **13**:1735, 1736
altitudes, high
  people living at **6**:*847*
  training at **15**:2052
altitude sickness **2**:283; **4**:502
alveolar processes **16**:2175
alveoli (air sacs) **2**:281; **4**:*563*
  COPD and **3**:370, *371*
alveolitis, fibrosing **13**:1751, 1752
Alzheimer's disease **1**:**82–83**; **4**:459, 552; **5**:693
  treatment **1**:82, 83
    development of smart drugs **14**:1989
amantadine **7**:927, 950
amblyopia *see* lazy eye
amenorrhea **9**:1205; **12**:1601
amino acids **4**:488; **12**:1701, *1702*
  dietary **10**:1381; **12**:**1701–1702**
aminoglycosides **1**:100
aminophylline **15**:2085
amnesia **9**:1192
  post-traumatic **6**:762
  retrograde **6**:762
amniocentesis **1**:84; **2**:207; **3**:367; **4**:506, 508; **5**:677, 686; **12**:1664, 1676
  miscarriage after **1**:84; **3**:368
  sex of the baby and **5**:638; **12**:1675
  spina bifida and **15**:2038
amnioscopy **4**:571
amniotic sac **9**:1188, 1189
amoebas **11**:1510
amphetamines **1**:**85–87**; **4**:*527*; **13**:1737; **15**:2083
  abuse **4**:524, 526, 527; **15**:2084
  causing schizophrenic symptoms **14**:1882
  used to lose weight **10**:1385
  withdrawal **17**:2417
ampicillin **1**:99
amputation
  phantom pain and **11**:1477
  reattachment of body parts **5**:709; **9**:1218, *1219–1221*; **12**:**1614–1615**
  severed fingers **6**:747
Amsler grid **8**:1119
amylase (ptyalin) **4**:*494*, 495; **5**:702; **8**:1149; 1261; **11**:1487, *1487*; **13**:1853; **15**:2063, *2064*
amylobarbital **2**:170
amyloid precursor protein (APP) **1**:83
amyotrophic lateral sclerosis (ALS) **9**:**1256–1259**
anabolism **9**:1214
anal canal, hemorrhoids **6**:**807–808**
analgesics *see* aspirin and analgesics
Ancylostoma duodenale **6**:852, 853
androgens **1**:48; **2**:169
  acne and **1**:32
  see also testosterone
androgynous people **5**:672
anemia **1**:**88–90**; **2**:225; **9**:1205
  aplastic **1**:89–90
  blood transfusions for **2**:241
  of chronic diseases **1**:89
  effects of hemorrhage with **6**:805
  Fanconi's **5**:676
  hemolytic **1**:89, 90; **15**:2045
  with hookworm infection **6**:852, 853
  iron deficiency **1**:88–89, 90; **7**:977
    detection **7**:978; **11**:1514
    during pregnancy **1**:88
    Patterson Brown-Kelly syndrome and **16**:2211
  leukemia and **8**:1061

pernicious *see* pernicious anemia
sickle-cell *see* sickle-cell anemia
symptoms **1**:90
  blackouts **2**:215
  fatigue **5**:619, 620; **16**:2230
  in the hand **6**:747
thalassemia **1**:88, 89, 90; **16**:**2200–2201**
  detection **3**:367
vitamin B12 deficiency and **17**:2355
vitamin deficiency **1**:88
anencephaly **2**:207; **3**:401; **10**:1350
anesthesia, "glove and stocking" **7**:907
anesthesiologists **1**:91; **15**:2137
anesthetics **1**:**91–93**; **15**:2135
  aftereffects **1**:93
  dental uses **1**:92–93
  epidural **1**:92, 93
    for cesarean births **3**:*342*
    for labor **1**:93; **2**:201, 285; **8**:1093; **15**:*2041*
  general **1**:**91–92**, 93; **10**:**1405–1406**, **15**:2135
    recovery from **12**:1645
  local *see* local anesthetics
    premedication **1**:91, 93; **12**:**1670**; **14**:1902
  regional **15**:2135
  spinal **1**:92, 93; **15**:2134, 2135
  see also anesthetics, epidural
aneurysms
  aortic **1**:121; **6**:803
  berry, in the brain **6**:804; **15**:2107
angina **1**:121; **3**:**419–420**; **6**:783, 790; **15**:2067; **16**:2217
  exercise and **11**:1577
  pain **3**:348, 419–420; **6**:784, 786; **15**:*2149*
  pins-and-needles and **12**:1597
  shoulder or arm pain and **14**:1948
  treatment **15**:2151
    angioplasty **3**:421
    bypass surgery **3**:421; **10**:*1403*
    drugs **2**:157, 158; **3**:420; **16**:2260
    transdermal patches **16**:2260
angiography **4**:478; **10**:1356
  cardiac **6**:790
  carotid angiogram **17**:*2357*, 2431, *2434*
  fluorescein **8**:1119
angioplasty
  balloon **3**:346, 421; **9**:*1170–1171*, 1172
  cerebral **4**:557
angiotensin **2**:238, 239
animals
  diseases from **7**:935
  experiments on **12**:1718
  have minds **9**:1226, *1229*
  pets and hygiene **7**:887, *888*; **11**:1498, 1500
  phobias of **11**:*1561*, 1563
  quarantine **13**:1763
  sense of taste **16**:2169
  transgenic **4**:503; **5**:681
ankles
  edema **4**:*544*, 545; **6**:790; **15**:2146
  fractured **5**:661
  ligaments **8**:1070
  osteoarthritis **10**:1437
  sprained **6**:764; **15**:*2057*, 2145
  stiffness **15**:2079
ankylosing spondylitis **1**:123; **2**:161, 163
  cause **1**:123, 126
  the ribs and **13**:1834
  symptoms **1**:126; **8**:1094
  treatment **1**:126
anodontia **16**:2178

anorexia and bulimia 1:*94–96*
    anorexia nervosa 1:*94–96*; 4:487;
        6:846; 17:2398
    constipation 3:405
    bulimia 1:94, *95*, 96; 10:1384;
        17:2391
anosmia (loss of sense of smell)
    14:1993; 16:2169, *2170*
antacids 6:787; 7:930
anthrax 1:97
    a biological weapon 1:97; 2:185, 186
    vaccination 1:97
anthroposophical medicine 1:79
antianxiety drugs *see* tranquilizers
antibiotic-resistant bacteria 1:98, 100;
    2:164; 9:1174; 11:1527, 1529; 13:1744;
    16:2199
    MRSA 1:98; 11:1508; 15:2062
antibiotics 1:*99–100*; 2:165; 7:940;
    9:1174
    ineffective against viruses 11:1528;
        17:2369
    side effects 1:100; 14:1959;
        17:2364
    see also penicillin; tetracycline
antibodies (immunoglobulins) 2:165,
    227; 7:908, 940; 8:1113; 17:2330
    allergies and 1:72–73, 140
    antilymphocyte 7:914
    antinuclear 8:1107
    antiphospholipid 8:1107
    classes of 7:909
    from donated blood 2:232
    treatment for Guillain-Barré
        syndrome 6:728, 729
anticoagulants, side effects 14:1959
anticonvulsants 5:585
antidepressants 4:464, 466;
    13:1737–1738; 14:1903–1904;
    15:2084
    side effects 14:1958, 1959
antidiuretic hormone (ADH) 4:566,
    567; 5:597; 6:858; 7:898–899;
    8:1018–1020; 12:1599, 1601
antifreeze poisoning 12:1631
antihistamines 1:72, 74; 6:756, 831
    rashes and 13:1784
    sedative 7:893
    side effects 7:893; 14:1956, 1959
antioxidants 1:101; 7:946; 9:1187;
    10:1328, 1382; 17:2379, 2384, 2387
antiperspirants 2:249; 5:596; 11:1544
antipsychotic drugs 12:1720, 1722;
    13:1737; 14:1905
    side effects 14:1959
antiretroviral agents 17:2372
antiseptics
    garlic 6:*814*
    Lister and 15:2135, *2137*
antivenin 14:2000, *2001*
antiviral drugs 17:2369
    see also aciclovir
ant stings 2:211
anus 1:*102–103*; 13:1787
    bleeding from 1:102
    boils 1:*102*, 103
    damage to, and constipation
        3:405
    fissures 1:*102*, 103; 6:808
        treatment 6:808
        use of laxatives and 8:1046
    fistulas 1:*102*, 103; 6:808
    hemorrhoids 6:*807–808*
        constipation and 3:405
        during pregnancy 5:637; 12:1662,
            1675
        external (prolapsed) 1:103; 6:*808*;
            15:2095, *2096*

strangulation of 15:2095
    internal 1:103; 6:*808*; 15:*2096*
        treatment 6:808
        use of laxatives and 8:1046
    itching 1:103
    rectal prolapse 1:*103*; 12:1686,
        1687, 1688
    skin tags 6:808
anxiety 1:*104–106*; 10:1343, *1357–1358*;
    12:1713; 15:2150
    disorders 10:*1357–1358*
    nervous breakdown and
        10:*1341–1342*
    reactive 10:1357
    symptoms 1:106; 10:1357; 12:1724
        cold sores 3:382
        dry mouth 9:1262; 13:1852, 1854
        gastrointestinal problems 7:980
        insomnia 7:959
        stomachache 1:11, 13
        tremor 16:2275
        ulcers 4:531
    treatment 2:*176*; 9:1178;
        13:1737–1738; 14:1905;
        15:2150; 16:2256
    see also complexes and
        compulsions; hypochondria;
        obsessive-compulsive disorder;
        phobias; stress
anxiety complex 3:398
anxiolytic drugs *see* tranquilizers
aorta 1:118; 3:372, 419
    aneurysms 1:121; 6:803
    coarctation of the 9:1289
    dissection of the 1:121; 13:1754
    valves 3:320
aphasia 1:*107–108*; 10:1308; 15:2030
apnea
    in babies 15:2117
    sleep 16:2236
apocrine glands 5:*700*; 11:1544; 14:1970
apothecaries 11:1551
appendicitis 1:*109–111*; 11:1512
    "left-sided" *see* diverticulitis
        peritonitis and 1:111; 11:1532,
            1534–1535
        symptoms 1:110, 111; 11:1535
appendix 1:*109*, 110
    appendicitis 1:*109–111*; 11:1512
        "left-sided" *see* diverticulitis
        peritonitis and 1:111; 11:1532,
            1534–1535
        symptoms 1:110, 111; 11:1535
    gangrenous 5:669
    "grumbling" 1:21, 109, 110
    on the left side 2:252
    perforated/ruptured 1:111;
        11:*1532*, 1534
    removal 1:110, 111; 11:1512
        discharge from the scar 5:644
        flatulence after 1:109, 111
        as a preventative measure 1:109
        scar 1:109
appendix mass 11:1535
appestat 1:113
appetite 1:*112–113*
appliances, orthodontic 10:*1426*,
    1428–1429; 16:*2175*, 2177
aqueous humor 5:701
arboviruses 17:2406, 2439
ARDS (adult respiratory distress
    syndrome; shock lung; wet lung)
    14:1943, 1946
armpits, swollen lymph nodes 8:*1109*,
    1111
arms
    artificial 1:127, *128*; 12:*1696*, *1697*,
        1698

bionic 2:*191*
    body language and 2:*247*
    broken, treatment 15:*2048*, *2049*
    reattached 9:1218
    stiffness 15:2078
    swollen after lymph node removal
        8:1109, 1112
Arnold-Chiari malformation 7:*879*
aromatherapy 1:79, 114–117; 6:837
arrhythmias 2:215; 3:421; 11:1472
    sinus 6:781
arteries and artery disease 1:*118–121*
    arteries
        bleeding from 1:18, 20; 6:803
        bypassing blocked arteries 9:1221;
            10:*1403*; 17:2341, 2357
        clearing blocked arteries 3:421;
            9:*1170–1171*, 1172
        fatty degeneration and
            hemorrhaging 6:803, *804*
        grafting 5:711
        pulse and 13:*1753–1754*
        structure 1:119, 121
    atherosclerosis 1:119; 2:214; 3:372, 419;
        10:1382; 16:2215
        cholesterol and 1:119–120; 3:366;
            6:783
        coronary artery 1:121; 3:419–420
            development of 1:*121*
            epileptic seizures and 5:583
            gangrene and 5:669
            men and 1:118
            obesity and 10:1385
            prevention 5:600; 17:2387
            smoking and 1:118; 6:783
            strokes and 1:121; 15:2107
            transient ischemic attacks and
                16:2261
            treatment 3:345, 346
        coronary arteries and
            thrombosis 1:118; 3:419–421;
                6:783–784
        coronary artery surgery 3:420–421;
            10:*1403*
        coronary disease 3:421; 6:789
        coronary thrombosis 3:419–420;
            6:783–784; 16:2215–2216, 2217
        hardening & loss of elasticity
            (arteriosclerosis) 1:119; 15:2121
        limping and 8:1075
        smoking and 1:101, 118; 5:669;
            6:783
    arteriograms 1:118
        cerebral 2:265, 266
    arteriosclerosis 1:119; 15:2121
    arteriovenous anomaly 15:2108
    arteriovenous malformation
        6:804
    arteritis
        temporal 15:2150
            treatment 15:2073
    arthritis 1:*122–126*
        in the back 2:163; 7:1002
        dysentery and 4:533
        the feet and 12:1628
        fibrositis and 5:643
        flitting 13:1818
        fractures and 5:662
        from gonorrhea 5:705, 706
        from Lyme disease 8:1108
        from rubella 1:124
        from tuberculosis 1:124
        help available 1:*124*, 126
        reactive *see* reactive arthritis
        rheumatoid *see* rheumatoid
            arthritis
        septic 1:124
        traumatic 1:123–124

treatment 1:124–126
    heat 6:797, 799
    hydrotherapy 7:881, 882
    meditation 9:1178
    rehabilitation 13:1795, *1798*, 1799
    splints 15:2049
    see also gout; osteoarthritis
arthrodesis 1:126
arthrograms 17:2432
arthroplasty, hip 2:189
arthroscopy 1:125; 4:571; 10:*1432*, 1434
artificial insemination 1:*129*, 130;
    15:2141
    by donor (AID) 1:129, 130; 7:942, 945
    by husband (AIH) 7:945
artificial limbs 1:*127–128*; 8:1076;
    10:*1344*; 12:*1696–1699*
    arms 1:127, *128*; 12:*1696*, *1697*, 1698
    bionic 2:*191*
    legs 1:127; 12:*1696–1698*
    physical therapy and 11:1580
    see also bionics; prostheses
artificial methods of conception
    1:*129–131*
    in vitro fertilization (IVF) 1:129, 131;
        7:*971–974*; 11:1520
artificial respiration (kiss of life;
    mouth-to-mouth resuscitation)
    1:*132–135*; 3:*321*; 4:522, 555; 13:*1809*
    for a baby or child 1:*134*
    cardiopulmonary resuscitation
        (CPR) 1:134, 135; 3:320, *321*; 13:1807,
        1808, *1809*, 1810
art therapy 3:390
arytenoid cartilages 17:*2389*
asbestos 12:*1639*
    an occupational hazard 10:1391,
        1395
asbestosis 1:136; 12:*1639*; 13:1751
ascariasis 11:1501; 17:2419
Ascaris 11:*1499*, *1500*, 1501; 17:*2420*
ascites 4:545; 11:1533
ascorbic acid 17:2378
aseptic techniques 15:*2135–2136*
aspartame 5:654
Asperger's syndrome 4:536
asphyxia 1:132–135
aspirin and analgesics 1:*137–138*
    analgesics (painkillers) 1:*137–138*;
        11:*1478–1480*, *1481–1482*
    see also acetaminophen; codeine;
        ibuprofen; morphine
    aspirin 1:137, 138; 11:1478–1479, 1482,
        1554
        allergy 10:1370
        damage to the esophagus 6:787
        damage to the kidneys 8:1020
        dangerous to suck 16:2235
        deafness and 1:122; 4:455
        dosage 1:137; 11:1460
        gargle 14:2013; 16:2213
        heart attacks and 6:785; 11:1478
        interaction with warfarin
            14:*1957–1958*
        overdose 4:562; 11:1460; 12:1629
        Reye's syndrome and 5:641;
            11:1478, 1479; 13:*1813–1814*
        side effects 14:1959
        stomach irritation 7:1002
        gastric ulcers and 1:122; 11:1479
        stroke prevention 15:2111;
            16:*2261*, 2262
        treatment for arthritis 1:122
        treatment for stiffness 15:2079
    see also painkillers
assertiveness training 15:2104
assisted living programs 6:841
asthma 1:*139–141*; 8:*1103–1104*; 11:1464;

asthma (cont'd)
13:1751
avoidance of beta-blockers 3:419,
420
breast-feeding and 13:1750
causes 1:140, 141; 8:1103
air pollution and 1:59, 60;
15:2050
anxiety as a trigger 8:1100
too much hygiene and 7:888
eczema and 4:542
pigeon chest and 12:1590,
1592
pneumonia and 12:1622
prevention 1:73, 141
symptoms 1:73, 140–141; 2:282; 3:348
phlegm 11:1560
wheezing 17:2407, 2408
treatment 1:73, 74, 141; 2:157, 158,
282; 8:1103; 17:2408
desensitization 14:1913
herbal remedies 6:814
inhalants 7:953–954
steroids 7:953, 954; 15:2072
astigmatism 1:142; 4:505; 5:608;
10:1413
after cataract removal 3:328
astrology 11:1542
ataxia 2:149; 3:335, 336
veganism and 17:2355
atheroma 1:118, 119–120; 3:419, 421;
6:783; 16:2215
atherosclerosis 1:119; 2:214; 3:372, 419;
10:1382; 16:2215
cholesterol and 1:119–120; 3:366;
6:783
coronary artery 6:783–784; 10:1403
angina and 3:419–420
heart attack and 1:121
development of 1:121
epileptic seizures and 5:583
gangrene and 5:669
men and 1:118
obesity and 10:1385
prevention
exercise 5:600
using antioxidants 17:2387
smoking and 1:118; 6:783
strokes and 1:121; 15:2107
transient ischemic attacks and
16:2261
treatment
chelation therapy 3:345, 346
surgery 3:346
athetosis 3:335, 336
athlete's foot 2:150; 7:886, 937; 13:1763,
1838; 14:1975
affecting nails 2:150; 13:1837, 1838
Candida as cause of 17:2436
treatment 2:150; 13:1838
atopy (atopic syndrome) 1:70; 4:542;
6:756; 14:1975
ATP (adenosine triphosphate) 5:703
atrial fibrillation 4:551
atrophic vaginitis see vaginitis,
atrophic
atropine 2:158
as a medication 7:1004; 12:1670
allergy to 12:1670
attention deficit disorder (ADD) 2:152
attention deficit hyperactivity
disorder (ADHD) 1:86; 2:151–152;
4:536; 8:1051
audiometers 6:778
aura, color therapy and 3:390
auriscopes 15:2157
Australopithecus, skeleton
14:1967–1968

autism 2:153–155; 8:1051–1052
speech difficulties and 10:1308,
1309
autoanalyzers 15:2025
autogenic training 2:183
autografts 5:709, 710
autoimmune diseases 8:1113
Crohn's disease as 4:442
diabetes as 4:472
Guillain-Barré syndrome 6:728
lupus 8:1105–1107; 11:1565
pernicious anemia as 11:1536–1537
rheumatoid arthritis 1:122; 7:1002
scleroderma 14:1888–1889; 15:2148
treatment, immunosuppressive
drugs 7:914; 8:1113
vitiligo 17:2388
see also glomerulonephritis;
myasthenia gravis
autonomic nervous system 2:156–158;
9:1268; 10:1345
labile 5:612
autopsies 11:1511, 1512, 1514
on stillborn babies 15:2080
avascular necrosis, of the head of the
femur see Perthes' disease
aversion therapy 2:176, 177; 7:969
awareness 5:696
Awareness Through Movement (ATM)
5:630, 631, 632
axons 10:1344, 1347
ayurvedic medicine 1:75, 79, 80
azathioprine 4:443
azoospermia 1:130
AZT 2:230

B

babies
abdomen 1:11
accident prevention 1:23–25
anxiety 1:104
appetite 1:112
balance 2:167
blue 2:242–243; 6:788
bonding with 2:204
burping 3:306
choking 1:135
colic 3:356; 4:444, 445; 5:702
constipation 1:69
convulsions 5:413
coordination 3:415
cradle cap 14:1972–1973
crying 4:444, 445; 6:758; 10:1366
dangers of shaking babies 11:1515
development 3:354–355, 356
diarrhea 1:69; 4:485, 486; 7:1004;
13:1856
drooling 9:1262
of drug addicts 4:524
eczema 4:542, 543
erections 5:589
exchange transfusions 2:240; 7:992
eye color 5:639, 682
feces 4:486; 5:623
feeding
breast milk 2:272–274; 4:486;
9:1186
cow's milk 4:494
formula milk 4:494
solid food 3:354
feet 5:626
fontanelles (fontanels) 2:257;
14:1967
gastroenteritis 4:486; 5:671
gestational limits and viability
10:1336

handicapped 6:749
head injuries 6:762
head lifting 10:1332
head shape 7:878
heat loss 7:900, 901, 902
hiccups 1:67
hygiene and 7:886
hypertonic 4:444
illness diagnosed in 15:2149
infantile acne 1:32
inherited immunity in 7:908;
13:1763
meningitis 9:1196
middle-ear infection 11:1453
mouth
putting things into 9:1260
thrush (Candida) 17:2437, 2438
newborn
begin to breath 8:1102–1103
brain damage at birth 2:267
can sense pain 10:1338
with a caul 9:1188
hips checked 6:829–830
jaundice 3:336; 6:810; 7:990, 991,
992; 8:1087
oxygen therapy 2:266
pediatrics and 11:1515–1516, 1517,
1518
PKU heel-prick test 11:1559
screening 14:1893
skeleton 14:1967
sucking reflex 13:1789, 1792
teeth already in the mouth
16:2175
tests for congenital diseases
3:401; 11:1518, 1559; 14:1893
vitamin K for 17:2385, 2386
overweight 4:488
period 17:2328
premature 2:204, 279; 7:933;
10:1338; 11:1516, 1517;
12:1666–1669
giving oxygen to 11:1464, 1466
rashes 12:1685
diaper rash 1:102, 103; 4:481–483;
5:598; 14:1973, 2009; 17:2438
reflexes 13:1789, 1790, 1791, 1792
screening 14:1893
eye tests 10:1407
hearing tests 4:454
sense of touch 16:2239
shyness 3:356
skull 14:1967
sleep 3:354; 14:1976, 1980
sleeping position 15:2116, 2117
spitting out food 9:1262
sudden infant death syndrome
(SIDS) 15:2116–2117
suffocation 1:135
teeth 16:2175, 2176, 2177
teething 9:1262; 16:2177, 2178
temperature 15:2116
test-tube see in vitro fertilization
vaccinations, diphtheria 4:497
vision 11:1515
vomiting 1:69
projectile 1:67, 69
weaning, flatulence and 5:645
see also children; fetus
Babinski's sign 6:763
baby blues 9:1247; 12:1649
see also postpartum depression
and psychosis
Bach flower remedies 1:79
bacilli 2:164; 5:670
Bacillus anthracis 1:97
backache, see also chiropractic;
osteopathy

back and backache 2:159–163, 258
back injuries, hydrotherapy and
7:883
causes of backache 2:160, 161–163;
8:1094
ankylosing spondylitis 1:126;
2:163; 8:1094
arthritis 2:163; 7:1002
cancer 2:161; 8:1094
chills 2:160
crush fractures 8:1094
fibrositis 5:643
gallstones 2:161
gynecological disorders 2:161
muscular spasm 2:163; 5:643
osteoporosis 2:163
pregnancy 2:159, 163; 11:1526;
12:1662
psychosomatic 2:161
sciatica 2:161–163; 8:1078, 1094,
1095; 10:1349; 14:1885–1887, 1983
shingles 2:161
slipped disks 14:1983
strains or sprains 2:160, 161;
8:1072, 1094, 1095
tuberculosis of the spine 2:161
wear and tear 2:160–161
exercises to avoid backache 2:162
humpback 11:1450, 1451
lower-back pain (lumbago) 2:160,
161; 8:1094–1095
treatment 2:163; 5:630
manipulation 8:1135
stiff back 15:2078
heat treatment 15:2076
treatment of backache 2:163;
8:1094, 1095; 13:1796
heat 6:797, 798
spinal fusion 7:1002
yoga 17:2442
see also spine
backbone see spine
bacteria 2:164–166; 7:935, 936–939
antibiotic-resistant 1:98, 100; 2:164;
9:1174; 11:1527, 1529; 13:1744;
16:2199
antibiotics and 1:99–100
causing fever 5:641
infections, incubation period 7:928
intestinal, and vitamin K 17:2385
toxins 7:936–939, 940
"baker's cyst" 1:122
Balamuthia mandrillaris 12:1703
balance 2:167–168; 4:453, 454; 17:2364
dizziness/vertigo and 4:502;
17:2364–2365
physical therapy and 11:1581
balanitis 10:1368; 11:1531; 17:2437
balantidiasis 12:1704
baldness (alopecia) 2:169; 5:709; 6:736;
17:2387
male pattern (androgenic alopecia)
2:169; 6:737; 14:1969
in patches (alopecia areata)
2:169; 6:736; 14:1969
"ballet dancer's toe" 1:122
bandages see dressings and bandages
barbiturates 2:170; 4:527; 7:892–893;
14:1903, 1904
abuse 4:525, 526
overdose 2:170; 3:395
withdrawal 5:583; 17:2417, 2418
barium liquids 2:171–172; 4:443, 475,
478; 17:2433, 2434
enemas 4:478, 572; 15:2096
Bartholin glands 5:690; 7:964; 9:1269;
17:2394
abscess 6:733; 17:2335, 2394

blocked 17:2333, 2335
  infection 17:2394
Bartholinitis 17:2394
basal metabolic rate (BMR) 2:173;
  17:2401
basophils 2:227
BCG vaccine 7:912; 16:2287, 2290
bedbugs 2:174, 175
bedsores (decubitus ulcers) 2:175;
  11:1490, 1494; 14:2008–2009;
  17:2310, 2314
bed-wetting (enuresis) 2:217–218;
  7:925, 926
bee stings 2:210, 211–212
behavior therapy 2:176–177; 10:1358;
  11:1482, 1541; 12:1712, 1714–1715;
  13:1734–1736
  see also biofeedback techniques
Behçet's disease 17:2311–2312
belladonna 2:158
belle indifférence, la 7:907
Bell's palsy 3:403; 5:610
  sense of taste and 16:2171
Bell's phenomenon 5:610
belly button, pierced 11:1515
bends 2:178
bentonite 9:1273
benzene 1:59
benzene poisoning 10:1393
benzodiazepines 7:892, 893; 14:1903,
  1904, 1905, 1978; 16:2256–2258
  see also chlordiazepoxide;
    diazepam; nitrazepam
benzoyl peroxide 1:33
bereavement see grief, bereavement
beriberi 17:2375, 2376
beta-blockers 2:158
  effect on blood pressure 2:239
  side effects 14:1959
    in asthmatics 3:419
      sedative action 14:1904
    as tranquilizers 16:2257
  treatment for angina 3:420
beta-carotene 1:101
beta thalassemia 16:2200–2201
Bhopal disaster 4:574
bicalutamide (Casodex) 12:1694–1695
bicarbonate of soda 7:929
bile 2:179–180; 3:366; 4:494; 5:597, 598,
  667; 7:991
  digestion of fats and 5:621
  gallstones and 5:667–668
  lack of 4:495
  vitamin K absorption and 17:2385
bile duct, common, obstruction 5:668
bilharzia see schistosomiasis
bilious attacks 5:596
bilirubin 2:180; 5:598, 623
  jaundice and 7:990, 991; 11:1581
biliverdin 2:180
bill of rights, a patient's 7:873
BioChips 3:334
bioenergetics 9:1222; 13:1735
biofeedback techniques 2:181–184;
  5:648, 650; 9:1232, 1266; 11:1482
  see also feedback
biofuels 5:674
biological and chemical warfare 1:97;
  2:185–186; 4:440
biological clocks 2:187–188; 9:1187
  jet lag and 7:993–994
  sleep and 14:1976, 1977
biomedical engineering 2:189–190
  see also diagnostic imaging; kidney
    dialysis; pacemaker; prostheses
bionics 2:191
biopsy 2:192–193; 4:570; 8:1029;
  15:2025–2026

heart muscle 6:794
  for malignancy 6:726
    breast 8:1132
    skin 9:1184
biorhythms 2:194–197; 8:1055
bioterrorism, emergency departments
  and 4:557
bipolar disorder 2:198–199; 9:1207,
  1209, 1247; 12:1713
  hypochondria and 7:895
  treatment 2:198, 199; 9:1209;
    12:1710, 1720; 13:1738
bird fancier's lung 13:1751
birds, catching psittacosis from 12:1705
birth 2:200–205
  "baby blues" following 9:1247;
    12:1649
  biological clock and 2:187
  breathing exercises during 12:1679
  breech 2:205, 284–285; 3:342
  cesarean 2:204–205; 3:340–342;
    7:931, 932
  development of PMS after 12:1671
  emergency delivery 2:205
  episiotomy 2:203, 285; 5:586;
    8:1030; 10:1322, 1324
  father at the 12:1676
  forceps delivery 2:201, 208
  lack of libido and difficulties with
    sex after 8:1062; 14:1921, 1928
  men can experience pain of 11:1476
  multiple 9:1277
  natural childbirth 2:200;
    10:1321–1325
  pain relief
    acupuncture 1:39
    drugs 10:1319, 1324
    epidural anesthesia 1:93; 2:201,
      285; 8:1093; 15:2041
    postnatal sessions 11:1580
  postpartum depression and
    psychosis 4:465; 8:1062; 9:1247;
      10:1322; 12:1648–1651
  puerperal sepsis following
    17:2338–2339
  umbilical-cord accidents 15:2094
  vaginal discharge after
    17:2338–2339
  vaginal lacerations and 8:1031;
    17:2333
  see also babies, newborn; labor
birth control see contraception;
  rhythm method
birth defects 2:206–207; 4:574
  of the brain and spine (neural tube
    defects) 2:207
    anencephaly 2:207; 3:401; 10:1350
    hydrocephalus 2:207; 7:878–880;
      9:1197; 10:1350
    meningocoele 10:1351; 15:2037,
      2039
    myelomeningocoele 10:1351
    see also spina bifida
  clubfoot 2:207; 3:379; 12:1594
  detection 2:207
    amniocentesis 1:84
    chorionic villus sampling 2:207;
      3:367–368; 5:638; 7:877
    ultrasound 2:207, 285; 4:477, 479,
      480; 12:1664, 1676; 13:1869, 1870;
      14:1893, 1894; 15:2143; 17:2315,
      2316–2317
  eye 2:207
  genetic see genetic diseases and
    disorders
  heart 2:206–207, 242–243
  hip dislocation 3:402; 4:499;
    6:829–830

thalidomide and 2:206; 3:402;
  6:749; 9:1170; 11:1550;
  16:2203–2204
  of the urinary tract 2:207
  see also cleft palate; congenital
    disorders
birthmarks 2:208–209; 12:1613; 14:1972,
  1974
  see also moles
bisacodyl, suppositories 15:2133
bisexuality 6:851; 14:1929
bites and stings 2:210–212; 7:887;
  15:2145, 2147
  ants 2:211
  bedbug 2:174, 175
  bee 2:210, 211–212
  blisters and 2:223, 224
  dog 2:210, 211, 236
  first aid 2:210, 211; 4:556
  fleas 2:211; 5:646–647
  itching 7:988, 989
  jellyfish and similar creatures 2:210,
    211; 16:2272
  lice 2:211; 8:1065
  mosquito 2:210, 211; 5:646; 12:1703;
    16:2272
  rabies and 13:1766–1767
  sea urchin 2:212; 16:2272
  snakebites 2:212; 14:2000–2001;
    16:2280
  ticks 2:211
  wasp 2:210, 212
Black Death 12:1606, 1607
black eye 2:213; 5:604; 17:2424
blackheads (comedones) 1:31, 32;
  14:1901
blackouts 2:214–215
  in the elderly 5:691
  see also fainting; unconsciousness
blackwater fever 8:1123; 12:1704
bladder and bladder problems, cystitis
  2:217, 218; 3:409; 4:449–450;
  6:857; 7:886; 17:2324
  bladder capacity 17:2324
  bladder control 2:217–218
  cystoscopy 4:570; 9:1236
  problems
    cancer 3:316; 13:1776; 17:2325
    incontinence 2:218; 5:693;
      7:925–926; 12:1687; 15:2040
    prolapse (cystocele) 7:925;
      12:1686, 1687
    stones 17:2325
    tumors 2:217
bleach, swallowed 4:562;
  5:592
bleeding see hemorrhage
blepharoplasty 17:2427
blindness and braille 2:219–222
  blindness 10:1411
    color 3:388–389; 5:606
    glaucoma and 5:701
    hallucinations and 6:742
    hearing and 6:777
    hysterical 7:906, 907
    night 10:1362; 17:2373, 2374
    the senses and 14:1990,
      1993–1994; 16:2239, 2242
    toxins and 10:1411
  braille 2:220, 221–222; 16:2242
blind spot 5:606, 607; 10:1410
blinking 13:1789, 1792
blisters 2:223–224
  blood 13:1756
  cold sore 3:382
  from burns 3:304
  from impetigo 7:918
  over bunions 3:300

blood 2:225–228
  "blue" 2:225
  clotting 1:17; 2:226, 227; 6:801–802
    thrombus formation and 16:2214
  clotting disorders 2:228; 6:804
    hemophilia 2:206, 228;
      5:685–686; 6:801–802; 7:922;
      10:1306
    purpura 2:228; 13:1756
    vitamin K deficiency and 2:228;
      17:2385–2386
    von Willebrand's disease 17:2392
  manufacture of blood cells 2:226,
    227–228
  pH 1:26
  plasma 2:227; 12:1611
    burns or scalds and 2:227;
      13:1867, 1868
    transfusions 12:1611; 13:1867
  platelets 2:226, 227, 228; 3:298;
    13:1755
  red blood cells 2:225, 281
    anemia and 1:88
    broken down 7:990–991
    sickle-cell anemia and 14:1954, 1955
    sugar 15:2121
    tests 2:225; 4:475; 8:1029;
      15:2024–2025
    "tired" 2:225
  umbilical-cord 5:676, 677
  white blood cells 2:165, 225–227;
    7:946
    disorders 2:228
    inflammation and 7:948
    leukemia and 8:1059, 1060–1061
    see also eosinophils; lymphocytes
blood-brain barrier (BBB) 2:229–230;
  3:318–319
  cellular phones and 3:334
blood donors 2:231–232; 6:810; 7:977,
  990; 12:1611
blood groups 2:233–235
  blood transfusions and 2:234, 240,
    241
  see also rhesus (Rh) factor
blood poisoning 2:236; 14:1914
blood pressure 2:237–239; 3:373
  biofeedback techniques and 2:183
  changes in a day 2:188
  control 2:239; 6:847
  low (hypotension) 2:237
    postural hypotension 2:215;
      17:2364
  measurement 1:119; 3:373; 15:2036
    in the heart 14:1945, 1947
  raised (hypertension) 1:46;
    2:237; 12:1724–1725
    effect on the kidneys 8:1017, 1021
    headaches and 6:759
    the heart and 4:551
    hemorrhoids and 6:807
    hypertensive retinopathy and
      13:1812
    "malignant" 8:1124
    ongoing treatment 9:1173
    proteinuric see preeclampsia
    salt and 13:1861
    self help for 2:238
    stroke and 15:2107, 2111
    treatment 2:181, 183, 183–184, 237,
      239; 4:500; 5:611, 650
blood transfusions 2:240–241; 6:806;
  7:970
  before transplant surgery 16:2265
  blood groups and 2:234, 240, 241
    rhesus factor 2:233; 13:1815
  exchange transfusions 2:240; 7:992
  malaria and 11:1500

blood transfusions (cont'd)
plasma 12:1611; 13:1867
blue baby 2:242–243; 6:788
blushing 2:244; 14:1974
body language 2:245–248; 12:1712
body mass index (BMI) 11:1577; 17:2399, 2400, 2401
body odor 2:249
body piercing 2:250–251
ears 2:250, 251
keloid scars and 14:1880
infected 11:1515
body plethysmography 3:371
body structure 2:252–254
body wraps, marine algae 6:776
boils 2:255–256; 13:1757
bone marrow see marrow
bone marrow puncture 8:1061
bones 2:257–260
in the back 2:159
bent 3:352
cancer 2:161, 163, 260; 14:1966
pain relief 8:1093; 12:1692
in ribs 13:1834
thermography and 16:2208
chipped 5:662
congenital diseases 2:259
cracked 5:662
cysts 4:447; 11:1503
fractures 2:258, 259; 5:660–664; 14:1964, 1968
avulsion 8:1072
Colles' 5:660; 17:2430
comminuted (crushed) 5:660, 661, 664
compound 5:660, 662; 10:1432–1433
dangers 5:663
first aid 4:556; 5:663; 10:1393
greenstick 5:660, 662; 14:1964
hairline 15:2048
healing 5:660
and infection 5:660
manipulation 8:1135
march 5:662
osteoporosis and 2:161; 3:310; 5:660; 6:828; 8:1078
pathological 5:660; 14:1964
Pott's 5:661
recovery 5:664
repair 2:260
simple 5:660, 661
spontaneous 14:1964
sports 15:2050–2051, 2054
stress 15:2050–2051, 2054
treatment 5:663–664; 8:1135; 10:1430–1433; 15:2048, 2049; 16:2253, 2254, 2255
untreated 5:664
grafts 5:709, 711; 10:1430, 1432; 12:1616, 1617
growth 5:698, 717–718
gigantism or acromegaly and 5:698
infections (osteomyelitis) 2:258, 260
movement and 9:1265
osteomalacia 2:259; 13:1835, 1836
osteoporosis 2:258, 260; 3:310, 311; 5:693; 6:854, 855; 9:1199; 11:1450–1451; 14:1968
backache and 2:161, 163
causing limping 8:1078
fractures and 2:161; 3:310; 5:660; 6:828; 8:1078
HRT and 2:260; 6:855, 856; 9:1199; 11:1450, 1451

immobilization 2:260
Paget's disease 2:260
tumors 2:258, 260
rib 13:1834
vitamin deficiencies and 2:260; 3:311; 13:1835, 1836
see also joints; skeleton
borage 6:814
Bordella pertussis 17:2412, 2414
Borrelia vincentii 2:166
botox injections 17:2428
botulism 2:261; 4:485; 5:657, 659
a biological weapon 2:185, 186
bovine spongiform encephalopathy (BSE) 4:438
bowel 5:597
cancer 3:316
intussusception 5:624; 15:2095–2096
obstruction 11:1533; 15:2094
see also colon; small intestine
Bowman's capsule 8:1018
BR-16A 14:1989
bracelets, medical alert 16:2270
braces 15:2048
dental
invisible 10:1428
sports injuries and 15:2050
brachydactyly 5:684
brachytherapy 10:1400; 12:1693
braille 2:220, 221–222; 16:2242
brain 2:262–264; 6:761; 10:1345
blood circulation, monitored 16:2208
cerebrospinal fluid circulation 7:879
circulation of cerebrospinal fluid 7:879
communication and 1:108
consciousness and 17:2318
coordination and 3:414, 415
electroencephalograms (EEGs) 2:263, 266; 4:552; 10:1356; 14:1892
biofeedback and 2:183, 184
epilepsy and 4:552; 5:584
unconsciousness and 3:394–395; 17:2319
layered, and flotation therapy 5:650
the mind and 9:1228
movement and 9:1265
pain and 11:1475–1476
scans 10:1354, 1355; 11:1547; 12:1713; 13:1869
speech and 15:2029
survival time without oxygen 4:555
temporal lobes, and epilepsy 5:583, 585
touch and 16:2241–2242
transplants 16:2263
visual cortex 5:606
waves 5:648–649
during meditation 9:1179
brain damage and disease 2:265–268
aphasia 1:107–108; 10:1308; 15:2030
ataxia and 2:149
at birth 2:267
blood clots 2:266, 271; 6:759
brain damage, causing mental illness 9:1206, 1208, 1209
cancer 2:268, 271
coma and 3:395
concussion 2:266, 267; 6:762; 17:2318, 2321
Creutzfeldt-Jakob disease 2:231; 4:438–439; 12:1709

embolisms 1:107; 15:2107–2108
fracture of the skull 2:267; 5:663; 6:760
from head injuries 6:760
fracture of the skull 2:267; 5:663; 6:760
hemorrhage 1:107; 2:266–267, 271; 3:395; 4:457; 6:803; 5:2108, 2109
hydrocephalus and 7:879
subarachnoid 8:1097
herniation of the brain 15:2096
hydrocephalus 2:207; 7:878–880; 9:1197; 10:1350
injuries 2:266–267, 268
and life support 2:266
memory loss and 2:267
psychiatric brain disorders 12:1712
recoveries from 2:268
speech difficulties and 10:1308, 1309
symptoms 2:268
tests for 2:266
thrombosis in the arteries 1:107; 15:2107
transient ischemic attack 16:2261–2262
tumors 2:222, 268, 271; 6:727; 10:1347, 1356
coma and 3:395
dementia and 4:459
headaches and 6:758; 15:2150
hydrocephalus and 7:879
see also Alzheimer's disease; brain death; cerebral palsy; dementia; encephalitis; epilepsy; meningitis; multiple sclerosis; Parkinson's disease; stroke
brain death 2:265, 269–270; 3:394; 4:503, 504; 10:1356
organ donation and 4:503, 504; 16:2264
brain stem 2:263; 10:1345
damage to, vertigo and 17:2366
sleep-wakefulness center 14:1977, 1978
unconsciousness and 17:2318–2319
vomiting and 17:2391
brain surgery 2:271; 8:1092; 10:1354, 1355, 1356; 15:2134
psychosurgery 12:1715
Braxton Hicks contractions 2:201
bread 6:772
breastbone see sternum
breast-feeding 2:272–274, 275–276; 3:311
allergies and 13:1750
eczema and 4:542, 543
foods to avoid while 4:485
lactation 8:1032
medications taken while 11:1461; 12:1648
passing on immunity and 7:908
premature babies 12:1668
when suffering from mastitis 9:1158, 1159
breasts 2:275–277; 8:1032
biopsies 2:192; 3:315; 8:1132, 1147
cancer 2:277; 3:316; 8:1098, 1130; 9:1187
deaths from 10:1399
family history of 8:1124
histopathology 11:1512–1513
hormone replacement therapy and 6:856; 7:875
mastitis and 4:446
risk of 8:1129–1130
screening for 8:1129–1132
self-checking for 12:1680
staging 8:1098–1099, 1132

thermography and 16:2208
treatment 2:176; 3:315; 8:1098–1099, 1145–1148; 1172
changes in 2:276–277
cosmetic surgery 3:424, 425
cysts 2:277; 4:446, 447; 9:1159
effect of the Pill on 10:1417; 14:1956
examination 2:276, 277; 8:1098, 1147; 15:2148
external prostheses 8:1145, 1146, 1148; 12:1698, 1699
implants 12:1614, 1615, 1616, 1700
following a mastectomy 8:1145; 10:1421; 12:1614, 1698
mastitis 9:1158–1159, 1284
chronic 2:276–277; 4:446
microcalcification 8:1131
pregnancy and 2:276; 12:1663, 1664
prevention of mastitis 9:1159
problems 2:275, 276
reduction 12:1615, 1617
thermography 16:2207, 2208
tumors 2:277; 16:2292
unequal size 13:1739
breath
bad see halitosis
shortness of 13:1751–1752
breath holding 1:132; 2:278; 3:413; 17:2320
breathing 2:279–283; 4:484; 8:1101–1102; 13:1833
deep 11:1578
how babies begin 8:1102–1103
hysterical overbreathing 3:311; 11:1504
problems, crooked nose and 10:1372
reflex 13:1790, 1792
tests 13:1752
through the mouth 1:40; 9:1262; 16:2209
breathlessness 15:2151
breech birth 2:205, 284–285; 3:342
breeding, selective 5:674, 675
bridges, dental 4:463
Briquet's syndrome 10:1357
bromides 14:1903
bromocriptine 12:1601
Brompton cocktail 6:861
bronchi 2:281
wheezing and 17:2407–2408
bronchiectasis 6:741; 12:1623–1624; 13:1750, 1751
bronchioles 4:563
bronchitis 3:294–296, 348; 12:1623
acute 2:282; 3:295, 296; 13:1751; 15:2151
chronic 2:282; 3:294, 295, 296; 8:1103; 11:1464; 13:1751; 15:2151
colds and 7:936
emphysema and 4:564
smoking and 2:279; 3:294, 426
treatment 13:1751; 15:2151
wheezing and 17:2407, 2408
bronchodilators
as drugs 1:74, 139, 141; 7:953, 953–954
natural 1:139–140
bronchopneumonia 8:1104; 12:1623, 1624–1625
bronchoscopy 4:571; 8:1100, 1104; 13:1752
Broselow tape 4:560
Brucella spp. 3:297
brucellosis (Malta fever; undulant fever) 3:297
bruises (contusions) 3:298, 319; 17:2422, 2423, 2424
black eyes 2:213; 17:2424

cervix and cervical smears *(cont'd)*
 6:733; 11:1488, 1489;17:2327, 2368
  circumcised men and 3:374
  genital herpes and 6:825; 14:1933
  see also cervix and cervical smears,
   Pap smear
  cervical erosion 3:338; 6:733; 11:1488;
   17:2327
  cervicitis 3:337
  dysplasias and carcinoma in situ
   6:733; 11:1488, 1489; 17: 2327
  incompetent or abnormal cervix
   3:338; 9:1238, 1239; 17:2326
  mucus 9:1203, 1269
    the rhythm method and 13:1829,
     1830
  Pap smear (cervical smear) 3:313,
   314, 337, 338; 6:734; 7:966, 967;
   8:1126; 11:1488–1489, 1513;
   14:1894
    after sterilization 15:2071
    detecting infection 17:2336
    during pregnancy 12:1676
    polyps 3:339; 5:642; 6:733; 11:1488;
     17:2327
cesarean birth 2:204–205; 3:340–342;
 7:931, 932
  preeclampsia and 12:1659
CFCs *see* chlorofluorocarbons
Chagas' disease 12:1704
Chang San-Feng 16:2168
chat room 3:343–344
checkups 4:474; 6:766; 12:1680, 1684
  for children 11:1518–1519
  see also physical examination
cheilosis 9:1263
chelation therapy 3:345–346
chemical dependency units 4:528
chemical pathogens 11:1510
chemical warfare 2:186
chemosurgery 3:424
chemotherapy 3:314, 316–317; 10:1400;
 13:1775
  for leukemia 8:1061
  resistance to 3:312
  side effects 3:317; 8:1145
Chernobyl disaster 4:574; 6:821; 8:1110
chest 3:347–348
  bandaging 4:519
  barrel chest 3:295; 4:564
  concavity 13:1832
  infections, after flu 7:950
  pains 3:347, 348; 15:2151
    ECGs and 4:550
    pleurisy and 12:1619–1620; 15:2151
  pigeon chest 3:347; 12:1590–1592
  steering-wheel injury to 4:556
  strapping 13:1832
  see also coughing; ribs; sternum
chewing *see* mastication
chi 1:35, 37; 6:776
chicken pox 3:349–350; 6:825; 7:927,
 938; 13:1814
  in adults 7:935
  rash (blisters) 2:223, 224; 3:349;
   13:1782, 1783
  Reye's syndrome and 13:1814
  scars 2:223, 224; 3:349; 13:1782, 1783
  shingles and 3:349, 350; 6:825;
   14:1938
  vaccination 3:350; 7:912
chi kung *see* qigong
chilblains 6:746; 7:988, 989; 12:1596;
 14:1973
child abuse 3:351–353; 5:660
  whiplash injury 17:2409
  see also incest; sexual abuse
childbirth *see* birth

child development 3:354–357;
 11:1518–1519
  speech 15:2028, 2030–2031
children
  abdominal pain 1:11, 13, 111
  accident prevention and 1:23–25
  alimentary problems 1:69
  allergies 1:70
  aphasia 1:107, 108
  appendicitis 1:111
  attending funerals 4:457
  attention deficit hyperactivity
   disorder (ADHD) 1:86; 2:151–152;
   4:536; 8:1051
  autism 2:153–155; 8:1051–1052
   speech difficulties and 10:1308,
    1309
  avoiding car sickness in 9:1254
  bed-wetting 2:217–218; 7:925, 926
  blindness 2:219–220
  breath holding 1:132; 2:278; 3:413;
   17:2320
  bullied 12:1710
  checkups 11:1518–1519, 1568
  choking 1:132
  clumsiness 3:414
  constipation 1:69
  convulsions 3:413; 5:583, 585, 641
  cross-eye 8:1047; 10:1407
  deafness 4:453
   hearing tests 4:454
  death of a child 4:458
  diarrhea 1:69; 4:486; 7:1004
  diet 4:488
   milk 3:310
   protein 4:489
   spicy foods 4:494
  dwarfism 4:532; 5:684
  dyslexia 4:534–535, 536
  dyspraxia 4:536
  eczema 4:542, 543
  educational psychology and 12:1716,
   1717, 1718
  emergency care of 4:560
  emotional outbursts 7:907
  exercise 5:600
  eye tests 10:1407
  fears 11:1563
  feet 5:626
  fever 5:641
  flat feet 5:628
  food 11:1516
  fractures 5:660, 662, 663, 664
  gastroenteritis 5:671
  giving medicines to 9:1173, 1175
  grieving 5:712
  growing pains 5:715, 716
  growth 5:716–717; 9:1186–1187
  hallucinations 6:742
  handicapped 6:748, 749–751
  heart murmurs 6:788; 9:1289
  homesickness 6:848, 849
  in hospitals 7:870, 871;
   11:1516–1517, 1518
  hydrocephalus 7:878, 879–880
  incontinence 7:925, 926
  independence 6:848
  lead poisoning 8:1049
  lethargy 8:1058
  leukemia 8:1060, 1061
  lisping 8:1081–1082; 11:1483;
   15:2060
  mastoiditis 9:1160, 1161
  mentally retarded 9:1210–1213
  middle-ear infection 11:1453
  Munchausen syndrome by proxy
   and 9:1285, 1286
  mutism 10:1307–1308, 1309

  nosebleeds 10:1371
  of one-parent families 3:397
  overdose and 11:1460–1461, 1462
  overweight 10:1383
  personality 11:1538
  pigeon toes 12:1593–1594
  rheumatoid arthritis (Still's disease)
   1:123
  scarlet fever (scarlatina)
   14:1878–1879
  screening 14:1893–1894
  sex education 6:768, 769
  sexual abuse of 3:353; 14:1926–1927
  skeleton 14:1967
  skin conditions 14:1972–1974
  sleep 9:1186–1187
   needing little 1:85
   nightmares 4:511; 14:1978
   sleepwalking 14:1981
  speech problems 8:1081–1082;
   15:2028, 2030, 2032, 2033
   stammering and stuttering
    15:2058–2061
   therapy for 15:2032, 2033
  squint 4:505
  sunburn 15:2128, 2129
  teeth 16:2176, 2177, 2178
  temper tantrums 3:356, 413; 7:906
  thumb sucking 8:1081
  urination reflex 13:1791
  vaccination/immunization 5:641;
   11:1519
  vomiting 1:69
  worms 5:623
  see also babies
Chinese medicine 3:358–361
  cupping 6:835
  dietary therapy 3:358, 361
  herbal medicine 1:80; 3:359–360
  qigong exercises 1:81; 3:358,
   360–361
  see also acupressure; acupuncture
chiropractic 1:77–78; 3:362–364; 6:836;
 11:1446
chives 6:813
chlamydia 1:22; 2:161; 11:1520, 1531
  causing STDs 14:1931–1933, 1935;
   16:2192
   vaginal discharge and 17:2338
  Chlamydia psittaci 12:1705
   reactive arthritis and 13:1786
chloasma 8:1090, 1091; 11:1564
chloracne 1:32
chloral hydrate 7:892, 893
chloramphenicol 16:2295, 2297
chlordiazepoxide (Librium) 14:1903,
 1904; 16:2257
chlorofluorocarbons (CFCs) 1:60; 4:574;
 11:1468, 1471; 12:1636
chlorofluoroquine 8:1123
chlorpromazine (Largactil) 11:1565;
 13:1738; 15:2126; 16:2256
choking 1:132, 135; 16:2212, 2252
  babies 1:135
cholecalciferol 17:2380
cholecystectomy (gallbladder
 removal) 2:179, 180; 5:667; 6:764;
 9:1236
cholecystitis 5:668; 15:2152
cholecystokinin 2:180; 11:1487
cholera 3:365; 4:485, 573; 5:624;
 16:2285; 17:2320–2321
  vaccination 3:365; 16:2272, 2282,
   2285
cholesterol 3:366
  in the body 1:120; 5:622; 7:991
   atherosclerosis and 1:119–120;
    3:366; 6:783

  dietary 1:120; 3:366; 5:621–622
   reduction 17:2379
  cholinesterase 10:1313
  chordae tendineae 17:2341
  chorionic villus sampling (CVS) 2:207;
   3:367–368
   Huntington's disease and 7:877
   sex of the baby, and 5:638
  chromium 9:1235; 16:2250
   dangers of working with
    10:1392–1393, 1395
  chromosomes 3:331; 5:682
   abnormalities, and mutations
    10:1305
   division 3:331–332
    aging and 1:55
   extra 5:676, 683; 10:1305
    Down syndrome and 3:368;
     4:507, 508
    Philadelphia 8:1061
   sex and 3:331; 5:672, 683
   structure 3:332
  chronic fatigue syndrome (CFS) 3:369;
   5:619; 10:1311, 1353
  chronic obstructive pulmonary
   disease (COPD) 3:370–371
   oxygen therapy for 11:1465, 1467
   see also emphysema
  chyme 1:67, 68, 69; 4:494; 15:2088
  cimetidine 11:1486
  cinchona bark 13:1765
  ciprofloxacin 16:2295, 2297–2298
  circadian clock 2:187–188; 7:993; 9:1187
  circulation, poor
   biofeedback and 2:183
   cramps and 4:437
   gangrene and 5:669
   massage to treat 8:1142
   numbness and 10:1378
   pins and needles and 12:1596, 1597
  circulatory system 3:372–373
   William Harvey and 17:2358
   see also arteries and artery disease;
    capillaries; heart; pulse; veins
  circumcision 3:374; 5:688; 14:1918
   female 5:687–688
  circumoral pallor 14:1878
  cirrhosis 2:228; 3:375; 6:727; 7:968, 991;
   8:1087
   hemochromatosis and 6:800;
    7:978
  CJD *see* Creutzfeldt-Jakob disease
  clang associations 12:1722
  claudication 8:1075–1076
   intermittent 8:1075; 11:1577
   treatment 8:1078
   venous 8:1075
  claustrophobia 11:1562–1563
  cleft palate 2:207; 3:376, 401; 11:1483,
   1484, 1485; 12:1612–1613
   speech and 15:2030
  climacteric 9:1198
  Clinical Risk Index for Babies (CRIB)
   10:1338
  clitoris 5:690; 7:964; 14:1919; 17:2393,
   2394
  clonidine 2:152; 6:824; 16:2259
  cloning 3:377–378
   humans 3:378; 9:1166
   see also genetic engineering
  clostridia, and gas gangrene 5:669
  Clostridium spp.
   C. botulinum 2:261; 5:659
   C. tetani 2:166; 8:1030; 16:2197
  clotrimazole 16:2220
  clotting factors 6:804
  clubfoot 2:207; 3:379; 12:1594
  clumsiness, in children 3:414

cobalt, in high doses 16:2249, 2250
cocaine and crack 3:380–381; 4:526, 527; 6:770
   withdrawal 17:2417, 2418
coccyx 2:159; 11:1522
cochlea 6:777
   damage, and tinnitus 16:2228
cochlear implants 2:191; 6:780
codeine 1:137, 138; 9:1250; 10:1319; 11:1479–1480
cod liver oil 13:1835
coffee 15:2083, 2084
cognitive enhancers see smart drugs
cognitive reappraisal 15:2104
cognitive therapies 13:1734–1736
cold, the common see common cold
cold sores 2:223; 3:382; 6:825; 9:1263; 14:2008
   eczema and 3:382; 4:543
   sunlight and 14:1970
cold therapy 11:1579
colic 3:356; 4:444, 445; 5:702
   biliary 5:668
collagen 14:1896–1897; 17:2378, 2427, 2428
   in skin creams 17:2427
collarbone, broken 14:1948–1949
collars
   cervical 10:1334, 1430
   tight 2:214
colon and colitis 3:383
   colitis 3:383, 404; 15:2152
      acute 3:383
      chronic (ulcerative) 3:383; 4:443, 485; 17:2311
      treatment 3:383; 4:486; 15:2152
   colon
      cancer 3:386, 387; 4:442; 5:624; 15:2022
      colonic irrigation 3:384–385
      colonoscopy 3:386–387; 4:501, 570, 571; 12:1643
      colostomy 3:392–393; 5:644; 13:1787, 1788
      constipation and 3:404, 405
      diverticulitis 3:384, 386; 4:501
      halitosis and 6:741
      perforated 11:1535
      feces in 5:623
      polyps 3:386, 387; 12:1642, 1643
      sigmoidoscopy 4:501, 570; 14:1960
      spastic colon 15:2022–2023
      tumors 16:2291
      ulceration 3:387
      see also Crohn's disease
colonic irrigation (colonic hydrotherapy; colonic lavage) 3:384–385
colonoscopy 3:386–387; 4:501, 570, 571; 12:1643
color blindness 3:388–389; 5:606
color therapy 3:390–391
colostomy 3:392–393; 5:644; 13:1787, 1788
colostrum 2:273, 276; 8:1032; 12:1663, 1664
colposcopes 11:1489
coma 3:394–395; 5:611; 17:2321
   diabetic 1:26; 3:395; 4:473; 7:1006; 17:2321
   hypoglycemic 4:473
   resembling death 2:270
comedones see blackheads
common cold 3:396; 7:938; 9:1170; 10:1374
   antibiotics ineffective against 1:99
   deafness with 4:453
   leading to pneumonia 12:1624

symptoms 2:282
   runny nose or nasal congestion 10:1371; 13:1825, 1826
   treatment 2:157, 282; 10:1374
      herbal remedies 6:812
   vaccination useless against 7:936
   vitamin A deficiency and 17:2373
complementary medicine and therapies 1:76; 16:2206
   see also alternative medicine
complexes and compulsions 3:397–398
compulsions 3:397, 398; 9:1208, 1209; 12:1713
   obsessive-compulsive disorder 3:398; 10:1342, 1358, 1387–1388
compresses
   cold 15:2056
   hot 13:1757
   for sties 15:2113
   see also poultices
compulsions 10:1387
   see also complexes and compulsions
computerized (axial) tomography see CT scans
computerized ultrasound fetal cardiotocography (CTG) 3:340
computers
   working with
      hazards of 10:1391, 1396; 13:1803
      posture 13:1804, 1846
conception 3:399–400; 5:634; 13:1828; 15:2035
   artificial methods of 1:129–131
   in vitro fertilization (IVF) 1:129, 131; 7:971–974; 11:1520
   lovemaking positions and 14:1916
   menstruation and 9:1201
   while breast-feeding 12:1600
concussion 2:266, 267; 6:762, 17:2318, 2321
conditioning, operant 2:177
condoms 3:407, 408, 410; 14:1934–1935; 16:2273
conduct disorder 2:152
confabulation 12:1722
congenital disorders 3:401–402
   bone 2:259
   cleft palate 2:207; 3:376, 401; 11:1483, 1484, 1485; 12:1612–1613
   clubfoot 2:207; 3:379; 12:1594
   cataracts 2:207, 219; 3:326
   cysts 4:446
   deafness 4:455
   genetic see genetic diseases and disorders
   Gilbert's syndrome 7:989
   heart defects and blue babies 2:242–243; 3:401, 402; 6:788
   hip dislocation 3:402; 4:499; 6:829–830; 10:1434;15:2048; 16:2254
   hydrocephalus 7:879
   of the kidney 17:2325
   pyloric stenosis 15:2067
   tests for 3:401; 11:1518
   tracheoesophageal fistula 5:644
   of the uterus 17:2327, 2328–2329
   in vitro fertilization and 7:971
   see also birth defects; Down syndrome; spina bifida
conjunctivitis 3:403; 5:588, 607
connective tissue, massage 8:1144
consent forms 8:1035

constipation 3:385, 404–405; 5:596, 619, 624
   in babies 1:69
   before menstruating 9:1201
   causing anal fissures 1:102
   in children 1:69
   during pregnancy 3:404; 8:1045; 12:1662, 1675
   flatulence and 5:645
   hemorrhoids and 6:807
   spurious diarrhea and 7:925
   treatment 3:405; 15:2152
      enemas 4:572
      laxatives 3:404, 405; 8:1045–1046
      suppositories 15:2132, 2133
contact lenses 3:403, 406; 10:1417
   astigmatism and 1:142
contagious diseases 7:935
contraception 3:407–411
   after menopause 6:732
   before penetration 7:964
   during breast-feeding 2:272; 3:407
   the Pill see oral contraceptives
   sterilization 15:2068–2071
      male see vasectomy
   vaginal douches ineffective for 17:2333
   withdrawal method 5:589
   see also rhythm method
contractions 2:201
   Braxton Hicks 2:201
contusions see bruises
convalescence 3:412
conversion disorder 7:906–907
convulsions 3:413
   febrile 3:413; 5:583, 585, 641
   see also epilepsy, seizures
coordination 3:414–415
   dyspraxia and 4:536
copper 9:1235; 16:2249, 2250
   poisoning 9:1235; 16:2249, 2250
   copper bracelets 13:1819
coprolalia 16:2244
copropraxia 16:2244
cordotomy 11:1481
cornea 3:416; 5:604
   grafting 3:416; 4:504; 5:710, 711; 10:1407
   passing on rabies 13:1766
   inflammation 5:607
   laser surgery on 8:1043–1044
   ulcers 13:1758
corns 3:417–418; 12:1627
   differ from verrucas 17:2362
coronary arteries and thrombosis 1:118; 3:419–421; 6:783–784
   coronary artery surgery 3:420–421; 10:1403
   coronary disease 6:789
      prevention 3:421
      risk factors 3:421
   coronary thrombosis 3:419–420; 6:783–784; 16:2215–2216, 2217
   see also angina; atherosclerosis; bypass surgery; heart attack; thrombosis
coronaviruses 3:396
   SARS and 13:1863, 1864
coroners 4:458
corpus callosum 2:264
corpus luteum 5:593; 9:1202; 11:1458, 1459, 1548
corticosteroids 1:74
   injections 13:1804
   the skin and 12:1706
Corti, organ of 6:777
cortisol 1:47–48; 6:858

cortisone 1:74; 4:566; 12:1598, 1601
   treatment using 1:46
Corynebacterium diphtheriae 4:497; 14:2013
cosmetics 3:422–423
cosmetic surgery 3:424–425; 12:1612, 1615
   see also plastic and reconstructive surgery
coughing 3:348, 426; 13:1751
   blood (hemoptysis) 3:371, 426; 11:1560
   causing purpura 13:1755
   croup 3:426
   food "going down the wrong way" 5:592; 8:1036
   needing medical attention 3:348, 426
   phlegm 11:1560
   smoker's cough 3:371, 426; 5:603; 8:1036
   treatment 3:426; 9:1177
      cough syrup 3:426, 427
      expectorants 3:426; 5:603
   whooping cough 3:426; 17:2412–2413
cough syrup 3:426, 427
   see also expectorants
counseling 3:428–430; 12:1712; 13:1733, 1735
   drug counseling 4:528–529
   genetic 5:683, 684, 686; 6:749
      for blood relatives 7:921, 922
cowpox, and smallpox vaccination 7:911; 14:1986, 1988; 17:2331
COX (cyclo-oxygenase) 10:1369
Coxiella burnetti 13:1762
CPR (cardiopulmonary resuscitation) 1:134, 135; 3:320, 321; 13:1807, 1808, 1809, 1810
crabs (pubic lice) 8:1066
crack see cocaine and crack
cradle cap 14:1972–1973
cramp 4:437; 5:599
   anaerobic exercise and 1:50
   during pregnancy 4:437; 12:1662
   heat cramp (stoker's cramp; miner's cramp) 6:796; 11:1544
   night cramps 4:437; 13:1764, 1861
   treatment 4:437; 13:1861
      quinine 13:1764, 1765
   see also stitch
cranberry juice 8:1018
cranioplasty (skull replacement) 10:1354, 1355, 1356
crash teams 13:1807–1808, 1810
creatinine 8:1020
creative therapies 13:1735
crepitus 10:1437
cretinism 16:2226
Creutzfeldt-Jakob disease (CJD) 2:231; 4:438–439; 12:1709
CRIB (Clinical Risk Index for Babies) 10:1338
cricothyroidotomy 16:2251, 2252
critical care unit (CCU) 4:440–441
   see also intensive care unit
Crohn's disease 4:442–443
   fistulas and 5:644
cross-eye 8:1047; 10:1407
croup (laryngotracheobronchitis) 2:282; 3:426; 8:1037, 1038, 1039; 17:2414
crowns, dental 4:462, 463
crying 4:444–445; 10:1373
   babies 4:444, 445; 6:758; 10:1366
cryotherapy 4:470; 12:1627; 17:2363
Cryptococcus infection 10:1409

cryptosporidiosis 12:1704
crystal therapy 1:80
CT scans (CAT scans) 2:266; 3:394; 4:477, 478; 10:1355; 17:2434–2435
   dyes used in 13:1869
cupping 1:80, 81; 6:835
Cushing's syndrome 1:46; 12:1601; 15:2152
cuts see abrasions and cuts; lacerations
cyanide poisoning 12:1631
cyanosis 2:242; 3:295, 371; 11:1464
   emphysema and 4:564
cyclic AMP 6:859; 15:2085
cycling, and the back 2:159
cyclosporine 7:913; 8:1022, 1024; 16:2265
   adverse effects 7:914
cyclothymia 10:1358
Cylert 2:152
cyst 4:446–447
   bone 4:447
   breast 2:277; 4:446, 447; 9:1159
   congenital 4:446
   Dandy-Walker 7:879
   eruption 16:2178
   eyelid (meibomian cyst) 4:447; 15:2112
   joint 4:447
   liver (hydatid) 4:446, 447
   ovarian 4:446, 447, 568, 569; 6:733; 11:1459; 16:2195
   polycystic kidney disease 2:207; 4:447; 8:1018; 17:2325
   polycystic ovary syndrome 1:32
   skin
      dermoid 4:446–447
      sebaceous 4:446, 447; 6:726; 14:1900; 15:2147, 2148
   testicular 4:447; 16:2191, 2193–2194
cysticercosis 11:1498
cystic fibrosis 2:192; 4:448; 5:678, 684; 11:1487
   detection 3:367
   pigeon chest and 12:1592
   treatment 4:448; 11:1581
      gene therapy 5:680
cystitis 2:217, 218; 3:409; 4:449–450; 7:886; 17:2324
   treatment 4:450; 6:857
cystocele (bladder prolapse) 7:925; 12:1686, 1687
cystoscopy 4:570, 571; 9:1236
   used in prostate surgery 12:1693
cystourethrography, micturating (MCU) 17:2324
cytokines 7:946; 8:1113, 1121–1122
cytology 11:1513
cytomegalovirus 5:587
cytoplasm 3:330, 331

D

D & C see dilatation and curettage
D & E (dilatation and evacuation) 1:16
Dacron 5:709, 711
dance therapy 9:1230, 1231–1233
dandruff 4:451–452
   sties and 15:2112
   see also dermatitis, seborrheic
Dandy-Walker cysts 7:879
danthron, suppositories 15:2133
daydreams 6:742
DDT 4:574; 13:1839
Dead Sea 9:1271–1272, 1273
deafness 4:453–456; 5:692; 10:1307
   causes 4:455–456

earwax 4:453, 537; 15:2156–2157
   loud noises 4:453, 455, 456; 6:777; 10:1363, 1365–1366
   measles 6:777
   Ménière's disease 2:168; 4:455; 9:1194
   otosclerosis 4:453, 456; 12:1696, 1700
   mutism and 10:1307–1308
   as plane takes off 4:454
   treatments 4:455, 456
      cochlear implants 2:191; 6:780
      hearing aids 6:779–780; 9:1194
      prosthetic earbones 12:1696, 1699, 1700
   see also hearing
death 4:457–458
   biological clocks and 2:187
   brain death 2:265, 269–270; 3:394; 4:503, 504; 10:1356 organ donation and 4:503, 504; 16:2264
   causes 4:457; 10:1399; 12:1682
      cancer 8:1125; 10:1399; 14:1998, 1999
      drowning 4:521
   mind still functions after 9:1226
   out-of-body experiences 9:1229
decompression sickness (the bends) 2:178
decongestants, nasal drops 1:40
deep heat lotions 6:797
deep vein thrombosis see thrombosis, deep vein defibrillators 13:1807, 1808; 17:2360
dehydration 13:1862
delirium tremens (the "DTs") 1:61
delusions 12:1719, 1720–1721
dementia 2:267; 4:459; 5:692, 693; 10:1347; 12:1719
   alcohol and 7:897
   hydrocephalus and 7:880
   see also Alzheimer's disease; Creutzfeldt-Jakob disease
Demerol 1:137
demyelination 9:1280–1281
dendrites 10:1347
dengue fever 16:2282
dental care 4:460–461; 6:740
   anesthetics 1:92–93; 8:1092; 10:1378
   avoiding plaque 4:461; 12:1610
   during pregnancy 12:1676
   fluoride 4:461; 5:651–652; 12:1636; 16:2176
   gums and gum diseases 4:461, 462; 6:730–731
   heart murmurs and 9:1287
   orthodontics 10:1425–1429; 16:2175, 2177
   while wearing orthodontic appliances 10:1425, 1426
dentine 16:2175, 2178
dentures, crowns, and bridges 4:462–463
dentures 4:462–463; 8:1149; 13:1760
deodorants 2:249; 11:1544
   vaginal 17:2334
Depo-Provera 3:411
depression 4:464–466; 9:1208, 1209, 1247; 12:1713
   in adolescence 1:44, 45
   dysthymia 10:1353
   in the elderly 14:1911
   fatigue and 5:618, 619; 8:1056
   hair loss following 6:735
   manic see bipolar disorder
   postpartum see postpartum depression and psychosis

sleeplessness and 7:957, 958; 8:1056–1057
   suicide and 15:2123, 2124
   treatment 4:466; 12:1712
      drugs 4:464, 466; 12:1710; 13:1737–1738
      electroconvulsive therapy 4:466; 9:1209; 10:1354
      occupational therapy 10:1397
      psychotherapy 13:1735
   unpleasant taste sensations and 16:2171
   see also seasonal affective disorder
dermabrasion (chemical abrasion) 1:31; 3:424; 17:2428
   for tattoo removal 16:2172, 2173
Dermagraft 2:190
dermatitis 4:467–468; 7:946; 13:1782; 14:1974
   ammoniacal 4:481, 482
   atopic see eczema
   contact 1:71, 73; 4:467, 468; 6:747; 14:1974
   industrial 14:1974
   perioral 7:948
   rubber 14:2009
   seborrheic 1:32; 4:468, 482, 483; 7:988, 989; 13:1783
   sties and 15:2112, 2113
   see also dandruff
   solar (photodermatitis) 4:468
dermatology 4:469–470
   see also skin and skin diseases
dermatomes, shingles and 14:1938, 1939
desensitization 1:74; 6:757; 14:1912
   systematic 2:177; 3:398
desferrioxamine 15:2093
Desipramine 2:152
detergents
   biological 5:581
   as pollutants 12:1638, 1639–1640
Detoxamin 3:346
Dexedrine 2:152
dextrocardia 2:252
dextromethorphan 10:1319
dhobie itch 13:1838
diabetes 3:323; 4:471–473; 5:703; 9:1215; 11:1487; 15:2121
   acidosis 1:27
   boils 2:255, 256
   breath smells 6:740, 741; 7:1006
   diabetes insipidus 4:471; 8:1018–1020; 16:2210
   diabetes mellitus 4:471
   diabetic coma 1:26, 27; 3:395; 4:473; 7:1006
   dietary sugar restricted 15:2120
   drowsiness and 4:523
   during pregnancy 7:960
   excessive urine secretion 16:2209
   eye changes 2:219; 3:327; 4:472; 5:609
      treatment 8:1040, 1041
   fatigue and 5:619
   foot problems 3:418; 5:669
   gum diseases and 6:731; 13:1760
   hypoglycemia 4:471; 7:896, 960
   itches 7:987
   juvenile 4:472
   kidney damage and 8:1017
   noninsulin-dependent (maturity-onset diabetes; type II diabetes) 4:472; 10:1367–1368
   pregnancy and 15:2082
   thirst and 15:2152; 16:2209, 2210
   thrush and (Candida) 10:1368; 16:2219, 2220; 17:2437

treatment
   herbalism 6:813
   insulin 4:472–473; 7:960
   pancreas transplants 16:2264
   weight and 10:1384
diagnosis 4:474–476
   see also specimens; symptoms
diagnostic imaging 2:190; 4:477–480
   potential risks 4:480
   see also CT scans; Doppler scans; MRI; PET scanning; radionuclide scanning; thermal imaging; ultrasound; X rays
dialysis, kidney see kidney dialysis
diaper rash 1:102, 103; 4:481–483; 5:598; 14:1973, 2009
   Candida and 17:2438
diaphragm 2:281; 4:484; 8:1102
   hiccups and 6:826, 827
   stitch and 15:2087
diaphragms (contraceptives) 3:408–410
   fitted after giving birth 17:2334
diarrhea 3:385; 4:485–486; 5:624; 15:2152; 16:2296
   in babies 1:69; 4:485, 486; 7:1004; 13:1856
   in children 1:69; 4:486; 7:1004
   incontinent 7:925
   spurious 4:485; 7:925
   travelers' 4:485; 7:887–888; 16:2272, 2280
   treatment 4:486; 7:1004; 9:1177; 15:2152
   while taking the Pill 4:485
   see also dysentery
diathermy, shortwave 11:1579
diazepam (Valium) 7:893; 14:1903, 1904; 16:2257
dichloralphenazone 7:893
diet 4:487–491; 17:2404
   acidic 9:1263
   calcium in 3:310–311; 10:1381; 11:1451; 12:1678
   Chinese 3:358, 361
   cholesterol and 1:120; 3:366; 5:621–622
   during convalescence 3:412
   during pregnancy 2:206; 3:402; 4:491; 8:1127, 1128; 10:1379; 12:1662, 1665, 1675, 1678
   elimination diets 1:73–74
   fats 4:489; 5:621–622; 8:1086; 9:1215; 10:1380; 12:1682
      cholesterol and 1:120; 3:366
      digestion 2:180; 5:621
      during pregnancy 12:1678
      malabsorption 5:624
   feces and 5:624
   fish 2:266
   gluten-free 3:329
   health foods 6:772–773
   high-fiber 5:645; 8:1045; 10:1382
      for irritable bowel syndrome 7:980
   importance of antioxidants 1:101; 10:1328
   iron in 1:89
   macrobiotics 8:1116–1118; 17:2353
   naturopathic 10:1326, 1327, 1328
   for patients on dialysis 8:1014
   of PKU-affected children 11:1559
   proteins 4:488–489; 6:772, 773; 10:1380; 12:1701
      during pregnancy 12:1678
   reducing see dieting
   roughage 1:102; 3:404; 4:490
   sugar-free 7:896

to avoid coronary disease 3:421
and tooth care 4:461
unhealthy 6:769–770
while breast-feeding 4:485
see also carbohydrates; minerals;
	nutrition; vegetarianism;
	vitamins
dieting 4:488, **492–493**; 6:768; 10:1385
basal metabolic rate and 2:173
constipation and 3:404, 405
diet clubs and 10:1386
diet pills 1:85; 4:493, 524
eating disorders and 1:94, 95, 96
in health spas 6:774
ketone production during 7:1006
using diuretics 4:500
yoga and 17:2441
diet pills 1:85; 4:493, 524
digestion 1:67–69; 4:487
aids to 1:68
drowsiness and 4:523
of fruit and vegetables 1:67
of starch 15:2063
see also digestive system
digestive system, stomach, cancer
	6:741; 15:*2090*; 16:2292
digestive system 4:**494–495**
appendicitis 1:**109–111**; 11:1512
	"*left-sided*" *see* diverticulitis
	peritonitis and 1:111; 11:1532,
		1534–1535
	symptoms 1:110, 111; 11:1535
celiac disease 1:71–72; 3:**329**;
	4:485
colitis 3:383, 404; 15:2152
	acute 3:383
	chronic (ulcerative) 3:383; 4:443,
		485; 17:2311
	treatment 3:383; 4:486; 15:2152
constipation 3:385, **404–405**;
	5:596, 619, 624
	in babies 1:69
	before menstruating 9:1201
	causing anal fissures 1:102
	in children 1:69
	during pregnancy 3:404; 8:1045;
		12:1662, 1675
	flatulence and 5:645
	hemorrhoids and 6:807
	spurious diarrhea and 7:925
	treatment 3:404, 405; 4:572;
		8:*1045–1046*; 15:*2132*, 2133, 2152
Crohn's disease 4:**442–443**
	fistulas and 5:644
diverticulitis 3:384, 386; 4:**501**
	constipation and 3:404, 405
	halitosis and 6:741
	perforated 11:1535
duodenal (intestinal) ulcers 4:495,
	530, *531*
	bleeding from 6:803–804;
		8:1042
	body weight and 15:2090
	excess salivation and 13:1854
	kissing ulcers 17:2313
	pain 17:2313
	perforated 11:1534, 1535; 17:2313
	treatment 2:157, 158; 4:531;
		8:*1042*; 15:2138; 17:*2340*
fistula 5:**644**
	anal 1:*102*, 103; 6:808
	for dialysis 8:1015
	from the bowel 4:443
	urinary 7:925
food poisoning 5:**657–659**,
	670; 7:928
	botulism 2:**261**; 4:485; 5:657, 659
	diarrhea 4:485; 5:657–658

from irradiated foods 7:979
	prevention 5:658; 7:886
	reactive arthritis and 13:1785,
		1786
	salmonella and 5:657, 659; 7:928;
		13:1855, *1856–1857*
	staphylococcus and 5:657, 659;
		7:928; 15:2062
	treatment 4:486; 5:657–659
	vomiting and 4:531; 5:657–658
gastritis 5:670, 671; 9:1269;
	15:*2088*, 2089
	viral 15:2090
gastroenteritis (gastric flu; summer
	flu) 4:485, 495, 573; 5:**670–671**;
	15:2089, 2152
	in babies 4:486; 5:671
	prevention 5:671
	treatment 5:671; 15:2151
indigestion 7:**929–930**; 9:1189, 1269;
	10:*1331*
	on eating fatty foods 5:667
	hiatus hernia and 4:484
	persistent 15:2090
	treatment 7:929; 9:1177
intestinal obstruction 3:405
irritable bowel syndrome (IBS)
	4:501; 7:980; 15:2022
	spastic colon 15:**2022–2023**
membranes 9:1269
peritonitis 1:111; 4:501; 9:1189;
	11:1532, 1533–1535
	problems 4:495
stomach (gastric) ulcers 1:11; 4:495;
	5:581; 15:*2088*, 2089–2090;
	17:*2313*, *2314*
	aspirin and 1:122; 11:1479
	asymptomatic 17:2312
	biopsy 2:192
	bleeding from 6:803–804;
		8:1042; 14:1945
	body weight and 15:2090
	causes 15:2089; 17:2313
	gastroscopy and 4:570, 571;
		8:1042
	stomach or arm pain and 14:1948
	treatment 2:157, 158; 5:581;
		8:*1042*; 15:2090
	see also alimentary canal; colon;
		duodenum; stomach
digitalis 14:1957, *1958*
digoxin 14:1957, *1958*; 15:2083
dilatation and curettage (D & C)
	4:496; 5:642; 9:1202; 17:2329
dilatation and evacuation (D & E) 1:16
dilaudid 1:137
dill water 6:*813*
dimercaprol 3:346
dimethylaminoethanol (DMAE)
	14:1989
diphenhydramine 7:893
diphtheria 4:**497**; 7:938, 939; 8:1037,
	1039; 14:2011, *2013*
	vaccination 4:497; 7:911, 912;
		14:2011–2012
diplegia 3:336
diplococci 11:1510
diplopia, binocular and monocular
	4:505
dipyramidol 16:2262
disability, physical *see* handicaps
disaccharides 15:2120, *2121*
disclosing agents, dental 4:*461*;
	12:1608, *1609*
discoid lupus erythematosus (DLE)
	8:1105, 1107
dislocation 4:**498–499**; 8:1069;
	15:2055

hip 4:498, 499
	congenital 3:402; 4:499;
		6:829–830; 10:1434; 15:2048;
		16:*2254*
	traction for 16:2253, *2254*
	manipulation 8:1135
	repeated 10:1433
	wrist 17:2430
disodium cromoglycate 1:74; 7:954;
	14:2003
dispensers 11:1551
dissection, aortic 1:121; 13:1754
dissociation 12:1653–1654
dissociative disorders 10:1358
diuretics 4:**500**
	for high blood pressure 2:239
	for premenstrual syndrome
		12:1674
	side effects 14:1959
diverticulitis 3:384, 386; 4:**501**
	constipation and 3:404, 405
	halitosis and 6:741
	perforated 11:1535
divorce 5:615
dizziness 2:168; 4:**502**
	see also balance; fainting; vertigo
DMPS chelation 3:345, 346
DMSA chelation 3:345, 346
DNA 3:331, *332*; 5:**682–683**; 9:*1240–1241*
	mutations in 10:1304
	size 9:1240
DNR orders 7:961
doctors
	choosing 6:766
	emergency-room 4:561
	finding 6:766
Dolly (sheep) 3:*377*
donors 4:**503–504**; 6:791; 16:2264–2265
	blood 2:231–232; 6:810; 7:977, 990;
		12:1611
	bone marrow 8:1139, 1140
	kidney 8:1017, 1022, 1023–1024
	"do not resuscitate" (DNR) orders
		7:961
dopamine 11:*1507*
	amphetamines and 1:85–86
	antipsychotic drugs and 12:1720;
		13:1737
Doppler scans 4:479
double vision 4:**505**
douching 14:1935
	vaginal 5:689
	douching (contraceptive method)
		3:411
dowager's hump 11:1450
dowapram 15:*2085*
doxycycline 6:787
dreaming 4:**511–512**; 5:620; 9:1190,
	1228; 13:1781; 14:1978–1979; 15:2114
	wet dreams 5:589; 14:1906
dressings and bandages 4:**513–520**;
	17:*2425*
	bandages 1:17; 4:**516–520**
		allergies to 4:513, 516
		when not to bandage 4:520
	dressings 1:17; 4:*513–515*, 516
driving
	relaxation while 13:1800
	while pregnant 5:638
	while using cellular phones
		3:333
	see also road rage
drooling 9:1262, 1263
dropsy 4:500

drowning 1:135; 4:**521–522**, 556
	secondary 4:522
drowsiness 4:**523**
	after a meal 2:156; 5:618
	biological clock and 2:187
	see also fatigue
drug abuse 4:**524–527**, 528; 6:770
	in adolescence 1:43, 44, 45
	amphetamines 4:524, 526, 527;
		15:2084
	barbiturates 4:525, 526
	drug counseling 4:**528–529**
		hallucinations and 6:742; 8:1096
	health education and 6:770
	treatment, rehabilitation
		13:1798–1799
	see also alcohol; cocaine and crack;
		ecstasy; heroin; LSD; marijuana;
		overdoses; smoking
drug automatism 2:170
drug counseling 4:**528–529**
drugs
	abuse *see* drug abuse
	acetylation 14:1958–1959
	affecting the autonomic nervous
		system 2:156
	allergies to 9:1174; 14:1959
		penicillin 1:70, *99*, 100; 11:1527,
			1528, 1529; 14:1959; 16:2199
	antacid 4:531
	anticonvulsants 5:585
	antidepressant *see* antidepressants
	anti-inflammatory 4:468
	antiviral 17:2369
		see also aciclovir
	the blood-brain barrier and
		2:229–230
	central nervous stimulant (CNS)
		13:1737
	delivered via transdermal patches
		16:2259–2260
	dispensing 11:*1553*
	dosage 14:1957–1958
	first-pass metabolism 16:2260
	health risks associated with 13:1840
	hypnotic 7:**892–893**, 959
		see also sedatives; sleeping pills
	immunosuppressive *see*
		immunosuppressive drugs
	interaction with other drugs
		14:*1957–1958*
	manufacture 11:1550–1553, *1554*
	names of medications 11:1550, 1551
	new
		development 11:1552, 1554
		medical research and 9:1170–1172
		side effects and 11:1956
	nonsteroidal anti-inflammatory
		(NSAIDs) 6:787; 10:**1369–1370**;
		11:1482
		see also aspirin and analgesics
	overdose 11:**1460–1462**
		acetaminophen 11:1479; 12:1629
		amphetamine 1:87
		aspirin 4:562; 11:1460; 12:1629
		barbiturate 2:170; 3:395
		coma and 3:395
		suicide and 15:2124
		teenage "suicidal gestures"
			12:1630
		tranquilizers 16:2256, 2257
		treatment 2:170; 6:824; 11:1462,
			1479; 15:*2091–2093*
	photosensitizing 11:*1565*; 15:2126
	psychotropic 13:**1737–1738**
	smart 14:**1989**
	taken as suppositories 15:*2132–2133*
	testing 11:1552, 1554

drugs *(cont'd)*
 see also antibiotics; medicines;
  pharmacy; side effects
dry-cleaning fluid 4:526, *527*
DSM-IV 7:907
DTaP vaccines 17:2415
DTP vaccines 4:497; 17:*2413, 2414*, 2415
ductus arteriosus 8:1102, 1103
ductus venosus 8:1102
duodenum 1:68; 4:494–495, 530–531
 ulcers 4:495, 530, *531*
  bleeding from 6:803–804;
   8:1042
  body weight and 15:2090
  excess salivation and 13:1854
  kissing ulcers 17:2313
  pain 17:2313
  perforated 11:1534, 1535; 17:2313
  treatment 2:157, 158; 4:531;
   8:1042; 15:2138; 17:*2340*
 see also ulcers, peptic
Dupuytren's contracture 6:747
dusts, dangers of working with
  10:1391, 1393–1394, 1395
dwarfism 4:532
 achondroplasia 4:532; 7:922; 10:*1306*
dyes, Evan's Blue 11:1503
dysarthria 15:2031, 2033
dysautonomia 5:612
dyscalculia 4:536
dysentery 4:485, 533; 5:623; 16:2272
 amebic 4:485, *533*; 5:624; 11:1501;
  12:1704
 bacillary 4:*533*; 5:624
dysgraphia 1:108
dyshormonogenesis 16:2226
dyslexia 1:108; 4:534–535, 536; 15:2028
 inherited 6:816
dysmenorrhea 9:1202–1205
dysosmia 14:1993
dyspareunia (painful intercourse)
  4:568; 7:965; 8:1034; 9:1269;
  13:1860; 14:1924–1925, 1929
dyspepsia 15:2152
dyspraxia 4:536
dysthymia 10:1353, 1358
dystrophia myotonica (myotonic
  muscular dystrophy) 10:1302,
  1303

E

eardrums 4:453
 perforated 4:456; 11:1453; 15:2156
 caused by syringing 15:2157
ears 6:778; 11:*1452*
 balance and 2:*167*–168; 4:454
 bionic (cochlear implants) 2:191;
  6:*780*
 coordination and 3:414
 loud noises and 4:453, 455, 456;
  6:777; 10:1365–1366
 piercing 2:250, *251*
  keloid scars and 14:1880
 plastic surgery 12:*1612*
 "popping" 9:1262
 problems 2:168
  abscesses 1:21
  foreign bodies 4:456; 11:1452;
   15:2156
  glue ear 16:2236
  Hodgkin's disease lesions 6:*834*
  mastoiditis 9:1160–1161; 16:2171
  otitis 11:1452–1453
  otosclerosis 1:77; 4:453, 456;
   12:1696, 1700; 16:2228
  pain from throat infections 16:2212

perforated eardrums 4:456;
  11:1453; 15:2156, 2157
 skin tags 12:1613
 tinnitus 10:1365; 16:2227–2228
 tophi (chalk stones) 5:708
 vertigo and 17:2365–2366
 wax *see* earwax
 reconstruction 5:711
 syringing 4:454, 456, 537, 538;
  15:2156–2157
earwax 4:453, 537–538; 7:885
 deafness and 4:453, 537;
  15:2156–2157
 hearing aids and 6:779
 syringing 4:454, 456, 537, 538;
  15:2156–2157
 tinnitus and 16:2227
eating disorders 1:45; 5:673
 see also anorexia and bulimia
Ebola fever 2:186; 4:539–540; 7:*983*
eccentricity 9:1206
eccrine glands 11:1544, 1545
echocardiography 17:*2317*
E. coli see Escherischia coli
ecstasy 1:*85*, 87; 4:526, *527*; 6:770;
  13:1737
ECT *see* electroconvulsive therapy
ectomorphs 2:*253*
ectopic pregnancy 1:14; 4:541, 571;
  6:733; 11:1521
 after hysterectomy 7:903
 after sterilization 15:2068, 2069,
  2070; 16:2286
 the Pill and 10:1417
 salpingitis and 13:1860
eczema 2:224; 4:467–468, 542–543;
  14:1969, 1974–1975
 allergic 1:71, 73; 4:467, 468, 487, 542,
  543
 breast feeding and 13:1750
 in children 4:*542*, 543; 14:1973
 chronic atopic 4:*470*
 cold sore infection and 3:382; 4:543
 dandruff and 4:452
 itches 7:987, 989
 psoriasis and 12:1706, 1708
 smallpox and 14:1986
 stress and 12:1723
 sunshine and 4:542
 swimming and 4:542
 too much hygiene and 7:888
 treatment 4:467, 543
 vaccinia and 17:2331
 varicose 7:987; 17:2345
 see also dermatitis
edema 4:500, 544–545, 554
 angioneurotic 7:*947*; 15:2145,
  2147
 during pregnancy 4:544;
  12:1662–1663; 17:2399
 heart disease and 6:790
 nephrotic 15:2146
 pulmonary 2:283; 3:348; 4:545;
  17:*2407*, 2408
 weight gain and 17:2399
 see also swellings
EDTA 3:345–346
effleurage 8:1142–1143
eggs 3:399, *400*; 5:594; 11:*1458*, 1459
 chromosomes 5:683
 removed for in vitro fertilization
  7:972, 974
 see also conception
ejaculation *see* erection and
  ejaculation
elastase 4:*564*
elastin 17:*2427, 2428*

elbow 4:546–547; 7:*1002*
 bandaging 4:*518, 520*
 bursitis 3:307; 4:547
 dislocation 4:499
 injuries to 4:547
 ligaments 8:*1071*
 myositis ossificans 4:547
 osteoarthritis 4:547; 10:1437
 rheumatoid nodules 13:1821
 stiffness 15:2078
 structures 4:*546*
 tennis elbow 1:124; 4:547; 6:799;
  14:1968; 16:2187
 tophi (chalk stones) 5:708
elderly, the *see* aging
Electra complex 3:398
electrical skin resistance (ESR) 2:183
electric shocks 1:135; 4:548–549,
  556; 17:2321
 first aid 4:549, 556; 10:1393
 see also lightning strikes
electric shock therapy *see*
  electroconvulsive therapy
electrocardiograms (ECGs) 4:475,
  550–551, 559; 6:790; 17:*2341*
 fetal 10:*1390*
electroconvulsive therapy (ECT;
  electric shock therapy;
  electrotherapy) 4:466; 9:1209;
  10:1354; 11:1578, 1579; 12:1712, 1715;
  14:1884
electroencephalograms (EEGs) 2:263,
  266; 4:552; 10:1356; 14:*1892*
 biofeedback and 2:183, *184*
 epilepsy and 4:552; 5:584
 unconsciousness and 3:394–*395*;
  17:*2319*
electrolysis 4:553
electromyographs (EMGs) 2:181, 183
electromyography (EMG) 10:1356
electrosurgery 12:1628
electrotherapy *see* electroconvulsive
  therapy
elephantiasis 4:554; 8:1112; 11:1501;
  16:*2282*; 17:2419, *2420*
Elephant Man, the 2:209; 6:727
embolism 16:2215
 arterial 16:2217
 cerebral 1:107; 16:2215, 2217
 fat 8:1080
 pulmonary 13:1751, 1752; 16:2215
 transient ischemic attacks and
  16:2262
embryos
 cloning 3:377
 experiments on 9:1167
 from in vitro fertilization 7:972, 974
emergencies 4:555–556
emergency department 4:440,
  557–561; 11:1456
 see also trauma center
emergency medical technicians
  (EMTs) 4:561
emetics 4:562; 15:2092–2093
emotional holding 13:1846
emotions 9:1245
 the brain and 2:262, 264
 emotional outbursts 7:*907*
 hormones and 6:859
 puberty and 13:1741, 1742
 smell and 2:262; 14:*1993*
 see also moods
emphysema 3:295; 4:563–564; 11:1464;
  13:1752
 smoking and 2:279; 3:294, 296;
  4:563–564; 8:1103
 treatment 2:282; 5:681; 13:1752
 types 4:*563*, 564

 see also chronic obstructive
  pulmonary disease
enamel, tooth 16:2175, *2177, 2178*
encephalitis 2:267; 3:336; 4:565;
  9:1284; 11:*1513*
 a complication of measles 4:565;
  9:1164, 1165
 postviral 3:395
 rabies 13:1768
 St Louis 17:2406
 West Nile virus and 17:2406
encephalitis lethargica 16:2244
encephalocele 2:207
encephalopathy, Wernicke's 12:1722
endocarditis, infective 6:788, 789;
  17:2342, 2438
endocrine system 4:566–567; 5:699,
  700; 6:857–859
 homeostasis and 6:847
 see also hormones
endometriosis 4:568–569; 7:*904*, 905,
  943; 9:1204
 laparoscopy and 8:1034
endometritis 17:2327
endometrium 4:568; 5:594
 cancer 6:855; 17:2339
endomorphs 2:*253*
endoplasmic reticulum 3:331; 9:*1241*
endorphins 1:38; 3:363; 9:1231; 11:1477,
  1481
 opiates and 11:1482
endoscopy 4:570–571; 11:1455
 amnioscopy 4:571
 arthroscopy 1:125; 4:571; 10:*1432*,
  1434
 biopsy and 2:193
 bronchoscopy 4:571; 8:1100, *1104*;
  13:1752
 colonoscopy 3:386–387; 4:501, 570,
  571; 12:1643
 for Crohn's disease 4:443
 cystoscopy 4:570, 571; 9:1236
 of the duodenum 4:531
 gastroscopy 4:570, 571
 laparoscopy 4:568, 569, 570, 571;
  8:1033–1034; 9:1236; 11:1459,
  1520; 15:*2138*
  infertility investigation 7:945;
   8:1033–1034
 used in prostate surgery 12:1693
 sigmoidoscopy 4:501, 570; 14:*1960*
 telesurgery and 16:*2180*
endotracheal tubes 13:*1805*
enemas 3:384; 4:572
 barium 4:478, 572; 15:2096
energy
 emergency sources of 5:703
 energy from food 4:490–491;
  5:655–656; 9:1215
 glucose 5:702–703
entamebae 11:*1500*
Entamoeba histolytica 4:533; 11:1501;
  12:1704
enteritis 5:670
enterocele 12:1686
enterococci, vancomycin-resistant
  (VRE) 1:98
enuresis *see* bed-wetting
environmental hazards 4:573–574
 see also occupational hazards;
  pollution; sick building syndrome
enzymes 5:581; 9:*1241*
 digestive 4:494, 495, 530–531
 gene mutations and 10:1305
 trace elements in 16:2249
eosinophilia 2:228; 6:853
eosinophils 2:225–227; 8:1088
ephedra 6:813

ephedrines 4:493; 6:813
epidemics, of poisoning 12:1630
epidemiology 9:1172
epidermal nevus syndrome 2:209
epidermophyton 13:1838
epididymis 3:400; 5:689; 16:2191, 2192; 17:2347
epididymitis 16:2193
epidural injections 1:92
    for cesarean births 3:342
    for labor 1:93; 2:201, 285; 8:1093; 15:2041
epiglottis 1:67; 5:592; 8:1036; 9:1261; 16:2212
epilepsy 2:267; 5:582–585; 10:1347
    biofeedback and 2:184
    blackouts/unconsciousness and 2:215; 17:2320, 2321
    diet and 5:582
    flashing lights/television and 2:266; 5:582, 585
    inherited 5:684
    investigation 5:583–584
        electroencephalograms (EEGs) 4:552; 5:584
    seizures 2:267; 3:413; 4:555; 5:582
        differ from severe shivering 14:1940
        focal 5:585
        generalized (grand mal) 5:583, 584
    petit mal 5:584
    prevention 5:584
    unpleasant taste sensations before 16:2171
    what to do if someone has a seizure 5:585; 17:2321
    treatment 5:585
    twitching and 16:2293
    types
        acquired (secondary) 5:582, 583
        grand mal and petit mal 5:583, 584
        idiopathic 5:582, 583
        status epilepticus 5:585
        temporal lobe 5:585
epinephrine see adrenaline
epiphysis 5:698
episiotomy 2:203, 285; 5:586; 8:1030; 10:1322, 1324
epispadias 2:207
Epley maneuver 17:2366
Epsom salts 8:1046
Epstein-Barr virus 5:587–588; 6:834; 7:935
    infectious mononucleosis and 5:587; 7:941
erection and ejaculation 5:589–590; 11:1531
    ejaculation 5:590, 690; 7:965; 14:1907; 15:2035
        premature 5:589, 590; 14:1924, 1928
        retrograde 5:589; 12:1693, 1694; 14:1907
    impotence and 5:590; 7:919–920
    priapism and 12:1700; 14:1928; 16:2196
    see also penis and disorders; sperm
ergocalciferol 17:2380
ergotamines 9:1224
erosion 9:1202
    cervical 3:338; 6:733; 11:1488; 17:2327
erythrocytes see blood, red blood cells
erythropoietin 8:1015, 1016
Escherischia coli (E.coli) 4:449, 573; 5:624
    genetic engineering and 5:679

esophageal obturator airway 13:1808–1810
esophagitis
    pain 3:348
    reflux 5:592; 6:787, 820
esophagus 1:67; 5:591–592
    achalasia 6:787
    blocked 5:592
    cancer 3:316; 5:591
    Candida infection 17:2437
    esophageal speech 8:1036; 17:2389
    esophagitis
        pain 3:348
        reflux 5:592; 6:787, 820
    gastroesophageal reflux and 6:786; 17:2313
    narrowing (stricture) 6:787
    ulceration 17:2313
espundia 12:1703
essential (medical term) 4:474
Estraderm 16:2260
estradiol 16:2195
    skin patches 16:2259, 2260
estrogen 4:566; 5:593–594
    the bones and 3:310; 6:854; 11:1450
    the breasts and 2:275, 276
    in hormone replacement therapy 6:854; 11:1450
    menopause and 5:593; 6:854–855; 9:1199
    the menstrual cycle and 4:568; 5:593, 594; 9:1201; 11:1459; 12:1672
    in the Pill 17:2326
    pregnancy and 5:593
    puberty and 11:1459
    the skin and 8:1091
    urethral syndrome and 4:449
    vaginal cream 6:857
ethanol (alcohol) dehydrogenase 7:968; 8:1084
ethics, medical see medical ethics
ethyl chloride 13:1747
etiquette, medical 9:1166
eunuchism 16:2192, 2193
eustachian tubes 9:1262
    congestion 4:453, 456
    swollen adenoids and 1:40, 41
euthanasia 5:595; 9:1167; 15:2125
    see also suicide, assisted
evacuation of retained products of conception (ERPC) 17:2338
examinations, medical 4:474
    see also internal examination; physical examination
exams
    biofeedback and 2:182
    biorhythms and 2:194
excretory systems 5:596–598
exercise 5:599–602; 9:1230; 17:2404–2405
    aerobics 1:49–52; 7:995–997; 11:1573, 1575; 17:2401
        aerobic capacity test 11:1575
    anaerobic 1:50
    body temperature and 16:2181
    callisthenic 5:602
    cramp and 4:437
    during pregnancy 11:1570; 12:1665, 1677, 1678–1679
    effect on muscles 5:599; 9:1290
    effects of overtraining 1:50
    facial exercises 17:2427
    with a fever 5:640
    foot 5:628
    the heart and 6:781
    to improve posture 12:1658
    isometric 5:602, 664; 7:984–986
    isotonic 5:602

    lack of 6:769; 11:1574
    ligaments and 8:1069
    menstrual cycle and 15:2052
    for the pelvis 11:1524
    perspiration and 11:1544
    to prevent backache 2:162
    to prevent coronary disease or heart attacks 1:118; 3:419, 421
    qigong 1:81; 3:358, 360–361
    stitch following 15:2086, 2087
    for stroke patients 15:2111
    types, benefits 11:1572, 1573
    warm-ups before 15:2055, 2086
    yoga 17:2440–2445
    see also physical fitness
exercise testing 4:551
exercise tolerance 11:1575, 1576
existential therapy 13:1735
exotoses 2:257
expectorants 3:426; 5:603
    see also cough syrup
exposure 7:900
extrapyramidal system 8:1078
extroversion 11:1540, 1542
eye contact 2:245–246
eyelids, sty 2:256; 4:447; 6:799; 15:2112–2113
eye pads 4:515
eyes and eyesight 5:604–609
    affected by irritants 7:981
    artificial sight 2:191
    astigmatism 1:142; 4:505; 5:608; 10:1413
    after cataract removal 3:328
    bags under, removal 12:1613; 17:2427
    black eye 2:213; 5:604; 17:2424
    blind spot 5:606
    blows to 2:220, 221
    cataracts 2:219, 220, 222; 3:326–328; 5:609; 11:1470, 1471
        congenital 2:207, 219; 3:326
        treatment 3:326, 327–328; 5:609; 10:1408; 13:1811
    chemicals in 10:1393
    color blindness 3:388–389; 5:606
    conjunctivitis 3:403; 5:588, 607
    contact lenses 3:403, 406; 10:1417
        astigmatism and 1:142
    cornea 3:416; 5:604
        grafting 3:416; 4:504; 5:710, 711; 10:1407; 13:1766
        inflammation 5:607
        laser surgery on 8:1043–1044
        ulcers 13:1758
    cosmetic surgery 3:425
    cross-eye 8:1047
    cysts on the eyelids 4:447
    double vision 4:505
    eye color 5:605
        in babies 5:639, 682
        heredity and 6:818
        iridology and 7:976
    eye pads 4:515
    eyestrain, treatment 9:1233
    focusing 5:606
    foreign bodies in 5:606; 10:1393; 15:2047
    glaucoma 2:221, 222; 5:607–608, 701; 10:1362
        acute 5:608
        birth defect 2:207
        chronic 5:608
        treatment 2:157; 5:608, 701
    headaches and 6:758, 759
    hemianopia
        bitemporal 5:607
        homonymous 5:607; 16:2261

    hyperopia (hypermetropia; farsightedness) 5:604, 608; 10:1413
    injuries, NSAIDs dangerous for 10:1370
    lazy eye (amblyopia) 4:505; 8:1047
    loss of an eye, and coordination 3:414
    macular degeneration 2:220, 222; 8:1119; 13:1811, 1812
    microsurgery 9:1220
    muscles 5:607
    myopia (nearsightedness) 5:604, 608; 10:1413
    night vision 10:1362
    nystagmus 2:219
    optic nerve 2:220; 5:606; 10:1410–1411
    optometrists and 10:1412–1413
    presbyopia 5:608
    pupils, dilated 1:86, 87; 6:762
    rheumatoid arthritis and 13:1822
    scleral hemorrhage 6:804
    spots before the eyes 2:219
    squint 2:219; 4:505; 5:609
    sty 2:256; 4:447; 6:799; 15:2112–2113
    surgery 8:1092; 10:1407, 1408
        laser 2:221; 8:1041, 1043–1044
    tears 4:444–445
    tests 10:1407, 1413; 12:1681
    trachoma 2:220; 3:416; 16:2282
    transient ischemic attacks and 16:2261
    tunnel vision 2:219; 13:1812
    twitching eyelids 16:2293
    ultrasound examination 17:2316
    vision 2:220; 10:1411, 1412–1413
    yellowish tinge 6:811; 7:990, 992
    see also blindness and braille; retina and retinal disorders
eyesight see eyes and eyesight
Eysenck, Hans 11:1539

F

face
    facial exercises 17:2427
    massage 1:35; 8:1141
    puffiness on waking 15:2146
    trigeminal neuralgia 10:1347, 1348, 1349; 14:1939
face-lifts (rhytidectomy) 3:424, 425; 12:1612; 17:2428
    face-and-neck lift 12:1615
    scars 14:1880
face masks 9:1270, 1272
face packs or masks 3:422
facial palsy 5:610
Factor VIII 6:801; 17:2392
fainting, postural syncope 2:214, 215
fainting (syncope) 2:158, 167, 214, 215; 4:555; 5:611–612; 17:2319
    in adolescence 3:372
    differs from unconsciousness 17:2318
    pain causing 11:1474
    see also blackouts; dizziness
faith healing 5:613–614; 12:1603
fallopian tubes 3:399, 400
    blocked or damaged 6:733; 7:943; 13:1858
        diagnosis 7:945; 8:1033–1034
        IVF and 1:129, 131; 7:971, 972
    cancer, treatment 7:905
    ectopic pregnancy and 4:541; 6:733
    endometriosis of 4:569
    fibroids in 5:642

fallopian tubes (cont'd)
mucus 9:1269
salpingitis 3:400; 6:733; 7:943; 13:1858–1860
sterilization involving the 15:2069, 2070, 2071; 16:2286
Fallot's tetralogy 17:2342
false memory syndrome (FMS) 7:923, 924; 13:1734
familial Mediterranean fever 12:1619
familial polyposis coli 12:1643
families, one-parent 3:397
family planning
natural see rhythm method
see also contraception
family relationships 5:615–617
farmer's lung 13:1751
farsightedness see hyperopia
Fasciola hepatica 8:1088–1089; 17:2421
fasting 10:1327
fat, body
the body mass index and 11:1577
broken down for energy 1:26, 50; 5:703; 11:1577
laid down in the body 10:1384
reduction, cosmetic surgery 3:424, 425
fat embolism 8:1080
fathers 5:617
fatigue 5:618–620; 10:1352–1353
chronic fatigue syndrome (CFS) 3:369; 5:619; 10:1311, 1353
exercise and 5:601–602
lethargy and 8:1056
see also drowsiness; tiredness
fats 4:489; 5:621–622; 8:1086; 9:1215; 10:1380; 12:1682
cholesterol and 1:120; 3:366
digestion 2:180; 5:621
during pregnancy 12:1678
malabsorption 5:624
types 4:489
monounsaturated 4:489
polyunsaturated 4:489; 17:2382
saturated 4:489; 5:621–622; 10:1382
unsaturated 4:489; 5:621, 622
fatty acids 5:621, 622
in the diet 10:1382
favism 14:1958
fear 2:156
fecal softeners 8:1046
feces 5:623–624
of babies 4:486; 5:623
blood in 5:624
testing for 8:1028
color 5:597, 623, 624; 7:991
black 4:531; 5:623, 624; 7:977
loss of 5:624, 668; 7:991
enemas and 3:384; 4:572
samples 15:2025
worms in 5:623
see also diarrhea
feedback
homeostasis and 6:846, 847
thyroid gland and 4:567; 12:1599
see also biofeedback techniques
feet 5:625–628
Achilles tendon damage 5:625
aching 5:626; 12:1628
amputated 10:1344
artificial 1:128
athlete's foot 2:150; 7:886, 937; 13:1763, 1838; 14:1975
affecting nails 2:150; 13:1837, 1838
Candida as cause of 17:2436
treatment 2:150; 13:1838

ballet and the 12:1628
blisters 2:223
prevention 2:224; 3:417
bunions 3:299–300; 12:1627
corns over 3:417, 418
calluses 3:417, 418; 12:1627; 17:2362
children's 5:626
clubfoot 2:207; 3:379; 12:1594
cold feet in bed 5:669
corns 3:417–418; 12:1627; 17:2362
edema 4:545
evolution 14:1968
exercises 5:628
fetal development 5:639
flat 5:627, 628; 12:1626–1627
foot strain 12:1658
fractures 5:662; 12:1626
fungal infections 12:1628
general diseases and 12:1628
gout 3:299; 5:707
hammertoe 12:1628
hard skin 3:417
hygiene 5:625, 627
infections 12:1626, 1627
injuries 5:627
massage 5:625; 8:1141, 1143
reflexology 1:78, 80; 6:837; 8:1143; 13:1793–1794
osteoarthritis 10:1437
pigeon toes 5:625, 628; 8:1076; 12:1593–1594
pins and needles 12:1596
rheumatoid nodules 13:1821
smelly 5:625
stiffness 15:2079
sweaty 11:1543
swollen, on long air journeys 15:2145, 2147
tarsal tunnel syndrome 3:322
tendons and tendon sheaths 16:2186
thrush 16:2220
toenails see nails
verruca (plantar wart) 3:418; 5:625; 7:886; 12:1627; 17:2361–2363, 2395
Feldenkrais method 5:629–632
female genital mutilation (FGM) 5:687–688
femoral anteversion 12:1593, 1594
femur 14:1967
fractured 6:805
traction for 16:2253, 2254, 2255
fennel 6:812; 10:1329
Fentanyl 12:1670; 16:2259, 2260
fertility drugs 7:972, 974
multiple births and 7:942; 9:1274, 1275
fertilization 3:399, 400
in vitro (IVF) 1:129, 131; 7:971–974; 11:1520
fertilizers, as pollutants 12:1640
FES (functional electrical stimulation) 2:191
fetal alcohol syndrome 5:633
fetus 5:634–639; 12:1662
cartilage 3:324
development 5:634–639
feet 5:639
hands 5:638
the palate 11:1484–1485
respiratory system 2:279
teeth 16:2177
thalidomide affecting 16:2203
manipulation of 8:1136
oxygen supply 8:1102
placenta and the 12:1604–1605
sex determined 5:638; 12:1675; 17:2315

feverfew 9:1222
fevers 5:640–641; 6:759; 9:1214; 11:1545; 15:2150
shivering with 14:1940, 1942
treatment 5:641; 9:1177; 15:2150
fiber, dietary see roughage
fibrillation 7:900
atrial 4:551; 17:2359
ventricular 17:2359–2360
fibrin and fibrinogen 2:226; 16:2214
fibroadenosis see mastitis, chronic
fibroblasts 7:948; 8:1070; 17:2423
fibroids 5:642; 6:733; 7:905; 12:1643; 17:2327
fibromyalgia syndrome (FMS) 10:1310–1311
heat treatment 6:798, 799
fibrosing alveolitis 13:1751, 1752
fibrosis, pleural 16:2289
fibrositis 5:643
"fight or flight" response 1:46–47; 2:158, 182
a reflex 13:1790, 1792
suppressed 12:1652–1653
filariasis 11:1501; 16:2283
filoviruses, and Ebola fever 4:539, 540
fingernails see nails
fingerprints 6:745
fingers
anesthetized 10:1378
arthritic 8:1135; 10:1435; 13:1823, 1824
bandaging 4:517
broken 6:746
chalk stones (tophi) 5:708
clubbing 6:747
congenital disorders 3:401
cracking the joints 7:1000
cut, numbness above 10:1376
dislocated 4:498, 499
extra (polydactyly) 2:257; 10:1305; 12:1613
fused (syndactyly) 12:1613, 1614
movement 6:745
Raynaud's syndrome 5:669; 6:747; 8:1105
reattachment 9:1218, 1219, 1220
severed 6:747
first aid 10:1393
spindle 2:257
splints 15:2049
stiffness 15:2078
tingling in 9:1280
vibration white finger 10:1394, 1395, 1396
webbed 10:1304, 1305
fire, rescue from 3:305
first aid 10:1393
after a traffic or other accident 4:556
bites and stings 2:210, 211; 4:556
bleeding/hemorrhaging (external) 6:804; 16:2246; 17:2422
burns 3:304; 4:556; 10:1393
chemical 10:1393
chemicals in the eye 10:1393
choking 1:132, 135; 16:2212, 2252
common emergencies and their treatment 4:556
convulsions 3:413
CPR (cardiopulmonary resuscitation) 1:134, 135; 3:320, 321; 13:1807, 1808, 1809, 1810
drowning 4:521, 522, 556
elbow injuries 4:546
electric shock 4:549, 556; 10:1393
fevers 5:641
foreign body in the eye 5:606; 10:1393; 15:2047

fractures 4:556; 5:663; 10:1393
frostbite 5:666
gas inhalation 4:556; 10:1393
heart attack 6:784
the home medicine chest 9:1175–1177
lacerations 8:1031
minor injuries 1:18
multiple injuries 17:2426
nosebleeds 10:1374
poisoning 4:556
rabies 13:1769
requirements for overseas travel 16:2272
shock 14:1947
sports injuries 1:50
sprained ankle 15:2057
sties 15:2111, 2113
suffocation 15:2119
for suspected drug overdose 6:824; 11:1462
tongue, swallowing the 15:2118; 16:2232
vomiting 17:2390, 2391
see also dressings and bandages
fishhooks, embedded in the skin 15:2047
fistula 5:644
anal 1:102, 103; 6:808
treatment 6:808
artery to vein, for dialysis 8:1015
from the bowel 4:443
urinary 7:925
fitness, physical see physical fitness
fits, epileptic see epilepsy
flatulence 5:645
from foods 4:494
flaviviruses 17:2406
flavonoids 1:101; 10:1382
flavor enhancers, food 5:656
fleas 2:211; 5:646–647
Fleming, Alexander 11:1527, 1528
flexibility 11:1577
floss, dental 4:461; 6:731; 12:1610
flotation therapy 5:648–650
flu see influenza
flucloxacillin 11:1528
fluconazole 16:2220
fluid retention 4:500; 12:1672–1673, 1674
fluids
body 2:254
not to be given to accident victims 4:555
fluoride 4:461; 5:651–652; 9:1235; 10:1381; 12:1636; 16:2176
fluorine 12:1636, 1639
fluoxetine see Prozac
flushing 2:244
folic acid see vitamin B, folic acid
follicle-stimulating hormone (FSH) 5:593, 594; 9:1200, 1201, 1202; 11:1459; 12:1599–1600
folliculitis 1:34
fontanelles (fontanels) 2:257; 14:1967
food
additives 4:574; 5:653–654, 656
color 5:653, 654, 655
monosodium glutamate 5:653, 654; 9:1244
preservatives 5:654
allergies 1:73; 4:485, 487, 562; 5:657
causing angioneurotic edema 7:947; 15:2145
causing migraine 9:1224
diagnosis 1:73–74
fish 1:72
hives and 6:831
itches and 7:989

milk 1:72
monosodium glutamate 5:653
prostaglandin involvement 12:1689
soy 5:675
antioxidants in 1:*101*; 10:1328, 1382
appetite and 1:*112*
canned 2:*261*
causing diarrhea 4:*485*, 486
dreaming and 4:511
energy from 4:490–491; 5:655–656; 9:1215
glucose 5:702–703
genetically altered (GA) 5:**674–675**; 10:1420
gluten-free 3:329
hazards 4:574
health foods 6:**772–773**
high-fiber 5:*645*; 8:1045
for irritable bowel syndrome 7:980
hygiene 2:166; 5:671; 7:884, 886–887
intolerance, celiac disease 1:71–72; 3:**329**; 4:485
iron in 7:*977*, 978
irradiated 7:979
labeling 5:**655–656**
irradiated food 7:979
listeriosis from 8:1083
organic 10:1328, **1418–1420**
pesticides in/on 4:574; 5:657, 659; 10:1418, 1420
public health and 13:*1743, 1745*
purine-rich, gout and 5:707
raw 10:1326
salty 11:1484
toddlers spitting out food 9:1262
types 4:487–490
unpasteurized 3:297
use in the body 9:*1215*
Food and Drug Administration (FDA) 5:655; 13:1745; 14:1956
smart drugs and 14:1989
food poisoning 5:**657–659**, 670; 7:928
botulism 2:261; 4:485; 5:657, 659
diarrhea 4:485; 5:657–658
from irradiated foods 7:979
prevention 5:658; 7:886
reactive arthritis and 13:1785, 1786
salmonella 5:657, 659; 7:928; 13:1855, *1856–1857*
shellfish poisoning 8:1086
staphylococcus and 5:657, 659; 7:928; 15:2062
treatment 4:486; 5:657–659
vomiting and 4:531; 5:657–658
foot drop 8:1075
foramen magnum 6:761
forced expiratory volume (FEV) 3:296, 371
forensic science 11:1513
hair analysis 6:739
formication 7:987
fractures 2:*258, 259*; 5:**660–664**; 14:*1964*, 1968
avulsion 8:1072
Colles' 5:660; 17:2430
comminuted (crushed) 5:660, *661*, 664
compound 5:660, *662*; 10:1432–1433
dangers 5:663
first aid 4:556; 5:663; 10:1393
greenstick 5:660, *662*; 14:1964
hairline 15:2048
healing 5:660
infection and 5:660
manipulation 8:1135
march 5:662

osteoporosis and 2:161; 3:310; 5:660; 6:*828*; 8:*1078*
pathological 5:660; 14:*1964*
Pott's 5:661
recovery 5:664
repair 2:*260*
simple 5:660, *661*
spontaneous 14:*1964*
sports 15:2050–2051, 2054
stress 15:2050–2051, 2054
treatment 5:*663–664*; 10:*1430–1433*
realignment 8:1135
splinting 15:*2048, 2049*
traction 10:1431–1432, *1433*; 16:2253, *2254*, 2255
untreated 5:664
fragile-X syndrome 2:206
freckles 8:1090; 14:*1971*
free radicals
antioxidants and 1:101; 9:1187; 10:1328; 17:2379, 2384, 2387
chelation therapy and 3:345
inflammation and 7:946, 948
freeze-fixing, biopsy samples 2:193
frenulum 16:2232; 17:2394
freon 12:1636
Freud, Sigmund 3:397–398; 4:511–512; 7:923; 12:1653, *1711*
cocaine and 3:380–381
theory of personality 12:1711
Friedrich's ataxia 2:149
frigidity 14:1920
frostbite 5:**665–666**; 16:2271
frostnip 5:665
fructose 15:*2121*
fruit and vegetables, antioxidants in 1:*101*
FSH *see* follicle-stimulating hormone
functional electrical stimulation (FES) 2:191
Functional Integration 5:*631–632*
fungal infections 7:936; 11:1510
dermatological investigations 4:469
of the foot 12:1628
see also athlete's foot
itching 7:989
ringworm 7:938, *939*; 10:1315; 13:**1837–1838**; 14:*1974*
whitlow (paronychia) 6:747; 10:1314; 17:**2411**, 2438
see also thrush; yeast infections
funny bone 4:546; 10:1344
furuncles *see* boils

G

galactorrhea 12:1601
galactosemia 3:327; 5:685
gallbladder and stones 5:**667–668**
gallbladder 5:597, 667–668
inflammation (cholecystitis) 5:668; 15:2152
removal (cholecystectomy) 2:179, *180*; 5:667; 6:764; 9:1236
operation time 15:2134
shoulder or arm pain and 14:1948
gallstones 2:*180*; 5:*667–668*
back pain and 2:161, 163
biliary colic and 5:668
blood clotting and 2:228
causing jaundice 7:991–992
diagnosis 5:668
feces and 5:624
treatment 5:668
typhoid and 16:2295

gamma rays, radiotherapy and 13:1773–1774, *1775*
gangliosides, Tay-Sachs disease and 16:2174
gangrene 1:120; 5:**669**
after frostbite 5:*665*, 666
blood clots and 16:2216
diabetes and 5:669
gas gangrene 5:669
typhus and 16:2299
gardener's knee 3:307
Gardnerella vaginalis 17:2336, 2338
gargling, for a sore throat 14:*2010*, 2013; 16:2213
garlic 6:814, *815*; 10:1329
gas dilution 3:371
gas inhalation, emergency treatment 4:556; 10:1393
gastrectomy, partial 17:2314
gastric flu *see* gastroenteritis
gastric lavage *see* stomach pump
gastrin 4:494
gastritis 5:670, 671; 9:1269; 15:*2088*, 2089
viral 15:2090
gastroenteritis (gastric flu; summer flu) 4:485, 495, 573; 5:**670–671**; 15:2089, 2152
in babies 4:486; 5:671
prevention 5:671
treatment 5:671; 15:2151
gastroenterostomy 17:2314
gastroesophageal reflux disease (GERD), and halitosis 6:740
gastroscopic laser coagulation 8:1042
gastroscopy 4:570, 571
gate theory 1:38
Gattefosse, René-Maurice 1:115
gender
body structure differences 2:252
height 4:532
chromosomes and 3:331; 5:672, *683*
influencing the sex of a child 3:399
gender and health 5:**672–673**
sex changes 5:672, 673
transsexuals 5:672, 673; 16:2196
genes 3:331; 5:678, 682; 6:816
defective 5:678
see also genetic diseases and disorders
dominant and recessive 5:682, 683–685; 6:816–817
inbreeding and 7:922
expression 15:2066
mutations 10:1305
numbers 5:678
polygenes 6:817, *818*
see also genetics
gene therapy 5:677, 679
cancer treatment 10:1400
germ-line 5:679
somatic 5:679–680
genetically altered (GA) food 5:**674–675**; 10:1420
genetic diseases and disorders 2:206; 5:**676–677**, 683; 11:1508, 1509; 13:1840
celiac disease 1:71–72; 3:329; 4:485
color blindness 3:**388–389**
dementia as 4:459
dominant and recessive 5:683–686
Fanconi's anemia 5:676
fragile-X syndrome 2:206
galactosemia 3:327; 5:685
genetic counseling and 5:683, 684, 686; 6:749
hemochromatosis 6:*800*; 7:978
Huntington's disease (Huntington's

chorea) 5:677, 678, 684; 7:**877**, 922
motor neurone disease as 9:1259
muscular dystrophy as 7:922; 10:1301
phenylketonuria (PKU) 3:401; 5:581, 654, 684; 11:**1558–1559**
psoriasis 12:1706
risks of inbreeding 7:*922*
sickle-cell anemia 1:89, 90; 14:**1954–1955**
Tay-Sachs disease 16:2174
testing for 8:1028
see also amniocentesis; chorionic villus sampling
thalassemia 1:88, 89, 90; 16:**2200–2201**
treatment 5:677, 679–680
X-linked inheritance 10:*1302*
see also birth defects; congenital disorders; cystic fibrosis; hay fever; hemophilia
genetic engineering 5:**678–681**
see also cloning; genetically altered (GA) food
genetics 5:**682–686**
genetic code 5:683
genitals 5:**689–690**
female 5:*690*
see also hymen; uterus; vagina; vulva
itches 7:988
male 5:*689–690*
see also erection and ejaculation; penis; sperm
mutilation 5:**687–688**
male (MGM; circumcision) 3:374; 5:688
sex-change operations and 5:673
George VI, King 15:*2061*
geriatric medicine 5:**691–694**
physical therapy and 11:1581
German measles *see* rubella
germs 2:164; 11:1509–1510
portals of entry 7:928
Gestalt therapy 5:**695–696**; 13:1735
gestures 2:*245*, 246–248
giardiasis 12:1704
giddiness 4:502
gigantism 5:**697–698**, 718; 12:1601
Gilbert's syndrome 7:990
ginger 10:1329
gingivectomy 13:1759, *1761*
gingivitis *see* pyorrhea and gingivitis
gingivostomatitis 17:*2312*
ginkgo biloba 14:*1989*
glands 5:**699–700**
adrenal 1:46–48; 9:1246
overactive 6:858
pituitary gland and 4:567; 12:1598
underactive 6:858
apocrine 5:*700*; 11:1544; 14:1970, *1971*
endocrine 4:566–567; 5:699, 700
exocrine 5:699, *700*
lachrimal 4:444, 445; 5:*700*
lymph *see* lymphatic system, lymph nodes
mammary 5:*700*
mucous 5:*700*
parathyroid 5:*700*; 10:1335; 11:**1503–1505**
bones and 2:259; 11:1505; 13:1836
removal 11:1503, 1504
tumor 3:311; 11:1505
underactive 11:1504, 1505
pineal 2:187–188; 5:*700*; 9:1186, *1187*; 14:1899
pituitary *see* pituitary gland
salivary 5:*700*

glands (cont'd)
 sebaceous 5:700; 14:1900–1901, 1971
  acne and 1:32
  cysts 4:446, 447; 6:726; 14:1900;
   15:2147, 2148
  sties and 15:2112
 sweat 2:249; 5:596, 699, 700;
  11:1543, 1544; 14:1970, 1971
  prickly heat and 12:1685
  "swollen" 5:699
 thymus 5:700; 8:1113; 9:1187;
  16:2221–2222
  tumors 16:2222
 thyroid see thyroid
glandular fever see infectious
 mononucleosis
glasses 5:604; 10:1412, 1413
glaucoma 2:221, 222; 5:607–608, 701;
  10:1362
 acute 5:608
 birth defect 2:207
 chronic 5:608
 treatment 2:157; 5:608, 701
glenoid cavity (glenoid fossa) 14:1948
glial cells 2:229
glomeruli 8:1017, 1018
glomerulonephritis 8:1020; 15:2097;
  17:2325
glottis 8:1036
glucagon 7:960; 11:1487; 15:2064
glucose 5:702–703; 9:1215
 dietary 5:702; 15:2120
  levels controlled 5:703; 6:847;
   15:2121
  stored as glycogen 4:488; 5:702;
   6:847; 15:2064, 2120
glue ear 16:2236
glue-sniffing 4:526, 527; 14:2006, 2007
gluten 3:329
glycerol 5:621, 622
 suppositories 15:2132, 2133
glycerol monostearate (GMS) 5:654
glyceryl trinitrate 16:2259
glycogen 4:488; 5:702; 6:847; 15:2064,
  2120
goat's rue 6:813
goiter 5:704; 10:1334; 16:2224, 2225,
  2226
"golden hour" 4:560
gold injections 13:1820, 1821, 1823
Golgi apparatus 3:331; 9:1240
gonadotropins 4:439; 12:1599–1600
gonococci 2:164
Gonococcus spp. 2:166
gonorrhea 2:161; 5:705–706; 7:938;
  8:1018; 11:1531; 14:1930, 1931
 pregnancy and 12:1675; 14:1932
 salpingitis and 13:1859
 statistics 14:1935
 vaginal discharge 17:2334, 2338
goose pimples 6:735; 14:1942
gout 3:299, 307; 5:707–708; 10:1306
Graafian follicles 9:1201
grafting 5:709–711
 blood vessels 5:711; 10:1403
 bone 5:709, 711; 10:1430, 1432
 cartilage 5:711
 corneal 3:416; 4:504; 5:710, 711;
  10:1407
  passing on rabies 13:1766
 graft-versus-host and (GVH) disease
  5:677
 hair 5:709; 6:739
 heart valves 5:711
 rejection and 5:710
 skin 5:709, 710–711; 9:1221; 12:1612,
  1615–1616
  after burns 3:302, 304

 tendons 5:711
 see also bypass surgery; transplants
graft-versus-host (GVH) disease 5:677
 thalidomide and 16:2204
Granuflex 4:515
granulation tissue 7:951
granuloma 4:443
grass see marijuana
Graves' disease 5:704; 16:2225–2226
grazes see abrasions
grief 5:712
 after miscarriage 9:1239
 bereavement 4:458, 464, 465; 5:712;
  9:1206; 17:2446
  hallucinations 6:742; 12:1719
 shock and 14:1943, 1944
grommets 4:456
ground itch 6:852–853
group therapy 5:713–714; 13:1736
growing pains 5:715, 716
growth 4:532; 5:716–718
 control of 4:532
 gigantism and 5:697–698
 psychosocial short stature and
  4:532
 spurts 5:716–717
 see also height
growth hormone (somatotropin)
 4:439, 532, 566; 5:718; 6:858;
 7:899; 12:1600
growths 6:726–727
 malignant 6:726–727
 see also cancer; malignancy
Guillain-Barré syndrome 6:728–729;
  7:882
guinea worm 11:1501
gullet see esophagus
gumboils 1:21
gums and gum diseases 4:461, 462;
  6:730–731
 bleeding gums 6:730, 731; 10:1426;
  12:1608
 halitosis and 6:740, 741
 ulcers 17:2311
Guthrie test 3:401
gynecology 6:732–734
 laparoscopy used in 8:1034

H

Haemophilus influenzae 12:1623
Hageman factor 6:801–802
Hahnemann, Dr. Samuel 6:842, 844
hair 6:735–736; 14:1971
 analysis 6:739
 bleached in sunlight 15:2126
 dermatologists and 4:469
 drying 6:737
 on face and body of women 4:566
 grafts 5:709; 6:737–739
 growth 6:738; 14:1971
 how hair color is inherited 5:682
 lanugo 5:638; 12:1664
 puberty and body hair 5:689; 13:1742
 removal
  electrolysis 4:553
   folliculitis on regrowth 1:34
  "standing on end" 2:156; 6:735
hair and scalp disorders 6:737–739
 cradle cap 14:1972–1973
 dandruff 4:451–452
  sties and 15:2112
 excessive facial hair in women
  16:2196
 hair loss 6:737
  alopecia areata 2:169; 6:736;
   14:1969

baldness 2:169; 5:709; 6:736;
  17:2387
 following chemotherapy 8:1145
 following depression 6:735
 normal rate of 6:737
 psoriasis 6:739; 12:1706
 ringworm 13:1837–1838
halitosis (bad breath) 4:460;
  6:740–741; 9:1263; 12:1608
hallucinations 6:742; 12:1713, 1721;
  15:2150
 drug abuse and 6:742; 8:1096
 during bereavement 6:742; 12:1719
hallux rigidus 15:2079
hallux valgus 3:299, 300
halzoun 8:1088
hammers, rubber (patellar) 4:475
hammertoe 12:1628
hamstring injuries 6:743–744
handicaps 6:748–751
hands 6:745–747
 accidents to 6:746
 anesthetizing 8:1093
 arthritis 6:746, 799; 10:1437; 13:1820,
  1821, 1823, 1824
  physical therapy and 13:1799
 artificial 1:128; 12:1697, 1698
 athlete's foot and 2:150
 bandaging 4:518, 520
 blisters, prevention 2:224
 body language and 2:246
 bone fractures 6:746
 carpal tunnel syndrome 1:124;
  3:322–323; 6:747; 10:1344, 1396;
  13:1804
 chalk stones (tophi) 5:708
 cold
  chilblains and 6:746
  numbness 10:1376
  Raynaud's syndrome and 8:1105;
   10:1378
  sense of touch and 16:2239
  warming 5:665; 6:746
 congenital disorders 3:401
 contact dermatitis 4:468
 cracks on the skin 6:746
 cramp 4:437
 dermatitis 6:747
 Dupuytren's contracture 6:747
 fetal development 5:638
 fractures 5:662
 liver palms 6:747
 pigmented creases 6:747
 pins and needles 12:1595
 rheumatoid nodules 13:1821
 stains on 6:746
 sweaty 6:746
 synovial joints 13:1823
 tremor 6:747; 11:1506
 warts 17:2396
 washing 5:657; 7:884, 887
  compulsive 3:397, 398; 10:1387,
   1388
 see also fingers; nails
hangover 6:752–753
 cures for 1:62
Hansen's disease (leprosy) 6:754–755;
  11:1474; 16:2282–2283, 2284
 treatment 6:755; 16:2204
haptics 2:246; 16:2180
harelip (cleft lip) 3:376, 401; 11:1485;
  12:1612–1613, 1614
Harris-Benedict equation 2:173
Harvey, William 17:2358
Hashimoto's disease 5:704
Hawking, Stephen 9:1256, 1258, 1259
hay fever 1:70, 73; 3:396; 6:756–757;
  13:1749, 1826; 14:2003

eczema and 4:542
the eyes and 7:946
 conjunctivitis 3:403
increased mucus 9:1269
the nose and 10:1374
snoring and 14:2004
treatment 6:757; 14:1956
 desensitization 6:757; 14:1913
  self-help 1:74
Hayflick limit 1:55
headache 6:758–759; 9:1230; 15:2150
 defective eyesight and 10:1412
 meningitis 9:1196
 treatment 6:759; 9:1177; 11:1460;
  15:2150
  self-massage 9:1233
 see also migraine
head and head injuries 6:760–763
 bandaging 4:518
 injuries and blows to the head
  2:266–267, 268; 6:760, 761–762
  aphasia and 1:107
  brain herniation and 15:2096
  drowsiness or lethargy and
   4:523; 8:1058
  epilepsy and 5:583
  loss of sense of smell 14:1993
  mastoiditis and 9:1160
  unconsciousness and 17:2318,
   2320, 2321
  vomiting and 17:2391
healing 6:764–765
health care system 6:766–767
 home care 6:839–841
 managed care 8:1133–1134
 see also hospice care; hospitals
health education 6:768–771;
  12:1682–1684
 see also medical information
  highway
health foods 6:772–773
health spas 3:412; 6:774–776
hearing 6:777–778
 with one ear 6:777
 testing 4:454; 6:777–778; 11:1516
 see also deafness
hearing aids 6:779–780; 9:1194
heart 3:347–348; 6:781–782
 abnormal rhythms (palpitations
  and arrhythmias) 2:157, 215; 3:421;
  4:550; 6:781, 789, 790; 11:1472
 artificial 6:794
 birth defects 2:206–207
 dextrocardia 2:252
 electrocardiograms (ECGs) 4:475,
  550–551, 559; 6:790; 17:2341
 fetal 10:1390
 failure 3:348; 6:789, 790
  breathlessness 15:2151
  swollen ankles and 15:2146
  tiredness and 16:2231
  treatment 13:1861; 15:2083, 2151
 fitness and the 11:1576–1577
 heartbeat 6:781
  control 6:782; 9:1267, 1268
  exercise and 7:997
  pulse and 13:1754
  rate decrease during meditation
   9:1178
  smoking and 10:1360, 1361
  sneezing and 14:2002
  see also pulse, rate
 holes in the 2:242, 243; 3:402;
  9:1289; 10:1401; 17:2342
  closing on their own 6:788
  surgery 10:1402
 murmurs 8:1103; 9:1287–1289;
  15:2074

in children 6:788; 9:1289
muscle 9:1266, 1267, 1290, 1293
pacemaker
artificial 2:190; 3:421; 6:788;
11:1472–1473
natural (sinoatrial node) 6:782;
9:1267; 11:1472
pain, radiation of 15:2149
pericarditis
pain 3:348
tuberculous 16:2289
stops, and time before permanent
damage 13:1807
strangulation of 15:2096
stress and the 7:997
stroke volume 11:1576–1577
surgery
physical therapy after 11:1581
and ventricular fibrillation
17:2359
see also valves
heart attack (myocardial infarction)
1:121; 6:783–785; 11:1464
activity after 6:783
assesssment, blood tests 15:2024
a cause of shock 14:1944, 1945
coronary intensive care units and
7:962
diagnosis 6:785
ECGs 4:551
heart muscle scar tissue after
14:1881
menopause and 6:854, 855
pins and needles and 12:1597
prostaglandins and 12:1689
pulmonary edema following
17:2407, 2408
recovery after 6:764–765
reducing the risk of 1:118; 6:783;
11:1572; 16:2214
silent 3:419; 6:785
strokes associated with 15:2108
symptoms 3:348, 420; 6:784–785
pain 3:348; 15:2149
treatment 2:157; 6:785; 11:1472;
15:2151
ventricular fibrillation 17:2359, 2360
what to do if somebody has a 6:784
see also coronary arteries and
thrombosis
heart block 3:421; 6:789; 11:1472;
13:1753, 1754
heartburn 5:592; 6:786–787; 7:929
during pregnancy 5:592; 6:786, 787;
12:1661, 1662, 1675
heart disease 6:788–790
avoiding 3:366
cardiomyopathy 6:789
dilated 16:2231
hypertrophic 6:789
congenital heart disease and blue
babies 2:242–243; 3:401, 402;
6:788
detection 4:550
heart block 3:421; 6:789; 11:1472;
13:1753, 1754
hormone replacement therapy and
6:854, 855
infective endocarditis 6:788, 789;
17:2342
ischemic 1:121; 11:1472
menopause and 9:1200
palpitations 4:550; 6:789, 790
treatment 2:157
prevention, vegetarianism and
17:2354
risk of getting 13:1839
screening for 14:1892

valve disease 2:215; 6:788, 789;
9:1287–1289; 16:2215;
17:2341–2342
wheezing and 17:2408
see also angina; coronary arteries
and thrombosis; heart attack;
heart failure
heart failure 3:348; 6:789, 790
breathlessness 15:2151
swollen ankles and 15:2146
tiredness and 16:2231
treatment 13:1861; 15:2083, 2151
heart transplants 4:504; 6:791–794;
10:1422; 16:2263, 2264, 2266
repeated 16:2263
heat and heat disorders 6:795–796
heat cramp 6:796
heat exhaustion 6:796; 16:2270
prickly heat 6:795; 11:1545; 12:1685;
15:2130
sunstroke (heatstroke) 6:796;
11:1545; 15:2130–2131
heatstroke see sunstroke
heat treatment 6:797–799
for abscesses 6:797, 799; 13:1757
for stiffness 15:2076, 2079
Heberden's nodes 6:746; 14:1968
heel-prick test, PKU 11:1559
height 2:252; 5:716
aging and 1:53; 3:324
gigantism 5:697–698, 718; 12:1601
heredity and 6:817
inferiority complexes and 3:397
tallest man 14:1964
see also growth
Heimlich maneuver 1:132; 15:2119
Helicobacter pylori 4:531; 5:2089;
17:2313, 2314
Hellerwork 13:1846, 1847, 1848
hemarthrosis 6:802
hematology 11:1513–1514
hematoma 3:298; 15:2096
epidural 6:763
scrotal 17:2348
subdural 6:763
subungeral 3:298
hemianopia
bitemporal 5:607
homonymous 5:607; 16:2261
hemiplegia 3:336; 10:1411
physical therapy and 11:1579–1580
hemochromatosis 6:800; 11:1487;
16:2250
hemodialysis 8:1014–1015
hemoglobin 2:225; 11:1464; 14:1954
broken down 7:990–991
deficiency, and anemia 1:88
sickle-cell anemia and 14:1954
thalassemia and 16:2200
hemoglobin H disease 16:2201
hemophilia 2:206, 228; 5:685–686;
6:801–802; 7:922; 10:1306
detection 3:367
HIV from donated blood 1:57
treatment
genetically engineered protein
5:681
vitamin K ineffective as a
17:2385
Hemophilus 11:1453
hemoptysis (coughing blood) 3:371,
426; 15:2151
hemorrhage (bleeding) 6:803–806
brain 1:107; 2:266–267, 271; 3:395;
4:457; 6:803; 15:2108, 2109
external
dealing with 1:18; 6:804; 16:2246;
17:2422

tourniquets and 16:2245–2246;
17:2422
internal
leading to shock 6:805
leading to thirst 16:2210
nosebleeds 4:568; 6:803; 10:1371
treating 10:1374
postpartum 12:1605
hemorrhoids 6:807–808
constipation and 3:405
during pregnancy 5:637; 12:1662,
1675
external (prolapsed) 1:103; 6:808;
15:2095, 2096
strangulation of 15:2095
internal 1:103; 6:808; 15:2096
treatment 6:808
use of laxatives and 8:1046
hepadnaviruses 17:2371
heparin 2:227; 8:1015
hepatic portal system 17:2358
hepatitis 2:228; 6:809–811; 7:938;
11:1510; 16:2285
after acquiring a tattoo 16:2172, 2173
alcohol dangerous after 7:990;
8:1086
biopsy and 2:192
blood donation and 2:231
cirrhosis and 3:375
feces and 5:624
from shellfish 8:1086
hepatitis A (infectious hepatitis)
6:809, 810, 811; 17:2370, 2371
hepatitis B (serum hepatitis)
6:809–810, 811; 8:1016; 17:2371
hepatitis C (hepatitis non-A non-B)
6:809, 811; 8:1029
hepatitis D (delta hepatitis) 6:809
jaundice and 6:810–811; 7:991
an occupational hazard 10:1395
treatment 6:811
vaccinations 2:206; 6:811; 16:2285
hepatitis B (serum hepatitis)
5:681; 14:1935
hepatocytes 8:1084
herbs and herbalism 1:78; 6:812–815,
837
Chinese herbal medicine 1:80;
3:359–360
fragrant herbs 14:1991, 1993, 1994
for migraines 9:1222
naturopathy and 10:1327, 1329
heredity 6:816–818
nature versus nurture 6:817–818
see also genetics
hernia 6:819–821
brain 15:2096
femoral 6:819
hiatus 4:484; 5:592; 6:787, 819, 820;
7:930
incisional 6:819
inguinal 6:819, 820; 15:2148
paraumbilical 6:821
strangulated 6:820; 15:2094, 2095
treatment 6:821; 8:1136; 15:2095
umbilical 6:819, 821; 15:2148
ventral 6:819
heroin 4:524, 525, 526, 527; 6:822–824;
10:1319, 1320
withdrawal 6:823, 824; 10:1320;
17:2416, 2417–2418
herpes 6:825
family of viruses 5:587–588
genital 3:337, 341; 6:825; 11:1531;
14:1932, 1933, 2009
during pregnancy 14:1933
statistics 14:1935
herpes simplex

cold sores and 2:223; 3:382; 6:825;
7:928; 9:1263; 14:2008
facial palsy and 5:610
genital herpes and 6:825;
14:1933; 17:2394
lip ulcers and 17:2311
opportunistic infections 10:1409
herpes zoster
chicken pox and 14:1938
shingles and 6:825; 14:1938, 1939
mouth ulcers and 17:2310, 2311
rash 6:825; 13:1784
hexosaminidase 16:2174
hiccups 1:67; 4:484; 6:826–827
hip 6:828–830
arthritic 1:122; 10:1436, 1437
bandaging 4:518
damage, and limping 8:1077
dislocation 4:498, 499
congenital 3:402; 4:499;
6:829–830; 10:1434; 15:2048;
16:2254
traction for 16:2253
fractures 5:660–661, 693; 6:828,
830, 855; 9:1199; 17:2424
osteoporosis and 11:1450
ligaments 8:1071
pain 11:1578
Perthes' disease 6:830; 8:1076;
11:1546
replacement 1:122; 2:189; 6:829, 830;
7:998, 999, 1000; 10:1438;
12:1696, 1699
fitting a new 12:1696
hydrotherapy and 7:883
rehabilitation after 13:1798
see also pelvis
Hippocrates 10:1326
hirsutism 16:2196
histamine 1:72, 73; 6:756, 831
producing itches 7:988
histopathology 11:1512–1513; 15:2026
HIV see AIDS
hives (urticaria) 1:71, 73; 6:831; 13:1783;
14:1975; 15:2147
HLA-B27 13:1785, 1786
hoarseness 6:832; 8:1037
Hodgkin's disease 3:317; 6:833–834;
8:1114
holistic medicine 6:835–838; 17:2403,
2404
herbalism and 6:815
homeopathy and 6:843–844
see also alternative medicine
Holter machines 6:790
home care 6:839–841
homeopathy 1:78; 6:837, 842–845;
10:1326
homeostasis 6:846–847; 7:898
homesickness 6:848–849
homosexuality 6:850–851
"honeymoon disease" 4:449
hookworms 2:241; 6:852–853; 11:1499,
1500, 1501; 17:2419–2420
hormone replacement therapy (HRT)
2:260; 4:566; 5:594; 6:733,
854–856
osteoporosis and 2:260; 6:855, 856;
9:1199; 11:1450, 1451
the risk of breast cancer and 6:856;
7:875
skin patches 16:2259, 2260
hormones 6:847, 857–859
hormonal disorders 4:567
Addison's disease 1:48; 2:237;
6:747; 7:896; 9:1181; 13:1862;
15:2150
Cushing's syndrome 1:46; 12:1601;

hormones (cont'd)
   15:2152
   diabetes 4:471–473
   dwarfism 4:532
   gigantism 5:697–698
   goiter 5:704; 10:1334; 16:2224,
      2225, 2226
   hyperparathyroidism 11:1504,
      1505
   hypoglycaemia 7:896; 15:2121
   hypothyroidism see thyroid,
      underactive
   thyroid gland tumors 4:567
   thyrotoxicosis see thyroid,
      overactive
   moods and 9:1246
   substitutes 5:699
   see also endocrine system
hospice care 6:841, 860–861; 7:872,
   959
hospitals 6:767; 7:870–873
   children in 7:870, 871; 11:1516–1517,
      1518
   coronary care units 6:785
   crash teams 13:1807–1808, 1810
   day 11:1457
   emergency department 4:440,
      557–561; 11:1456
      see also trauma center
   occupational therapists 10:1398
   operating room 10:1404–1406
   outpatients 11:1454–1457
   patients as part of studies in 9:1170
   see also hospice care; intensive care
      unit
hot flashes 4:496; 6:855–856;
   7:874–875; 9:1198–1199
   acne rosacea and 14:1975
Houdini, Harry 11:1535
housemaid's knee 3:307
human chorionic gonadotropin (HCG)
   3:400; 15:2024
Human Genome Project 5:678
human papillomavirus (HPV) 1:22;
   3:339; 14:1933
human potential therapies 13:1734
human T-cell leukemia virus type II
   (HTLV II) 8:1059
humidifiers 7:876
Humulin 5:679
hunger 1:112; 6:846
Huntington's disease (Huntington's
   chorea) 5:677, 678, 684; 7:877, 922
hyaluronidase 7:936
hydatid disease 11:1500
hydergine 14:1989
hydraencephaly 2:207
hydramnios 2:284
hydrocele 16:2192
hydrocephalus 2:207; 7:878–880;
   9:1197; 10:1350
hydrocortisone 4:467, 468
   for eczema 4:543
   for joint pain and stiffness 15:2078,
      2079
   suppositories 15:2133
hydrophobia 13:1766, 1767, 1768
hydrops fetalis 13:1816
hydroquinone 8:1090, 1091
hydrosalpinx 13:1859
hydrotherapy 6:799; 7:881–883;
   10:1328; 11:1579; 13:1795; 16:2206
hydroxychloroquine 8:1107
hygiene 2:165, 166; 7:884–888; 11:1544
   in the bathroom 5:671; 7:888
   body odor and 2:249
   food and in the kitchen 2:166; 5:671;
      7:884, 886–887

foot 5:625, 627; 11:1543
   vaginal 17:2334
   vaginal douching and 5:689
   washing the hands 5:657; 7:884
hymen 5:690; 7:889; 17:2367, 2368,
   2393–2394
   imperforate 17:2335
hyoscine 9:1255
hyperactivity see attention deficit
   hyperactivity disorder
hyperglycemia 7:896
hyperhidrosis 2:249
hyperopia (hypermetropia;
   farsightedness) 5:604, 608;
   10:1413
hyperparathyroidism 11:1504, 1505
hyperpyrexia 14:1941
   malignant 8:1124
hypertension (high blood pressure)
   1:46; 2:237; 12:1724–1725
   effect on the kidneys 8:1017, 1021
   headaches and 6:759
   the heart and 4:551
   hemorrhoids and 6:807
   hypertensive retinopathy and
      13:1812
   "malignant" 8:1124
   proteinuric see preeclampsia
   salt and 13:1861
   self help for 2:238
   stroke and 15:2107, 2111
   treatment
      biofeedback 2:181, 183–184
      diuretics 4:500
      drugs 2:183, 237, 239; 5:611
      flotation therapy 5:650
      ongoing treatment 9:1173
hyperthyroidism see thyrotoxicosis
hypertrophy, muscle 11:1577
hyperventilation
   causing pins and needles 12:1595
   hyperventilation tetany 6:745;
      11:1504
   hysterical 1:26
hypnosis 7:890–891; 9:1229
hypnotherapy 1:79; 6:837; 12:1712;
   13:1735, 1736
hypnotic drugs 7:892–893, 959
   see also sedatives; sleeping pills
hypochondria 7:894–895; 10:1342
hypoglycemia 7:896; 15:2121
   blackouts and unconsciousness and
      2:214, 215; 17:2321
   coma caused by 4:473
   diabetic 4:471; 7:896, 960
hypoparathyroidism 11:1504, 1505
hypopyons 13:1758
hypospadias 2:207; 12:1613; 17:2323
hypotension 2:237
   postural 2:215; 17:2364
hypothalamus 2:263; 6:847;
   7:897–899
   appetite and 1:113; 7:897–898
   body temperature and 5:640, 641;
      7:897, 898; 9:1264; 14:1941, 1942;
      16:2182–2183
   effect on the pituitary gland 6:859;
      7:897
   heart rate and 9:1268
   narcolepsy and 7:897, 899
   water balance and 7:898–899;
      16:2209
hypothermia 4:523; 5:693–694;
   7:900–902; 8:1057; 14:1941
hypothyroidism (underactive thyroid;
   myxedema) 3:323; 5:699, 704;
   8:1055; 16:2223–2224, 2226
   coma and 3:395

congenital (cretinism) 16:2226
   growth and 4:532
   hair and 2:224
   Hashimoto's disease and 5:704
   heat production and 16:2182
hypovolemia 6:806
hysterectomy 7:903–905, 906; 10:1421
   abortion and 1:16
   cystitis and 4:450
   endometriosis and 4:568, 569;
      7:905
   fibroids and 5:642; 7:905
   Pap smears after 11:1488
   sex life after 6:732
   for sterilization 7:905; 15:2069, 2071
hysteria 7:906–907; 9:1208, 1209,
   1228; 10:1357
   hypochondria and 7:894–895
   hysterical neuroses 12:1713
   nervous breakdown and
      10:1340–1341
   overbreathing 3:311; 11:1504
      see also hyperventilation
   self-inflicted injury and 17:2310
hysterosalpingography 7:945; 13:1860

I

ibuprofen 1:138; 6:787; 10:1369
ice therapy 13:1804; 15:2051
idiopathic (medical term) 4:474
ileitis see Crohn's disease
ileum 4:495
ileus, paralytic 11:1534
ilium 11:1522–1523
imaging, diagnostic see diagnostic
   imaging
imidazopyridine derivatives 7:893
Imipramine 2:152; 13:1738
immune system 7:908–909, 940;
   17:2330–2331
   allergies and 1:72–73
   cellular immunity 17:2330–2331
   Crohn's disease and 4:442
   deficiency
      causes 10:1409
      opportunistic infections and
         10:1409; 16:2220
      see also AIDS
   inherited immunity 7:908; 13:1763
   natural immunity 2:227
   thymus and 16:2221, 2222
   UV radiation and 11:1470–1471
   see also antibodies; autoimmune
      diseases; lymphocytes
immunization 2:166; 7:910–912
   schedule for children 11:1519
   sudden infant death syndrome and
      15:2117
   WHO scheme 16:2283
   see also injections; vaccination
immunoglobulins see antibodies
immunohematology 8:1029
immunology 8:1029; 11:1514
immunosuppression 6:833
immunosuppressive drugs 7:913–914
   after transplant surgery 6:794;
      7:913, 914; 8:1022, 1024, 1139
   to treat autoimmune disorders
      7:914; 8:1113
immunotherapy 10:1400
impacted teeth 7:915–917; 14:2012
impetigo 2:223, 224; 7:918
impingement syndrome 3:308, 309
impotence 1:130; 5:590; 7:919–920;
   11:1531; 14:1924
inbreeding 7:921–922

incest 7:923–924
   denial of 5:615
incisions 17:2423
incontinence 2:218; 5:693; 7:925–926
   spinal cord damage and 15:2040
   stress 7:925; 12:1687
incubation period 7:927–928
incubators 10:1337; 11:1517; 12:1667, 1668
indigestion 7:929–930; 9:1189, 1269;
   10:1331
   on eating fatty foods 5:667
   hiatus hernia and 4:484
   persistent 15:2090
   treatment 7:929; 9:1177
indomethacin 1:138
induction of labor 2:201; 7:931–934;
   10:1322
   in the case of stillbirth 15:2082
infarction 1:120
infection and infectious diseases
   7:935–940
   incubation period 7:927–928
   infectious dose 7:928
   isolating patients with 7:982, 983
   opportunistic infections 10:1409
   portals of entry 7:928, 937
   subclinical infection 7:935
   tiredness and 16:2229–2230
   wound infections 17:2425–2426
   see also tetanus
   see also bacteria; fungal infections;
      protozoal infections; viruses
infectious mononucleosis (glandular
   fever) 5:699; 6:834; 7:941; 8:1087,
   1110, 1112; 15:2148
   cause 5:587; 7:941
   lymphocytes and 8:1113
   the spleen and 15:2044, 2046
   the tonsils and 16:2237
   treatment 7:941; 8:1112
inferiority complexes 3:397, 398
inferior vena cava 3:373
infertility 3:400; 7:942–945, 971–972
   artificial methods of conception
      1:129–131
   in vitro fertilization (IVF) 1:129,
      131; 7:971–974; 11:1520
   laparoscopic investigation 7:945;
      8:1033–1034
   salpingitis and 13:1860
   sperm and 1:129, 130; 7:943; 14:1907;
      15:2034, 2035
   STDs and 14:1932
infibulation 5:687
inflammation 2:165; 7:946–948
influenza 7:927, 938, 949–950; 11:1508;
   17:2369, 2372
   antibiotics not used against 1:99
   differs from colds 3:396; 7:949
   lethargy after 8:1057
   treatment 7:950
   vaccination 7:910, 912, 936, 949,
      950; 17:2332
infrasound 10:1364–1365
ingrown toenails 7:951–952; 10:1315,
   1318; 12:1626
inhalants 7:953–954
   drug-abuse see solvent abuse
inhalers 7:954; 13:1750
inhibitory factors (releasing factors)
   7:899
injections 7:955–956
inoculation see immunization;
   vaccination
insects, public health and 13:1744
insight-oriented therapy 10:1358
insomnia 7:957–959; 14:1980; 17:2446
   treatment 7:959; 14:1980

biofeedback 2:181
melatonin tablets 9:1186, 1187
sleeping pills 7:892, 958, 959
insulin 4:471–473; 6:858; 7:896, 960;
9:1215; 11:1487; 15:2064, 2121
administered 4:472–473; 7:960
genetically engineered 5:679
overdose 4:395
transdermal delivery possible?
16:2260
made by the body 4:472, 566;
5:702–703; 7:960; 10:1368
resistance 10:1368
insulinoma 7:960
insurance, medical 4:558; 6:766, 767;
16:2273
integrative therapies 1:76
Integra TM 3:301
intelligence 2:262
heredity and 6:817–818
memory and 9:1193
intensive care unit 7:961–962; 12:1646
neonatal 7:962; 10:1336–1338;
11:1516; 12:1667, 1669
physical therapy in 11:1581
respirators 13:1806
thermistors 16:2184
see also critical care unit
intensivists 4:441
intercourse 7:963–965; 14:1918–1919
abstinence 1:22, 45
periodic see rhythm method
bleeding during or after 11:1488,
1489
conception and 3:399
during adolescence 1:43
during pregnancy 5:634; 7:963;
12:1661, 1675
lack of interest in
after menopause 9:1200
since taking the Pill 7:963
painful (dyspareunia) 4:568; 7:965;
8:1034; 9:1269; 14:1924–1925,
1929
salpingitis and 13:1860
positions, and conception 14:1916
see also sex
interdental cleaners 4:461
interferon 7:927
cancer and 3:312
interleukin-2 7:914
internal examination 1:14; 6:732, 734;
7:966–967; 15:2027
Internet
Internet2 16:2179
medical information highway
9:1168–1169; 16:2180
interpubic disk 11:1523
interviews
body language at 2:246
relaxation during 13:1800
intestines 9:1268
enteritis 5:670
intussusception 15:2095–2096
obstruction 3:405
peristalsis 1:69; 15:2023
polyps 12:1642, 1643
strangulation 15:2094–2095
tumors 13:1774
removal 15:2136
see also bowel; colon; small
intestine
intoxication 7:968–969
intracytoplasmic sperm
injection/transfer (ICSI/T) 1:130,
131; 7:974
intrauterine devices (IUDs) 3:407,
410–411; 4:496; 7:972; 8:1033

ectopic pregnancy 4:541
morning-after pill 3:411
periods 9:1204, 1205
salpingitis 13:1859
intravenous infusions (IVs) 7:970;
12:1646
intravenous pyelograms (IVPs) 4:475;
8:1020
intrinsic factor 1:89; 11:1536
introversion 11:1540, 1542
in vitro fertilization (IVF) 1:129, 131;
7:971–974; 11:1520
iodine 9:1235; 10:1334; 16:2250
deficiency 5:704; 8:1128; 10:1334
radioactive (radioiodine) 13:1774;
16:2223
iontophoresis 4:470
ipecac syrup 4:562
iproniazid 13:1738
iridology 1:80–81; 7:975–976
iris 5:605
iridology and 7:975–976
iron 7:977–978; 9:1234–1235; 16:2250
blood donors and 7:977
deficiency 1:88–89, 90; 7:977; 8:1128
detection 7:978
dietary 7:977, 978; 10:1381
during pregnancy 12:1678
excess 6:800; 7:978
hemochromatosis 6:800
loss 7:977–978
supplements 6:787; 12:1675
black feces and 5:623; 7:977
children accidentally swallowing
4:555; 7:977; 9:1234
overdose 9:1234; 11:1460; 15:2093
vitamin E absorption and 17:2382
iron bacteria 17:2336
iron lungs 13:1805
irradiation (body), whole-body, bone
marrow transplants and 3:317
irradiation (food) 7:979
irritable bowel syndrome (IBS) 4:501;
7:980; 15:2022
spastic colon 15:2022–2023
irritants 7:981
see also poisoning
Ishihara cards 3:388
islets of Langerhans 7:960; 11:1486,
1487
isocyanates 10:1393, 1395
isolation 7:982–983
see also quarantine
isometrics 5:602, 664; 7:984–986
isosporiasis 12:1704
isotope scans see radioisotope scans
itches 7:987–989
anal 1:103
eczema 4:542–543
IUDs see intrauterine devices
IVF see in vitro fertilization
Ixodes ricinus 8:1108

J

jaundice 5:624, 668; 7:990–992
in babies 3:336; 6:810; 7:990, 991,
992; 8:1087; 13:1816
premature 12:1669
from hepatitis 6:810; 7:991
tattoos and 16:2172
itches 7:988
treatment 7:991, 992; 11:1581
types 7:990, 991
urine and 5:596
jaw
cancer of 14:1998

osteoarthritis 7:1002
wiring 10:1386
jellyfish stings 2:211
Jenner, Edward 7:911; 14:1986, 1988;
17:2331
jet lag 7:959, 993–994; 9:1186, 1187
Jews, Ashkenazi, and Tay-Sachs
disease 16:2174
Jocasta complex 3:398
jogging 5:599; 7:995–997
joints 2:259; 7:1000–1003;
9:1265–1266; 10:1435; 14:1968
being "double jointed" 7:1002;
13:1819
chiropractic and 3:363
effects of hydrotherapy on 7:882
injections into 15:2078
ligaments 8:1069, 1070, 1071
problems
bleeding (hemathrosis) 6:802
bursitis 3:307–309; 4:547; 6:799;
7:1002; 8:1025, 1027; 9:1189
clicking 3:324
cysts 4:447
dislocation 4:498–499; 8:1069;
15:2055
locked joints 8:1135
loose bodies in 8:1025, 1136
osteoarthritis 1:123, 123; 3:325;
5:691; 10:1435–1438; 11:1581;
14:1968
rheumatoid arthritis 1:122–123,
126; 3:323; 7:1002, 1003; 11:1581;
13:1820–1824; 16:2207, 2208
sports injuries 1:50; 15:2054–2055
sprains 6:764; 8:1072; 15:2048,
2051, 2055, 2056–2057, 2145
stiffness 8:1136; 15:2076,
2077–2079
replacement 7:998–999, 1003;
10:1434, 1438
hips see hip, replacement
knees 7:998, 999; 10:1430
synovial membranes 9:1188, 1189
types 1:100–103
Jung, Carl 3:397; 12:1711; 15:2115

K

kala-azar 12:1704; 15:2046
kaolin 7:1004
kaolin and morphine 7:1004; 9:1250,
1251
kaolin and pectin 7:1004; 9:1177
Kaposi's varicellum eruption 3:382
Keller, Helen 10:1308
Keller, Herbert 16:2202
keloids 7:1005; 14:1880, 1881
keratin, in the skin 14:1970
keratinocytes 8:1090
keratodermia blennorhagica 13:1786
keratometers 3:328
keratoses 6:726
solar 15:2127
keratosis pilaris 1:34
kernicterus 8:1087
ketones 1:26; 3:395; 4:473; 5:703;
7:1006
ketosis 1:26; 7:1006
kidney dialysis 2:190; 5:598;
8:1014–1016, 1020; 17:2322
treatment for poisoning 12:1632
kidneys and kidney diseases
5:596–597; 8:1017–1021; 17:2324
abscesses 17:2325
birth- and congenital defects 2:207;
17:2325

blood pressure 2:238, 239; 8:1017
cancer 17:2325
hormone production 11:1504
treatment 13:1772, 1776
cysts 4:450
polycystic kidneys 2:207; 4:447;
8:1018; 17:2325
function tests 8:1020
glomerulonephritis 8:1020; 15:2097;
17:2325
gout and 5:707
infections 8:1018, 1020–1021
kidney failure 8:1020; 12:1701
drugs and 11:1958
kidney dialysis 2:190; 5:598;
8:1014–1016, 1020; 17:2322
multicystic kidneys 17:2325
nephrectomy 10:1339
nephritis 5:707; 17:2325
nephrosis 17:2325
pain 2:161
pyelonephritis 17:2325
salt levels controlled 13:1862
stones (calculi) 2:217; 3:311; 4:450;
6:786; 8:1018, 1020, 1021; 11:1505;
17:2325
gout and 5:708
kidney removal for 10:1339
treatment 8:1020, 1021
uremia 15:2150; 17:2322
X rays 17:2432
kidney transplants 4:503, 504;
8:1022–1024; 16:2263, 2264–2266
ultrasound and 17:2315
kilocalories 5:655; 9:1214
see also calories
kinesiology 1:81; 6:836
kissing disease see infectious
mononucleosis
kiss of life see artificial respiration
Klebsiella 12:1625
Klein, Melanie 12:1711
Klinefelter's syndrome 10:1305
knee 7:1001–1002; 8:1025–1027
arthritic 1:123, 124, 125; 10:1436, 1437
arthrograms of 17:2432
"baker's cyst" 1:122
bandaging 4:520
bursitis 3:307, 309; 7:1002; 8:1025
cartilage
removed 3:324, 325; 10:1432, 1436
torn 3:325; 8:1026–1027; 10:1432,
1434; 15:2055
fluid in (knee effusion) 8:1025, 1026
kneecap (patella) 8:1026
dislocation 8:1027, 1136
manipulation 8:1135
knee-jerk reflex 8:1025; 9:1266, 1267;
13:1791
knock knees 5:628
ligaments and 8:1071
limping and 8:1075
loose bodies in 8:1024, 1136
osteoarthritis, hydrotherapy and
7:883
replacement 7:998, 999; 10:1430
stiffness 15:2079
twists and sprains 8:1026
knock knees 5:628
Koebner phenomenon 12:1708
Kohler, Wolfgang 5:696
Koplik's spots 9:1163, 1164
Korsakoff's syndrome 12:1722
Kunz, Wilhelm 16:2202
Kupffer's cells 8:1086
kwashiorkor 1:11; 16:2284
Kyoto Protocol 1:60
kyphosis 14:1968

L

LAAM (L-alpha acetyl methadol) 6:824
labia, inner and outer 5:690; 17:2393
labor 2:200, 201–204; 5:639
　accelerated 2:201
　breathing exercises 12:1679
　dry 7:932
　enema during 4:572
　induced 2:201; 7:931–934; 10:1322
　　see also induction of labor
　obstetricians and 10:1390
　premature 17:2326
　　see also premature babies
　see also birth
laboratory tests 8:1028–1029
　see also pathology
labyrinthitis 17:2365, 2366
lacerations 1:19, 20; 8:1030–1031;
　12:1615; 17:2422–2423
　treatment 8:1031; 17:2425
　see also abrasions and cuts
lachrimal glands 4:444, 445; 5:700
lactation 8:1032; 12:1598
　see also breast-feeding
lactic acid 1:49, 50; 11:1576; 15:2076
lactose, intolerance 15:2023
lactulose 8:1046
L-alpha acetyl methadol (LAAM) 6:824
laminectomy 14:1886, 1984, 1985
laparoscopy 4:568, 569, 570, 571;
　8:1033–1034; 9:1236; 11:1459, 1520;
　15:2138
　infertility investigation 7:945;
　8:1033–1034
　surgery see minimally-invasive
　surgery
laparotomy 8:1035
Largactil see chlorpromazine
large intestine see colon; rectum
laryngectomy 17:2389
laryngotracheobronchitis 2:282; 8:1037
　see also croup
larynx and laryngitis 8:1036–1039
　laryngitis 7:946; 8:1038, 1039; 10:1335;
　14:2011, 2013; 16:2212; 17:2389
　　acute 8:1036, 1037–1039
　　in children 16:2211
　　chronic 8:1036, 1037, 1039
　larynx 16:2212
　　blocked 10:1333; 16:2213
　　cancer 3:316; 6:832; 8:1036, 1037,
　　1038, 1039; 10:1335; 16:2212, 2213
　　cartilage 3:325
　　diphtheria and 8:1037, 1039
　　gastroesophageal reflux and
　　6:786
　　hoarseness and 6:832; 8:1039
　　injury to 8:1037
　　laryngotracheobronchitis (croup)
　　2:282; 8:1037, 1038, 1039
　　puberty and 13:1742; 17:2389
　　removal 8:1036; 16:2251–2252;
　　17:2389
　　stenosis 15:2067
　　vocal cord nodes or polyps 6:832;
　　8:1037, 1039; 10:1335; 17:2389
　see also vocal cords
lasers 8:1040–1042
　acne treatment 1:34
　argon 8:1041
　carbon dioxide (laser knife) 8:1042
　eye treatment
　　the cornea and see LASIK surgery
　　diabetic 8:1040, 1041, 1042
　　the retina and 2:221; 8:1041, 1042
　　tattoo removal 16:2173
LASIK surgery 8:1043–1044

Lassa fever 2:186
lateral geniculate body 10:1410
lathyrism 9:1259
laughter therapy 9:1232, 1233
lavage, gastric see stomach pump
laxatives 3:404, 405; 4:572; 5:598;
　8:1045–1046
　abuse 8:1045
laying on of hands 5:613, 614
lazy eye (amblyopia) 4:505; 8:1047
L-dopa 11:1506, 1507
lead poisoning 3:413; 4:573; 5:583;
　8:1048–1050; 10:1394, 1395;
　12:1630, 1638; 13:1746
　treatment 3:345; 8:1049
Lear complex 3:398
learning 2:264
learning disabilities 8:1051–1052; 12:1714
　mutism and 10:1307, 1308, 1309
　see also dyslexia
left-handedness correction, and
　stammering 15:2060
　dyslexia and 4:534
Legg-Calvé-Perthes' disease see
　Perthes' disease
Legionella pneumophila 8:1053, 1054
Legionnaire's disease 7:938;
　8:1053–1054
legs
　artificial (prosthetic) 1:127;
　12:1696–1698
　blood clots in the veins
　15:2146–2147; 16:2218; 17:2357
　cramps 4:437
　edema 4:544, 554
　fractures 5:661, 664
　　blood loss 6:805
　　leading to other problems 11:1581
　　leg shortening and 10:1430;
　　11:1448
　　limping after plaster removal
　　8:1076
　　osteoporosis following 11:1450
　　treatment 10:1430, 1431–1432,
　　1433; 15:2048, 2049; 16:2253;
　　17:2433
　movements 6:828–829
　one shorter than the other 5:664,
　709; 11:1448
　　causing spinal curvature 14:1890
　paralysis 11:1490, 1492
　pins and needles 12:1597
　rickets and 13:1836
　stiffness 15:2079
　ulcers 1:17; 17:2310, 2312
leishmaniasis 12:1703, 1704; 16:2283
lemon balm 10:1329
lepromin test 6:755
leprosy see Hansen's disease
leptins 1:113; 10:1384
Leptospira interrogans 17:2402
leptospirosis 17:2402
　see also Weil's disease
Leptothrix bacteria 17:2336
lesbianism 6:850, 851
lethargy 8:1055–1058; 11:1463; 13:1753;
　17:2446
leukemia 2:228; 3:316; 8:1059–1061
　enlarged spleen 15:2046
　from environmental hazards 4:574
　gum disease and 6:757
　treatment 3:316; 8:1061
　　radiotherapy 13:1774
leukocytosis 2:228
leukonychia 6:747
leukopenia 2:228
leukoplakia 17:2393
leukotrienes 1:139

Leydig cells 16:2195
LH see luteinizing hormone
libido 8:1062–1063; 14:1920–1921, 1922
　aging and 1:53
　the Pill and 7:963; 10:1414;
　14:1920–1921
　pituitary gland and 12:1598
Librium (chlordiazepoxide) 14:1903,
　1904; 16:2257
lice 2:211; 7:885; 8:1064–1066
　typhus and 8:1066; 16:2299, 2300,
　2301
lidocaine 1:92; 8:1092
Lieberkuhn, crypts of 4:495, 530
life, prolonging, ethics of 9:1166–1167
life expectancy 1:53; 4:458;
　8:1067–1068; 12:1682
　biological clock and life span 2:188
　of men and women 1:55
　obesity and 10:1385
life span
　biological clock and 2:188
　heredity and 6:818
　life-support systems 2:266
　　coma and 3:395
　　organ donation and 4:503
　　turned off 3:394; 5:595; 9:1167
lifting 2:163; 12:1688; 14:1985
ligaments 8:1069–1072; 9:1266
　peridontal 6:730, 731
　sprained 15:2056–2057
ligatures 15:2137
light
　acne and 1:34
　effect
　　on biological clocks 2:187–188
　　on the skin 15:2127
　ultraviolet and infrared 15:2127
lightning strikes 4:548; 8:1073–1074
light therapy (phototherapy)
　for jaundice 7:991; 11:1581; 12:1669
　for seasonal affective disorder
　14:1898, 1899
lignocaine 15:2078
limbic system 2:262, 263, 264
limbs
　artificial see artificial limbs
　bleeding
　　control 17:2422
　　tourniquets and 16:2245–2246;
　　17:2422
　cramps 4:437
　fractured 5:663
　　physical therapy and 11:1580
　growing pains 5:715
　paralysis 11:1490, 1492
　reattached 5:709; 9:1218, 1219–1221
　stiff 15:2076
　see also arms; legs
limping 8:1075–1078
linear accelerators 8:1115
linoleic acid 10:1382
linopirdine 14:1989
lipase 4:494, 495; 11:1487
lipectomy 3:424, 425
lipomas 6:726; 15:2147–2148
lipoproteins
　HDL 3:366
　LDL 3:366; 5:656
liposomes, used in gene therapy 5:680
liposuction 3:424, 425; 8:1079–1080;
　12:1615
　tumescent 8:1080
lips 9:1260
　bleeding from 9:1260
　blood blisters 13:1756
　blue 4:555, 564; 11:1463, 1464
　cheilosis 9:1263

cleft 3:376, 401; 11:1485; 12:1612–1613,
　1614
　tattooing pigments to 16:2173
　ulcers 17:2311, 2312
lisping 8:1081–1082; 11:1483; 15:2060
listeriosis 8:1083
lithium 4:466; 12:1720; 13:1738
　lithium carbonate 2:199
lithotripsy 11:1020, 1021
liver fluke 8:1088–1089; 11:1500, 1501;
　17:2420, 2421
liver and liver diseases 5:597;
　8:1084–1087
　diseases and disorders
　　abscesses 13:1757
　　cancer 6:811; 8:1087; 10:1399
　　cirrhosis 2:228; 3:375; 6:727;
　　7:968, 991; 8:1087
　　cysts 4:446, 447
　　hepatitis 6:810, 811; 8:1087
　　lacerations 8:1031
　　liver failure 8:1087; 13:1755;
　　14:1958
　　liver fluke 8:1088–1089
　　rupture 5:663
　　shoulder or arm pain and
　　14:1948
　　the spleen and 15:2046
liver
　biopsies 2:192, 193
　blood clotting and 2:228
　glycogen storage 15:2064, 2120
　jaundice and 7:991
　removal of part of 10:1421
　transplants 4:504; 8:1084; 16:2263,
　2265, 2266
liver spots 8:1090–1091
living wills 5:595; 15:2125
lobotomy, prefontal 12:1715
local anesthetics 1:92; 8:1092–1093;
　10:1378; 15:2135
　for fingers 10:1378
　topical 8:1092
lockjaw 1:17; 16:2197, 2198
longevity see life span
lordosis (swayback) 13:1848
Lou Gehrig's disease (amyotrophic
　lateral sclerosis) 9:1256–1259
lower-back pain (lumbago) 2:160, 161;
　8:1094–1095
　treatment 2:163
　　Feldenkrais method 5:630
lozenges, throat 14:2010, 2013
LSD 4:526, 527; 8:1096; 10:1320
lumbago see lower-back pain
lumbar puncture 2:266; 4:475, 565;
　8:1097; 9:1196
　myelography and 10:1355
lumpectomy 8:1098–1099, 1147, 1172;
　11:1513
　see also mastectomy
Lunelle 3:411
lung and lung diseases 2:281; 3:347;
　8:1100–1104
　abscesses 12:1625
　adult respiratory distress syndrome
　(ARDS; shock lung; wet lung)
　14:1943, 1946
　asbestosis 1:136; 12:1639; 13:1751
　asthma 1:139–141; 8:1103–1104;
　11:1464; 13:1751
　　avoidance of beta-blockers 3:419,
　420
　　breast feeding and 13:1750
　　causes 1:59, 60, 140, 141; 7:888;
　　8:1100, 1103; 15:2050
　　eczema and 4:542
　　pigeon chest and 12:1590, 1592

pneumonia and 12:1622
prevention 1:73, 141
symptoms 1:73, 140–141; 2:282;
3:348; 11:1560; 17:2407, 2408
treatment 1:73, 74, 141; 2:157, 158,
282; 7:953–954; 8:1103; 15:2072;
17:2408
bronchiectasis 6:741; 12:1623–1624;
13:1750, 1751
bronchitis 3:294–296, 348; 12:1623
acute 2:282; 3:295, 296; 13:1751;
15:2151
chronic 2:282; 3:294, 295, 296;
8:1103; 11:1464; 13:1751; 15:2151
wheezing and 17:2407, 2408
cancer 2:282; 3:294, 314; 6:727, 832;
8:1103, 1104, 1125; 13:1751
asbestos-related 1:136
in cities 12:1639
deaths from 10:1399
exposure to radon and 13:1839
hormone production 11:1504
smoking and 2:279, 283; 3:314;
8:1067, 1104; 13:1749; 14:1996,
1997–1998, 1999
symptoms 3:316; 13:1751
treatment 2:282; 13:1751, 1776
collapsed lung 13:1751
cystic fibrosis and 4:448
emphysema 3:295; 4:563–564;
11:1464; 13:1752
smoking and 2:279; 3:294, 296;
4:563–564; 8:1103
treatment 2:282; 5:681; 13:1752
types 4:563, 564
excretory organs 5:596
fibrosing alveolitis 13:1751, 1752
forced expiratory volume (FEV)
3:296, 371
gaseous irritants and 7:981
lung function tests 3:296; 13:1752
occupational hazards, from dusts
10:1391, 1394; 14:1961
pleural effusions 12:1618
pleurisy 2:281, 282; 3:426; 9:1189;
12:1618–1620; 13:1751, 1752
pain 3:348
pneumonia and 12:1625
treatment 12:1620; 15:2151
pneumoconiosis 2:282; 4:564;
12:1621; 13:1752
pneumonia 2:282; 3:347, 348; 7:937,
938, 940; 8:1103, 1104;
12:1622–1625; 13:1752
aspiration pneumonia 12:1624,
1625, 1631
bronchopneumonia 8:1104;
12:1623, 1624–1625
a complication of other diseases
3:350; 9:1165; 12:1625
double 12:1622
lobar 8:1104; 12:1622, 1623, 1624,
1625
pneumonic plague 12:1607
prevention 12:1624
treatment 2:282; 8:1103; 12:1624,
1625; 13:1752
pneumothorax 13:1751, 1752
pulmonary embolism 13:1751, 1752;
16:2215
removal of a lung 10:1421
shoulder or arm pain and
14:1948
small lungs 2:279
transplants 4:504; 13:1750
tuberculosis 16:2287–2289,
2290
volumes tested 3:371

wheezing 17:2407–2408
see also pulmonary disorders
lupus 8:1105–1107; 11:1565
discoid lupus erythematosus (DLE)
8:1105, 1107
systemic lupus erythematosus (SLE)
8:1105–1107; 12:1619
luteinizing hormone (LH) 9:1200, 1202;
11:1459; 12:1599–1600; 16:2195
Lyme disease 8:1108; 16:2199
lymph 8:1109
lymphangiograms 8:1112, 1114
lymphangitis 8:1111, 1112
lymphatic system 8:1109–1112
blockage 8:1111–1112
elephantiasis 4:554; 8:1112;
11:1501; 16:2282; 17:2419, 2420
cancer spread and 3:313; 10:1400
lymphangitis 8:1111, 1112
lymphatic vessels 8:1109, 1111
lymph nodes 3:313; 8:1109, 1111, 1130
removal in breast cancer 8:1098,
1109, 1146, 1147
secondary tumors in 16:2292
swollen 5:699; 6:833; 8:1109, 1114;
10:1335; 15:2145, 2148
lymphoma 8:1110, 1112, 1114–1115
B-cell 5:588
Burkitt's 5:588; 7:935
Hodgkin's disease 3:317;
6:833–834; 8:1114
non-Hodgkin's 6:833; 8:1114
the tonsils and 16:2237
see also adenoids; tonsils
lymphedema 8:1111, 1112
lymph nodes see lymphatic system,
lymph nodes
lymphocytes 2:226, 227, 228;
8:1109–1110, 1113
B lymphocytes 7:908, 909;
8:1109–1110, 1113; 16:2222
T4, AIDS virus and 1:57
T lymphocytes 7:908, 909;
8:1109–1110, 1113; 16:2222
lymphokines 7:914; 8:1113
lymphoma 8:1110, 1112, 1114–1115
B-cell 5:588
Burkitt's 5:588; 7:935
Hodgkin's disease 3:317; 6:833–834;
8:1114
non-Hodgkin's 6:833; 8:1114
the tonsils and 16:2237
lymphosarcoma 8:1112
lysosomes 3:331; 9:1240

M

macrobiotics 8:1116–1118; 17:2353
macrolides 1:100
macula 13:1811, 1812
macular degeneration 2:220, 222;
8:1119; 13:1811, 1812
macules 13:1783
mad cow disease 4:438
magical thinking 10:1388
magnesium 9:1235
magnesium sulfate 8:1046
magnetic resonance imaging see MRI
ma-huang 14:1989
makeup see cosmetics
malaria 5:640; 7:937, 938, 940;
8:1120–1123; 11:1500, 1501; 12:1704;
16:2285
Burkitt's lymphoma and 5:588
facts 16:2283
prevention 8:1123; 16:2272, 2281,
2284, 2285

thalassemia and 16:2200, 2201
treatment 8:1123
quinine 13:1764, 1765
malathion 8:1065
malaxone 1:138
malignancy 6:726–727; 8:1124–1126
see also cancer
malnutrition 8:1127–1128; 16:2284
obesity a form of 8:1127, 1128;
10:1382
Malta fever see brucellosis
mammography 2:192; 3:312;
8:1129–1132; 14:1895; 16:2292;
17:2432
managed care 8:1133–1134
manganese 9:1235; 16:2250
mania 4:464
of bipolar disorder 2:198, 199; 12:1713
manipulation 8:1135–1136; 11:1578–1579
chiropractic 3:364
see also massage; physical therapy
Marburg virus 4:539
Marfan's syndrome 14:1891
marijuana (cannabis; grass; pot) 4:526,
527; 6:822; 8:1137–1138
medicinal usage 8:1138; 9:1138
marjoram 6:815
marrow and transplants 2:258;
8:1139–1140
marrow
diseases 8:1139–1140; 13:1755
red blood cells and 2:226, 227
samples taken 8:1061; 11:1514, 1536
stem cells 15:2065
transplants (grafting) 3:317; 4:504;
5:711; 8:1139, 1140
Mary Tudor, queen of England 11:1548,
1549
massage 1:79–80; 8:1141–1144
aromatherapy 1:115, 117; 14:1936
around joints 3:363
cardiac 1:134, 135; 3:320–321; 4:555
Chinese (tui na) 3:360, 361
facial 1:35; 8:1141; 14:1936
foot 5:625; 8:1141, 1143
neck 10:1334
osteopathy and 11:1447, 1448
for pulled muscles 13:1747
reflexology 1:78, 80; 6:837; 8:1143;
13:1793–1794
rolfing 13:1846, 1847, 1848
scalp 6:739
self-massage 9:1233
shiatsu 1:80; 6:776; 8:1144;
14:1936–1937
to relieve stiffness 15:2078, 2079
to treat sprains 15:2056
see also acupressure; manipulation
mast cells 1:72; 6:756; 14:2003
mastectomy 8:1112, 1145–1148, 1172
breast implants following 8:1145;
10:1421; 12:1614, 1698
external prostheses following
12:1698, 1699
see also lumpectomy
mastication (chewing) 1:67, 68; 8:1149
mastitis 9:1158–1159, 1284
chronic 2:276–277; 4:446
mastoidectomy 9:1161
mastoiditis 9:1160–1161; 16:2171
mastoplexy 3:424
masturbation 9:1162, 1210; 13:1742
measles 7:938; 9:1163–1165; 13:1782,
1783
circumoral pallor 14:1878
complications
ear infections and deafness
6:777; 9:1165

encephalitis 4:565; 9:1164, 1165
hemorrhagic measles 9:1164
lung disease 8:1100; 9:1165
pneumonia 9:1165
German see rubella
inherited immunity to 7:908
rash 9:1163, 1164; 13:1782, 1783, 1784
sight and 5:604
spread 17:2371–2372
vaccination 7:910, 911, 912; 9:1163,
1164, 1165; 17:2331
mild reaction to 17:2330
mechanical percutaneous myocardial
revascularization (MPMR)
10:1403
meconium 4:486; 5:623
Medicaid 6:766, 767
medical alert bracelets 16:2270
medical ethics 9:1166–1167
brain death and harvesting of
organs 16:2264
embryonic stem cells and 15:2066
intensive care and 7:962
surrogacy and 15:2142–2143
medical etiquette 9:1166
medical information highway
9:1168–1169; 16:2180
see also health education
medical research 9:1170–1172
Medicare 6:766, 767
medicines 9:1173–1177
cough
cough syrup 3:426, 427
expectorants 3:426; 5:603
cure-all 11:1552
homeopathic 6:843–844
names of medications 11:1550,
1551
overdose 11:1460–1462
over-the-counter 11:1460
poisoning from 12:1629
reactions to medications 11:1550
see also drugs; pharmacy
meditation 1:75, 80; 9:1178–1179;
11:1477; 13:1802; 15:2104
transcendental 9:1178; 15:2104
Mediterranean fever, familial 12:1619
Medline 9:1168, 1169
meiosis 3:331–332; 5:683
melanin 6:736; 8:1090; 9:1180–1181;
11:1468, 1564–1565; 14:1971, 1972;
15:2127
melanocytes 8:1090, 1091; 9:1180,
1182–1183; 14:1971; 15:2127
melanocyte-stimulating hormone
(MSH) 9:1181
melanoma 9:1182–1185, 1242, 1243;
11:1470; 14:1975
acral lentiginous 9:1184
nodular 9:1183
superficial spreading 9:1183
melatonin 2:188; 9:1186–1187; 14:1898,
1899
medication 7:994; 9:1186, 1187
membranes 9:1188–1189
cell 9:1241
mucous 9:1188, 1189, 1269
serous 9:1189
synovial 7:1002; 9:1188, 1189
memory 2:262, 264; 9:1190–1193, 1229;
10:1345
absentmindedness 4:459
aging and 9:1190, 1192; 14:1908,
1909–1910
dementia and 4:459
false memory syndrome 7:923, 924;
13:1734
sense of smell and 14:1993

Ménière's disease 2:168; 4:455; 9:1194; 16:2228; 17:2366
meninges 9:1189
meningitis and 9:1195–1196
meningitis 2:267; 4:523; 6:759; 7:938; 9:1188, 1195–1197
in babies 3:336
cryptococcal 10:1409
diagnosis 8:1097; 9:1196
following mumps 9:1284
hydrocephalus and 7:878, 879
TB 16:2289
vaccination 7:912
West Nile virus and 17:2406
meningocele 10:1351; 15:2037, 2039
meningomyelocele 7:879; 15:2039
menopause 9:1198–1200
acne rosacea 14:1975
age at start of 9:1200
inherited 6:816
anxiety during 1:105
atheroma and 1:118
breast changes 2:276–277
contraception and 6:732
cystitis and 4:450
disappearance of PMS 12:1672
emotional changes 6:859
endometriosis during 4:569
estrogen and 5:593; 6:854–855; 17:2326
exercise 5:601
hair loss 2:169
hormone replacement therapy (HRT) 4:566; 5:594; 6:854–856; 7:875; 9:1199; 11:1450
hot flashes 4:496; 6:855–856; 7:874–875; 9:1198–1199
acne rosacea and 14:1975
menstruation stops 17:2326
osteoporosis and 2:260; 3:310, 311; 6:854, 855, 856; 9:1199
the ovaries and 11:1458
risk of breast cancer 6:856
risk of heart disease 9:1200
sterilization and 15:2070; 16:2286
sweats 11:1544
symptoms 6:855–856
tiredness 16:2230
the vagina and 17:2334
post-menopausal discharge 17:2339
vaginal atrophy 5:593; 6:856; 9:1198, 1199
menorrhagia (heavy periods) 4:496; 5:642; 9:1202, 1204, 1205
menstrual cycle 2:188, 194; 7:944; 9:1201–1203; 12:1671–1672; 17:2328
the breasts and 2:276
conception and 3:399
cramps 5:601
during puberty 13:1741
fluid retention and 4:500; 12:1672–1673, 1674
hormones and 4:567; 9:1200
estrogen 5:593, 594
lethargy 8:1058
libido and 14:1921
mid-cycle abdominal pain 1:13
pimples and 1:32; 14:1970
premenstrual syndrome (PMS) 6:859; 8:1056; 9:1201, 1202; 12:1671–1674
headaches 6:758
treatment 12:1674; 14:1898
swollen abdomen and 15:2148
weight gain during 1:112; 12:1672

menstrual regulation 1:15
menstruation 5:594; 9:1201–1205; 12:1671; 17:2329
cessation at menopause 17:2326
contraceptives and 3:407, 410
disorders 9:1204, 1205
failure to menstruate 17:2335
heavy periods (menorrhagia) 4:496; 5:642; 9:1202, 1204, 1205
period pains 9:1202–1205
during puberty 13:1739–1740
exercise during 1:49; 15:2052
first period 11:1458; 13:1739
hair condition during 6:737
newborn babies and 17:2328
use of tampons, and toxic shock syndrome 16:2247, 2248
see also menstrual cycle
mental illness 8:1051; 9:1206–1209
complexes and compulsions 3:397–398
compulsions 3:397, 398; 9:1208, 1209; 12:1713
obsessive-compulsive disorder 3:398; 10:1342, 1358, 1387–1388
fatigue and 5:619
neuroses 9:1207, 1208, 1227; 10:1357–1358; 11:1540; 12:1713
see also bipolar disorder; depression; hysteria; phobias; psychoses; psychosomatic problems; schizophrenia
mental retardation 9:1210–1213
Down syndrome and 4:507
epilepsy and 5:583
menthol 13:1825
meperidine hydrochloride 10:1319, 1320
mercury poisoning 2:230; 3:413; 4:574; 10:1392, 1394, 1395; 12:1640
chelation therapy for 3:346
meridian lines 1:35, 37, 38, 117; 6:776; 8:1144
mesenteries 1:11
mesomorphs 2:253
mesothelioma 1:136
metabolism 9:1214–1215
aerobic 1:49–50
anaerobic 1:49
basal metabolic rate 2:173; 17:2401
heat of 16:2182
metacarpals 6:745
metamorphic technique 13:1794
metastases 3:313; 8:1126, 1130
metatarsus varus see pigeon toes
methadone 6:824; 10:1320; 17:2418
methanol 10:1411
methicillin 1:98
methicillin-resistant Staphylococcus aureus see MRSA
methyldopa 15:2045
methyl prednisolone 7:914
metronidazole (Flagyl) 16:2279; 17:2337–2338
metrorrhagia 9:1205
microbiology 8:1029; 9:1216–1217; 11:1514
microcephaly 2:207
microorganisms 11:1509
identification 11:1514
microscopes, operating 9:1218, 1219
microsporidiosis 12:1704
microsurgery 5:709; 9:1218–1221; 10:1434; 15:2139
micturating cystourethrography (MCU) 17:2324
mifepristone 1:14

migraine 5:596; 6:758, 759; 9:1222–1225; 11:1479; 12:1723; 15:2150
lethargy following 8:1055
the Pill and 9:1222; 10:1417
premenstrual 12:1671
treatment 9:1224–1225
alternative medicine 9:1222
analgesics (painkillers) 1:137; 11:1480
biofeedback 2:184
visual disturbances 16:2261
milk
breast milk 2:273; 8:1032
drinking 3:310
penicillin in 14:1912
unpasteurized 3:297
mind 9:1226–1229
alters with age 14:1909–1910
over matter 9:1226, 1228, 1229
subconscious 9:1228; 15:2114–2115
see also memory
mind-body therapy 9:1230–1233
"mind mirrors" 2:183
minerals 4:490; 9:1234–1235; 10:1381
see also trace elements
minimally-invasive (keyhole/laparoscopic) surgery 6:764; 9:1236–1237; 15:2138, 2139
telesurgery and 16:2180
see also laparoscopy
minoxidil (Rogaine) 2:169; 14:1969
mirroring 2:247–248
miscarriage 1:16; 8:1083; 9:1204–1205, 1238–1239
abnormal sperm as cause of 15:2034
after amniocentesis 1:84; 3:368
after chorionic villus sampling 3:368
D & C after 4:496
due to cervical incompetence 3:338
vaginal discharge after 17:2338
mites
house (dust mites) 1:74, 140, 141; 5:646; 6:757
scabies and 13:1865, 1866
mitochondria 3:331; 9:1240, 1241
in muscle cells 11:1577
mitosis 3:331, 332
MMR vaccination 2:206; 7:911, 912
Mogadon (nitrazepam) 16:2257
moisturizers 3:423
molecular biology 9:1240–1241
moles 2:209; 6:726; 9:1242–1243; 11:1511; 14:1972
biopsies 2:192
congenital melanocytic nevi 9:1182
hairy 4:553; 9:1242
itching 9:1182
malignant 2:208; 6:726; 9:1182, 1183, 1184, 1242, 1243; 14:1974, 1975
see also melanoma
satellite 9:1243
Mongolian spots 2:209
Mongoloid race 2:252, 253
monoamine oxidase enzymes 9:1223
monoamine oxidase inhibitors (MAOIs) 4:466
monocytes 2:227, 228
monosaccharides 15:2120, 2121
monosodium glutamate (MSG) 5:653, 654; 9:1244
Montreal Protocol 11:1471
moods 9:1245–1247
in adolescents 9:1206, 1245, 1246

disorders 10:1358
see also bipolar disorder; depression; emotions
morning sickness 5:636, 645; 6:857; 9:1248–1249; 17:2391
morphine 1:138; 6:822, 861; 9:1250–1251; 10:1319; 11:1480
kaolin and morphine 7:1004; 9:1250, 1251
side effects 14:1959
withdrawal 6:823; 17:2417–2418
mosaics 4:510
mosquitoes
bites 2:210, 211; 5:646; 12:1703; 16:2272
elephantiasis and 4:554
malaria and 7:940; 8:1120, 1121, 1122; 11:1500; 16:2281
West Nile virus and 17:2406
yellow fever and 17:2439
mother and child relationship 5:617
single 5:616
mother complex 3:398
motion sickness 2:168; 9:1252–1255; 10:1330, 1331; 16:2271; 17:2390, 2391
motor neuron disease 9:1256–1259
Lou Gehrig's disease (amyotrophic lateral sclerosis) 9:1256–1259
mouth 9:1260–1263
breathing through 1:40; 9:1262
cancer 3:316
cleft palate 2:207; 3:376, 401; 11:1483, 1484, 1485; 12:1612–1613; 15:2030
cold sores 2:223; 3:382; 4:543; 6:825; 9:1263; 14:1970, 2008
drooling 9:1262, 1263
dry mouth 9:1262; 13:1852
halitosis (bad breath) 4:460; 6:740–741; 9:1263; 12:1608
irritants 7:981
problems 9:1263
accident to the palate 11:1485
acidic diet 9:1263
aphthous stomatitis (aphthous ulcers) 9:1263; 17:2311
pyorrhea (peridontal disease) and gingivitis 4:461; 6:731, 740, 759; 9:1263; 12:1610; 13:1759–1761
salivary duct stones 9:1263; 13:1854
speech and 9:1262–1263
stomatitis 9:1263
thrush 9:1263; 16:2219
ulcers 9:1260, 1263; 14:2008; 16:2234; 17:2310–2312
yeast infection 9:1263; 11:1484; 17:2436
see also lips; teeth and teething; tongue
movement 9:1264–1268
ligaments and 8:1071; 9:1266
muscles and 9:1264, 1265, 1294
moxibustion 1:39; 3:359
MRI (magnetic resonance imaging) 4:478, 479; 13:1869, 1870
of the brain 2:190, 230, 266, 269; 6:758; 10:1356
of the breasts 8:1132
of carpal tunnel syndrome 3:322
MRSA (methicillin-resistant Staphylococcus aureus) 1:98; 11:1508; 15:2062
MS see multiple sclerosis

MSH *see* melanocyte-stimulating hormone
mucolytics 5:603
mucoviscidosis *see* cystic fibrosis
mucus 9:1188, **1269**; 11:1560
  cervical 9:*1203*, 1269
  the rhythm method and 13:1829, *1830*
  nasal, smell and 14:1991, *1994*
mud therapy 9:**1270–1273**
Müllerian ducts 17:2328–2329
multiple births 3:400; 9:**1274–1277**
  fertility drugs and 7:942; 9:1274, *1275*
  from IVF 1:129
  see also twins
multiple myelomatosis 14:1966
multiple personality 9:1207, **1278–1279**; 11:1540
multiple sclerosis (MS) 2:267; 6:728; 9:1256, **1280–1282**; 15:2043
  bladder control and 15:2040
  distortions of the sense of touch 16:2242
  loss of vision 2:221; 9:1281; 10:1410, 1411
  slurred speech 15:2033
  tremor 16:2275
mummification 5:669
mumps 7:927, 938; 8:1110; 9:**1283–1284**; 13:1852
  in adults 7:935, 982
  affecting the testes 9:1284; 16:2193
  subclinical infection 7:935
  vaccination 7:911, 912; 9:1284
Munchausen syndrome 9:**1285–1286**
  by proxy 9:1285, *1286*
murmurs of the heart 8:1103; 9:**1287–1289**; 15:2074
  in children 6:788; 9:1289
muscae volitantes 2:219
muscles 9:**1290–1294**
  anerobic metabolism 1:49
  biceps and triceps 4:546; 9:*1265*
  building up 12:1701
  disorders 9:1292; 12:1724
    cramp 1:50; 4:437, *437*; 5:599; 6:796; 11:1544; 12:1662; 13:1764, *1861*
    enzyme defects 9:1292
    fibrositis 5:643
    hamstring injuries 6:743–744
    hot and cold treatment 6:797, 799
    hyperkalemic paralysis 9:1292
    hypokalemic paralysis 9:1292
    muscular dystrophy 9:1292; 10:**1301–1303**; 11:*1490*
    myalgia 10:**1310–1311**; 16:2248
    myasthenia gravis 5:619, 620; 10:**1312–1313**; 11:1491
    myopathies 9:1292, 1294
    myositis 9:1292, 1294
    paralysis 11:1491
    polymyalgia rheumatica 9:1292
    pulled or strained muscles 6:799; 9:1292, 1294; 13:*1747–1748*; 15:*2051*, 2054
    stiffness 15:2054, 2076–2077
    torn muscles 9:1290, 1292
  exercise and 5:599; 9:1290, 1294
  fitness and 11:1577
  injections into 7:955, 956
  intercostal, and stitch 15:2087
  movement and 9:1264, 1265, 1294
  postural 16:2182–2183
  spasms
    around joints 7:1000

  in the back 2:163; 5:643
  traction and 16:2253
  sports injuries, first aid 1:50
  structure 9:1291–1294
  types 9:1290
    cardiac (heart) 9:1266, 1267, 1290, *1293*
    smooth (involuntary) 9:1266, 1267, *1268*, 1290, *1293*
    striated (voluntary) 9:1290, *1291*, *1293*
  see also diaphragm; tendons
muscular dystrophy 9:1292; 10:**1301–1303**; 11:*1490*
  Becker's 10:1302, 1303
  Duchenne 10:1301–*1303*
    detection 3:367
  Landouzy-Dejerine (fasccioscapulohumeral dystrophy) 10:1302, 1303
  myotonic 10:1302, 1303
musculoskeletal system 14:1966
mushroom poisoning 5:657, *658*, 659
mussel poisoning 5:657, *658*, 659
mutation 10:1301, **1304–1306**
  beneficial 10:1306
  genetic disorders and 5:677
  nuclear radiation and 3:330
mutism 10:**1307–1309**
  elective 10:1307
myalgia 10:**1310–1311**; 16:2248
myalgic encephalomyelitis (ME) 3:369
myasthenia gravis 5:619; 10:**1312–1313**; 11:1491
  treatment 5:620; 10:1313
  thymus removal 16:2221
Mycobacterium leprae 6:754, 755
Mycobacterium tuberculosis 2:166; 16:2287
myelin 9:1280; 10:1347
myelitis 15:2040, 2043
myelography 10:1355
  myelograms 2:163; 14:1885, *1886*, 1887, *1984*
myelomatosis, multiple 14:1966
myelomeningocoele 10:1351
myocardial infarction *see* heart attack
myoclonic jerks 16:2293, 2294
myofibrils 9:1265, *1293*
myoglobin 11:1463
myomectomy 5:642
myopathies 9:1292, 1294
myopia (nearsightedness) 5:604, *608*; 10:1413
  index 3:327
myositis 9:1292, 1294; 11:1491, *1492*
myositis ossificans 4:547
myxedema *see* hypothyroidism

N

nails 10:1314–1318; 14:1970–1971
  athlete's foot affecting 2:150; 13:1837, 1838
  biting 10:1314, 1315–*1318*
  bruises under 3:*298*; 10:1314
  care 10:*1316–1317*, 1318
  cutting toenails 5:627; 10:*1317*
  dermatologists and 4:469
  flaky 10:1315
  ingrown toenails 7:951–952; 10:1315, 1318; 12:1626
  iron deficiency and 7:977; 10:1315
  koilonychia 6:747
  leukonychia 6:747
  loss 10:1314
  onycholysis 6:747

  psoriasis and 12:1708
  ridges 10:1315
  ringworm 10:1315
  splinter hemorrhages 16:2277
  thrush (Candida) 16:2220; 17:*2437*, 2438
  white spots 10:1315
  whitlow (paronychia) 6:747; 10:1314; 17:*2411*, 2438
naloxone 6:824
naproxen 11:1479
narcolepsy 7:897, 899; 15:2083
narcotics 10:1319–1320; 11:1481–1482
  addiction to 7:1004; 10:1319, *1320*
  see also heroin; opiates
nasal drops, decongestant 1:40
nasal spray or drops 13:1825; 14:2002
nasogastric tubes 15:2134
nasopharyngitis 16:2212
nasopharynx 11:1555–1557
natural childbirth 2:200; 10:**1321–1325**
natural family planning *see* rhythm method
natural healing 5:614
nature versus nurture (inherited versus acquired) 6:817–818; 11:1539–1540
naturopathy 1:81; 10:**1326–1329**
nausea 10:**1330–1331**
  motion sickness 9:1253–1254; 10:1330, 1331
  see also morning sickness; vomiting
navel, umbilical hernia 6:819, *821*
nearsightedness *see* myopia
Necator americanus 6:852, 853
neck 10:**1332–1335**
  Adam's apple 10:1332, *1335*
  arthritis 10:1335
    osteoarthritis 1:122
    vertigo and 17:2366
  broken 10:1332, *1334*; 15:2040
  bull neck 4:497
  cervical ribs 13:1832
  dislocation 4:498
  glands in *see* parathyroid glands; thyroid
  goiter 5:*704*; 10:1334; 16:*2224*, 2225, 2226
  pain and spasm, heat treatment 6:799
  stiff 10:1332; 15:2078, *2079*
  swollen lymph nodes 5:*699*; 6:*833*; 8:*1109*, 1114; 10:1335
  whiplash injury 10:1334, *1335*; 13:1747–1748; 17:**2409–2410**
  see also larynx and laryngitis; pharynx; throat; vocal cords
Neisseria gonorrhoeae 14:*1931*
neonatal intensive care unit 7:962; 10:**1336–1338**; 11:1516; 12:1667, 1669
  see also premature babies
nephrectomy 10:1339
nephritis 5:707; 17:2325
nephroblastoma 17:2325
nephrons 8:1017, 1020; 17:*2325*
nephrosis 17:2325
nerve block procedures 8:*1093*
nervous breakdown 10:**1340–1342**
nervousness
  tremor and 16:2274, 2275
  see also anxiety
nervous system 10:**1343–1347**
  autonomic *see* autonomic nervous system
  central 2:262; 10:1344–1345, *1346*
  see also brain; spinal cord
    disorders 10:1347

  function tests 10:1355–1356
  nerves
    cells (neurons) 2:157; 9:1256; 10:1343, 1344, 1345–1347
    of the spinal cord 15:2042
    cranial 10:1344
    facial 16:2169, 2171
    glossopharyngeal 16:2169, 2171
    growth 9:1221
    Guillain-Barré syndrome and 6:728, 729
    junction with muscles 10:*1313*; 11:1491, *1492*
    microsurgery and 9:1218, 1219, 1221
    multiple sclerosis and 6:728; 9:1280–1281
    numbness and 10:*1376–1378*
    olfactory 16:2169
    optic 2:220; 5:606; 10:**1410–1411**
    paralysis and 11:1491–1493
    pinched 10:1344
    polio and 6:728
    severed 1:20; 8:1030
    spinal 10:1344; 15:*2042*
    ulnar 10:1344; 11:1491; 12:1595
    vagus 11:1487
  pain from the 11:1476–1477
  parasympathetic 2:156, 158
  peripheral 10:1343–1344, *1346*
  somatic 10:1343, 1344, *1345*
  sympathetic 2:156, 158
nettle 6:*814*
neuralgia 10:**1348–1349**
  facial (trigeminal) 10:1347, *1348*, *1349*; 14:1939
  headaches 6:758, 759
  postherpetic 14:1938, 1939
  see also sciatica
neural tube defect 2:207; 10:**1350–1351**
  meningocele 10:1351
  myelomeningocele 10:1351
  see also anencephaly; hydrocephalus; spina bifida
neurasthenia 10:**1352–1353**
  see also chronic fatigue syndrome
neuritis 10:1377
  optic 2:222
neurofibrillary tangle 1:83
neurofibromatosis (Von Recklinghausen's disease) 6:727; 14:1891
neurology and neurosurgery 10:**1354–1356**
  physical therapy and 11:1579–1580
neuroma, acoustic 16:2228
neuronitis, vestibular 10:1347
neurons (nerve cells) 2:157; 9:1256; 10:1343, 1344, 1345–1347
  of the spinal cord 15:2042
neuropathy 10:1347
  peripheral 8:1049
  X-linked bulbospinal 9:1259
neuroses 9:1207, 1208, 1227; 10:**1357–1358**; 11:1540; 12:1713
  nervous breakdown and 10:1340
neurosurgery *see* neurology and neurosurgery
neurotransmitters
  Alzheimer's disease and 1:83
  myasthenia gravis and 10:*1313*
neutrophils 2:225, 227
nevi 2:208, 209
  blue 9:*1243*
  compound 8:*1091*; 9:*1243*
  congenital melanocytic 9:1182

2567

nevi (cont'd)
dysplastic 8:1091
giant melanocytic 9:1182
intradermal 8:1091
junctional 8:1091
strawberry 12:1613
see also moles
nicotine 10:1359–1361
poisoning 10:1361
skin patches 14:1995; 16:2259, 2260
night blindness 10:1362; 17:2373, 2374
nightmares 4:511, 512; 14:1978
nipples
extra 6:726
prenatal care 12:1675
nitrazepam (Mogadon) 16:2257
nitrogen oxides 1:28, 59, 60
nitroglycerine, skin patches 16:2260
nitroimidazoles 1:100
nocturia 2:218
nocturnal emissions (wet dreams)
5:589; 14:1906
noise 10:1363–1366, 1395
deafness and 4:453, 455, 456; 6:777;
10:1363, 1365–1366
tinnitus and 16:2227, 2228
noninsulin-dependent diabetes
(maturity-onset diabetes; type II
diabetes) 4:472; 10:1367–1368
nonspecific urethritis (NSU)
14:1931–1933
nonsteroidal anti-inflammatory drugs
(NSAIDs) 6:787; 10:1369–1370;
11:1482
interactions with other drugs
10:1370
see also aspirin and analgesics
noradrenaline (norepinephrine) 1:47;
2:158, 198–199; 5:622; 12:1724
normality 6:817
nose 10:1371–1375
adenoids 1:40–41; 2:281; 10:1372,
1375; 11:1557; 16:2212–2213
snoring and 14:2005
broken 10:1372, 1374
changing shape of (rhinoplasty)
3:424, 425; 12:1613
cocaine and 3:381
common cold 10:1374
congestion 10:1371, 1372, 1374
cosmetic surgery to 3:424, 425
crooked 10:1372
foreign bodies 10:1375; 14:1962,
2003
gaseous irritants and 7:981
hay fever 10:1374
nasal discharge 14:1962
nasal passages 2:279–281
nosebleeds 4:568; 6:803; 10:1371
treating 10:1374
picking 10:1371
polyps in 10:1372, 1375; 12:1642, 1643
rhinitis 11:1560; 13:1825–1826;
14:2002, 2003
vasomotor 14:2003
sinusitis 6:741; 9:1269; 10:1375;
13:1826; 14:1962–1963
headaches and 6:758, 759;
15:2150
nosebleeds 4:568; 6:803; 10:1371
treating 10:1374
novocaine 15:2078
NSAIDS see nonsteroidal anti-
inflammatory drugs
nuclear cell transfer 3:377, 378
nuclear disasters
radiation sickness 13:1771
see also Chernobyl disaster

nuclear medicine 2:190
numbness 10:1376–1378
see also local anesthetics; pins and
needles
nurses 7:871
emergency 4:561
home-care 6:840
postoperative care by 12:1644–1645
psychiatric 12:1712
nursing
barrier 7:982, 983
reverse barrier 7:982, 983
nutrition 10:1379–1382
see also diet; health foods
NuvaRing contraceptive rings
3:411
nystagmus 2:219

O

obesity 4:492; 5:655; 6:846;
10:1383–1386
atherosclerosis and 3:372
body mass index (BMI) and 17:2400
brown fat theory and 9:1171
diabetes and 10:1368
a form of malnutrition 8:1127, 1128;
10:1382
glands and 1:46; 4:566; 10:1383
Pickwickian syndrome 7:898
reflux esophagitis and 6:787
a symptom of Cushing's syndrome
15:2152
varicose veins and 17:2344–2345
yoga and 17:2444
see also weight, overweight
obsessions 7:894; 10:1387
obsessive-compulsive disorder 3:398;
10:1342, 1358, 1387–1388
obstetrics 10:1389–1390
physical therapy and 11:1580
occupational hazards 10:1391–1396
pneumoconiosis 2:282; 4:564;
12:1621; 13:1752
silicosis 10:1395; 14:1961
see also environmental hazards
occupational therapy 6:839;
10:1397–1398; 12:1715; 13:1796,
1797–1798
see also physical therapy
Oedipus complex 3:397–398; 7:923
oils, essential see aromatherapy
oil spills, detergents and 12:1638
old age see aging
olecranon 4:546
olfactory cells 14:1991
omentum 11:1532, 1533, 1534, 1535
Onchocerca 11:1500, 1501
oncology 10:1399–1400
integrative 10:1399
oncoviruses 3:314; 8:1126
onycholysis 6:747
oophoritis 9:1284
open-heart surgery 10:1401–1403
see also bypass surgery
operating room 10:1404–1406
operations see surgery
ophthalmia neonatorum 5:705
ophthalmology 10:1407–1408
ophthalmoscopes 4:475, 476; 5:604;
10:1408
opiates 1:137–138; 11:1482
abuse 4:525
see also codeine; morphine; opium
opioids 10:1320; 11:1481–1482
Opisthrocus viverina 17:2421
opium 9:1250, 1251; 10:1319; 11:1482

opportunistic infection 10:1409
oppositional defiant disorder 2:152
optical illusions 9:1227
optic disks 5:607
optic nerve 2:220; 5:606; 10:1410–1411
optometrist 10:1412–1413
tests for color blindness 3:388
oral contraceptives (the Pill)
10:1414–1417; 11:1458; 17:2326
age and 15:2107
antibiotics and 1:99
bleeding between periods and
9:1204, 1205
checkups while taking 10:1416
children swallowing 11:1462
coming off the 10:1416, 1417
common problems and solutions
10:1417
compared to HRT 7:874
D & C operation and 4:496
diarrhea and 4:485
during adolescence 1:42
forgetting to take 9:1202
internal examination before going
on 7:966
previous hepatitis infection and
6:809
side effects 5:593; 9:1158; 10:1415,
1417
on the breasts 10:1417; 14:1956
circulatory disorders 10:1417;
16:2214
cystitis 4:450
ectopic pregnancy 10:1417
on libido 7:963; 10:1414;
14:1920–1921
migraines 9:1222; 10:1417
premenstrual tension 9:1201
risk of stroke 15:2107
on sebaceous glands 14:1900
skin darkening 8:1091
skin pigmentation on the face
and 8:1090, 1091
weight 10:1416; 17:2398
taken during pregnancy 10:1416
taking a break from 10:1414
tanning and 9:1180
to treat acne 1:31; 14:1900
to treat endometriosis 4:569
to treat premenstrual syndrome
12:1674
types 10:1415, 1416–1417
varicose veins and 10:1414
while taking other medication
10:1414
orchiopexy 16:2192
orchitis 9:1284; 16:2193
organic brain syndromes 12:1722
organic food 10:1328, 1418–1420
organ removal 10:1421–1422
orgasm 7:964–965; 10:1423–1424
female 7:964–965; 10:1423;
14:1918–1919, 1921; 17:2394
multiple orgasms 14:1916
problems 10:1424; 14:1929
male 5:590; 7:965; 14:1919,
1921
problems 10:1423–1424
simultaneous 7:963
see also masturbation
orlistat 10:1385
oropharynx 11:1557
orthermography 16:2207
orthodontics 10:1425–1429; 16:2175,
2177
interceptive 10:1427
Ortho Evra patches 3:411
orthopantomography 17:2434

orthopedics 10:1430–1434
physical therapy and 11:1580
osmosis 4:544
ossification 3:324
osteoarthritis 1:123, 123; 3:325; 5:691;
10:1435–1438; 11:1581; 14:1968
cause 1:123, 126
causing lower back pain 8:1095
cysts and 4:447
dislocation and 4:498
of the elbow 4:547
of the hands 6:746; 14:1968
of the knee, hydrotherapy and
7:883
stiffness and 10:1436, 1437;
15:2077–2078
symptoms 1:123, 126
treatment 1:126
osteoid bumps 13:1836
osteomalacia 2:259; 13:1835, 1836;
17:2381
osteomyelitis 2:258, 260
osteopathy 1:78; 2:161; 3:362; 6:837;
11:1446–1449
cranial 11:1447, 1449
osteophytes 2:161
osteoporosis 2:258, 260; 3:310, 311;
5:693; 6:854, 855; 9:1199;
11:1450–1451; 14:1968
backache and 2:161, 163
causing limping 8:1078
fractures and 2:161; 3:310; 5:660;
6:828; 8:1078
HRT and 2:260; 6:855, 856; 9:1199;
11:1450, 1451
immobilization 2:260
osteotomy 10:1438; 12:1594
otitis 11:1452–1453
otitis externa 4:452, 456; 7:988;
11:1452–1452
otitis interna 11:1453
otitis media (middle ear infection)
4:453, 456; 6:758; 11:1453;
13:1826;16:2213
chronic 11:1453
mastoiditis after 9:1160, 1161;
16:2171
perforated eardrum and 15:2156
sore throat and 11:1555; 14:2011
tonsillitis and 16:2236
vertigo and 17:2366
otosclerosis 4:453, 456; 6:777; 12:1696,
1700; 16:2228
otoscopes 4:475, 476; 6:779
out-of-body experiences 9:1229
outpatients 11:1454–1457
ova see eggs
ovaries 3:399; 5:594; 11:1458–1459
cancer 11:1459
laparoscopy and 8:1034
treatment 7:905
cysts 4:446, 447, 568, 569; 6:733;
11:1459; 16:2195
as endocrine glands 11:1459
endometriosis of 4:568, 569
one removed 10:1422; 11:1458
pregnancy and 6:732; 10:1421
oophoritis 9:1284
salpingitis and 13:1860
sterilization involving the 15:2069,
2071; 16:2286
tumors 8:1124
overdoses 11:1460–1462
acetaminophen 11:1479; 12:1629
amphetamine 1:87
aspirin 4:562; 11:1460; 12:1629
barbiturate 2:170; 3:395
coma and 3:395

suicide and 15:2124
teenage "suicidal gestures" 12:1630
tranquilizers 16:2256, 2257
treatment 2:170; 11:1479; 15:2091,
    2092
    emetics 15:2092–2093
    first aid for suspected drug
        overdose 6:824; 11:1462
    stomach pump 15:2091–2093
overeating 3:397
    appetite and 1:112, 113
    during the menstrual cycle 1:112
ovulation 5:594; 7:945; 11:1459
    cervical mucus and 13:1829
    failure 7:943
    pain on 1:13
    the rhythm method and 13:1827,
        1828, 1829, 1830
oxygen 11:1463–1465, 1574–1575
    carried around the body 2:281;
        11:1464
    cycle 11:1465
    debt 11:1463
    gas exchange and 8:1102
    hyperbaric 3:302; 11:1466, 1467
    liquid 11:1467
    transtracheal 11:1464
    uptake during exercise 11:1573,
        1575–1576
oxygen chambers, hyperbaric 3:302;
    11:1465, 1467
oxygen cylinders 11:1467
oxygen masks 11:1463, 1464, 1466
oxygen tents 11:1467
oxygen therapy 11:1464–1465,
    1466–1467
oxytetracycline 15:2126
oxytocin 2:273; 4:566, 567; 6:857, 859;
    12:1599, 1605
    induced labor and 7:933, 934; 10:1322
    nicotine and 10:1361
ozone 4:573; 11:1468
    ground-level 1:59; 11:1465, 1468;
        12:1639
ozone layer 1:59; 11:1468–1471
    depletion 4:574; 11:1468, 1469;
        12:1636

P

pacemaker 11:1472–1473
    artificial 2:190; 3:421; 11:1472–1473
        failure 11:1472
        replacing 6:788
    natural (sinoatrial node) 6:782;
        9:1267; 11:1472
Paget's disease 2:260
pain 11:1474–1477
    analysis in the spinal cord
        16:2240–2241
    chronic 11:1474, 1477
    endorphins and 1:38; 11:1477, 1481
    function of 11:1474–1475, 1480
    the gate theory and 1:38
    hypnosis and 7:891
    radiation of 15:2149
    religious initiates and 11:1476
    tolerance to 2:188; 11:1474
    types 11:1476–1477
        from the nervous system
            11:1476–1477
        internal pain 11:1476
        phantom pain 1:127; 10:1344;
            11:1477
        referred pain 1:38; 11:1476;
            15:2149; 16:2212
        skin pain 11:1476

painkillers 1:137–138; 11:1478–1480,
    1481–1482
    see also acetaminophen; aspirin
        and analgesics; codeine;
        ibuprofen; morphine
pain management 11:1481–1482
    acupuncture 1:38; 11:1478
    cold therapy 11:1579
    electrical stimulation 11:1481, 1579
        transcutaneous electrical nerve
            stimulation (TENS) 11:1482, 1579
    flotation therapy 5:649
    in hospices 6:861
    pain clinics 11:1482
    painkillers (analgesics) 1:137–138;
        11:1478–1480, 1481–1482
        see also acetaminophen; aspirin
            and analgesics; codeine;
            ibuprofen; morphine
    skin patches 16:2260
    surgery 11:1481
    ultrasound 11:1579, 1580
    wax treatment 11:1579
palate 9:1260; 11:1483–1485
    accident to 11:1485
    cleft 2:207; 3:376, 401; 11:1483, 1484,
        1485; 12:1612–1613
        speech and 15:2030
    excessively concave 11:1485
    "falling" 11:1483
palatoplasty 14:2005
palilalia 1:108
palliative care 7:961
Palmer, Bartlett Joshua 3:362
Palmer, Daniel David 3:362
palpitations 4:550; 6:789, 790
    treatment 2:157
palsy
    pseudobulbar 9:1258, 1259
    see also Bell's palsy; cerebral palsy
pancreas and disorders 5:700;
    11:1486–1487
    cancer 5:624; 7:992; 11:1487
    cystic fibrosis affecting 11:1487
    diabetes and 4:471–472; 7:960;
        11:1487
    digestive function 4:495; 5:700;
        11:1486, 1487
    hemochromatosis affecting 11:1487
    injuries 11:1486
    pancreatitis 9:1283; 11:1486
    removal 11:1486, 1487
    shoulder or arm pain and 14:1948
    sugar levels and 7:960; 11:1486
    transplants 16:2264
    tumors 7:960
pancreatitis 9:1283; 11:1486
pandemics, flu 7:949, 950
panic attacks, treatment 2:182; 5:630
panic disorder 10:1358
papaverine 10:1319
papilledema 10:1411
papillomatosis 16:2213
Pap smear (cervical smear) 3:313, 314,
    337, 338; 6:734; 7:966, 967; 8:1126;
    11:1488–1489, 1513; 14:1894
    after sterilization 15:2071
    during pregnancy 12:1676
papules 13:1783
paraffin, liquid 8:1046
paralysis 8:1069; 11:1490–1493; 15:2150
    of cerebral palsy 3:336
    Guillain-Barré syndrome and 6:729
    hyperkalemic 9:1292
    hypokalemic 9:1292
    hysterical 11:1492
    spastic 10:1347
    treatment

    bionics and 2:191
    physical therapy 11:1579–1580
    splints 8:1048–1049
paralytic ileus 11:1534
paramedics 4:561
paraphimosis 11:1531
paraphrenia, late 14:1911
paraplegia 3:336; 11:1494–1497; 15:2043
parasites 11:1498–1502
    bedbugs 2:174, 175
    causing blindness 2:220
    causing malaria 8:1121
    cysts and 4:447
    fleas 2:211; 5:646–647
    lice 2:211; 7:885; 8:1064–1066
        typhus and 8:1066; 16:2299,
            2300, 2301
    mites, and scabies 13:1865, 1866
parathyroid glands 5:700; 10:1335;
    11:1503–1505
    bones and 2:259; 11:1505; 13:1836
    overactive 11:1504, 1505
    removal 11:1503, 1504
    tumor 3:311; 11:1505
    underactive 11:1504, 1505
parathyroid hormone (PTH;
    parathormone) 2:259; 3:310, 311;
    4:566; 6:858; 8:1020; 11:1504
    chelation therapy and 3:345
paratyphoid see typhoid and
    paratyphoid
Parkinson's disease 2:267; 9:1266;
    10:1347; 11:1506–1507, 1581
    speech and 15:2032
    tremor 11:1506; 16:2274, 2275
paronychia see whitlow
parotid glands 9:1261; 13:1853
patella see knee, kneecap
paternity testing 2:233
pathogens 11:1508–1510
    see also pathology
pathology 11:1508, 1511–1514
    chemical 11:1514
    forensic 11:1513
    see also biopsy; laboratory tests;
        microbiology; pathogens
pathomimicry see Munchausen
    syndrome
Patterson Brown-Kelly syndrome
    16:2211
peak flow meters 13:1752
peanut butter 6:772
peanuts 14:1912
pediatric medicine 10:1389;
    11:1515–1519
    physical therapy and 11:1580
pediculoses 8:1065
Pel-Ebstein fever pattern 1:114
pellagra 17:2376
pelvic inflammatory disease (PID)
    1:131; 2:161; 7:943; 11:1520–1521;
    14:1933
    from gonorrhea 5:706
pelvis 11:1522–1526
    fractured 11:1526
    see also hip
pemphigoid 2:223, 224
pemphigusis 2:224
Pendred's syndrome 16:2226
penetrance 6:818
penicillamine 13:1823
penicillin 1:99, 100; 10:1304; 11:1527–1529
    allergy to 1:70, 99, 100; 11:1527, 1528,
        1529; 14:1959; 16:2199
    semi-synthetic 11:1528
    sensitization to 14:1912
penicillin-resistant Streptococcus
    pneumoniae (PRSP) 1:98

penis and disorders 5:690;
    11:1530–1531
    disorders
        balanitis 10:1368; 11:1531; 17:2437
        cancer 11:1530; 17:2325
        discharge 11:1530, 1531
        hypospadias 2:207; 12:1613;
            17:2323
        impotence 1:130; 5:590;
            7:919–920; 11:1531; 14:1924
        pain 5:690
        paraphimosis 11:1531
        phimosis 3:374; 11:1531
        urethritis 11:1531
    penis
        circumcision 3:374; 5:688;
            14:1918
        prosthesis 12:1700
        size 14:1920
        see also erection and ejaculation
pentobarbital 7:893
pentothal (thiopental) 2:170
peppermint 6:812, 813; 10:1329
"pep pills" 1:86
pepsin 4:494, 531; 5:581
percussion 4:475
pericarditis
    pain 3:348
    tuberculous 16:2289
peridontal disease see pyorrhea and
    gingivitis
peridontal disease, see also gums and
    gum disease
peridontium 6:730
perineum 11:1525
period see menstruation
periodic abstinence see rhythm
    method
periosteum 8:1070
peristalsis 1:69; 3:404, 405; 5:592;
    15:2023
peritoneum 1:11; 11:1532–1535
    dialysis through 8:1014, 1016;
        17:2322
peritonitis 1:111; 4:501; 9:1189; 11:1532,
    1533–1535
Perls, Fritz and Laura 5:695
pernicious anemia 1:88, 89, 90; 11:1514,
    1536–1537; 17:2376
    vitiligo and 17:2388
peroxisomes 9:1240
persecution complex 3:398
persistent generalized
    lymphadenopathy (PGL) 1:57
persistent vegetative state 2:270;
    3:394
personality 5:682; 11:1538–1542
    A-type and B-type, and stress
        15:2101
    disorders 9:1207
        multiple personality 9:1207,
            1278–1279; 11:1540
    moods and 9:1247
    problems 12:1713
perspiration (sweat) 2:249; 5:597–598,
    699; 11:1543–1545; 14:1941–1942;
    15:2130–2131; 16:2183
    prickly heat and 12:1685
Perthes' disease 6:830; 8:1076; 11:1546
pessaries, ring 12:1686
pesticides 13:1839
    in/on food 4:574; 5:657, 659; 10:1418,
        1420
    as pollutants 12:1640
petechiae 13:1755
petrissage 8:1142, 1143
PET scanning 2:190; 4:480; 10:1355;
    11:1547; 13:1869, 1870

Peyer's patches, typhoid and 16:2295, 2297
Peyronie's disease 14:1929
phagocytes 1:17–18; 3:319; 7:946, 948
phalanges 6:745
phantom pregnancy 11:1548–1549
pharmaceutical companies 11:1550–1553
pharmacists 11:1551, 1552
pharmacology 11:1551, 1554
pharmacy 11:1550–1554
  see also drugs; medicines
pharyngeal web 16:2211
pharyngitis 11:1556, 1557; 14:2011; 16:2212
pharynx 11:1555–1557; 16:2211–2212
  cancer 16:2213
  grazed 11:1557
  pharyngeal web 16:2211
  pharyngitis 11:1556, 1557; 14:2011
  see also throat
Phenacetin 1:137; 8:1020
phenobarbital 2:170; 7:893
phenothiazines 14:1903
phenylalanine 5:581; 11:1558, 1559
phenylbutazone 1:138
phenylketonuria (PKU) 3:401; 5:581, 654, 684; 11:1558–1559
phimosis 3:374; 11:1531
phlebitis 16:2218; 17:2345
phlegm (sputum) 3:348, 426; 11:1560; 13:1757
  examination 13:1752
  expectorants and 5:603
  tests 15:2025
phobias 9:1209; 10:1358; 11:1561–1563
  treatment 9:1209; 11:1563; 12:1710
    flotation therapy 5:649
  see also agoraphobia
phonation 15:2029
phosphorus 9:1235
photocoagulation 8:1041
photodermatitis 4:468
photoic stimulation 5:583, 585
photosensitivity 11:1564–1565; 15:2126, 2129
photosynthesis 15:2063
phototherapy see light therapy
phrenology 6:760
physical examination 11:1566, 1566–1569
  for children 11:1518–1519, 1568
  see also checkups
physical fitness 11:1570–1573, 1574, 1575
  aerobics and 1:50; 11:1573
  jogging and 7:997
  pulse rate and 1:50; 11:1572, 1574
  see also exercise
physical fitness testing 11:1574–1577
physical therapy 11:1578–1581; 13:1797–1798; 16:2205, 2206
  after surgery 13:1795
  hydrotherapy 6:799; 7:881–883; 10:1328; 11:1579; 13:1795; 16:2206
  for stroke victims 11:1580; 15:2107, 2110
  see also manipulation; occupational therapy
physician assistants (PAs) 4:561
Pickwickian syndrome 7:898
picornaviruses 17:2371
piercing see body piercing
pigeon chest 3:347; 12:1590–1592
pigeons, infections from 10:1409
pigeon toes 5:625, 628; 8:1076; 12:1593–1594
piles 6:807
  see also hemorrhoids

Pill, the see oral contraceptives
pimples see acne and pimples
pineal gland 2:187–188; 5:700; 9:1186, 1187; 14:1899
Pinel, Philippe 12:1722
pin and plate operation 10:1431, 1433
pins and needles 3:372; 10:1343, 1377; 12:1595–1597; 16:2242
  with multiple sclerosis 9:1281
pinworms see threadworms
piracetam 14:1989
pituitary gland 4:567; 12:1598–1601
  direct influence 6:859
    antidiuretic hormone secretion 6:859; 12:1599
    on growth 4:532; 5:697–698
    oxytocin secretion 6:857, 859; 12:1599
    prolactin secretion 6:859; 8:1032; 12:1598, 1600
  effect of hypothalamus on 6:859; 7:897; 12:1598–1599; 13:1740
  effect on other glands 4:566, 567; 6:859
    adrenal glands 4:567; 12:1598
    pancreas 5:699
    sex glands 11:1459
    thyroid gland 4:567; 6:847; 12:1599; 16:2224
  failure 12:1598
  hormones 5:593; 7:899; 9:1201–1202; 12:1599–1600
  tumors 5:607; 7:899; 10:1411; 12:1598, 1600–1601
    gigantism or acromegaly and 5:697–698
  menstrual disorders and 9:1204
pituitary portal system 12:1599
Pityrosporum ovale 4:451
PKU see phenylketonuria
placebo effect 12:1602–1603
  ethical use of placebos 9:1167
  tonics and 15:2083; 16:2231
placenta 2:204; 8:1102; 12:1604–1605
  D & C and 4:496
  placenta previa 3:341; 9:1277; 12:1605
plague 12:1606–1607
  a biological weapon 2:185, 186; 12:1606
plants
  aromatic 14:1991, 1993, 1994
  contact photosensitivity and 11:1565
  as medicines 1:114
    see also herbs and herbalism
  a source of starch 15:2063
plaque 4:460, 461; 6:730, 731; 12:1608–1610
  gum diseases and 6:730, 731; 13:1759–1760
  testing for 4:461
Plaquenil 8:1105
plaques
  atheromatous see atheroma
  in the brain 1:83
plasma 2:227; 12:1611
plasma cells 8:1113
plasma exchange 6:729
plasmapheresis 12:1611
Plasmodium spp., and malaria 8:1121; 11:1500, 1501; 12:1704
plaster casts see casts, plaster
plastic and reconstructive surgery 12:1612–1617
  see also cosmetic surgery
platelets 2:226, 227, 228; 3:298; 13:1755
  deficiency 3:298

plethysmography, body 3:371
pleural rub 12:1620
pleurisy 2:281, 282; 3:426; 9:1189; 12:1618–1620; 13:1751, 1752
  pain 3:348
  pneumonia and 12:1625
  treatment 12:1620; 15:2151
PMS see premenstrual syndrome
PMS Escape 12:1674
Pneumococcus spp. 2:166
pneumoconiosis 2:282; 4:564; 12:1621; 13:1752
  treatment 2:282; 13:1752
Pneumocystis carinii pneumonia 12:1625
Pneumocystis jiroveci 10:1409
pneumonia 2:282; 3:347, 348; 7:937, 938, 940; 8:1103, 1104; 12:1622–1625; 13:1752
  aspiration pneumonia 12:1624, 1625, 1631
  bronchopneumonia 8:1104; 12:1623, 1624–1625
  a complication of other diseases 12:1625
    chicken pox 3:350
    influenza 7:950
    measles 9:1165
  double 12:1622
  lobar 8:1104; 12:1622, 1623, 1624, 1625
  pneumonic plague 12:1607
  prevention 12:1624
  secondary drowning 4:522
  treatment 2:282; 8:1103; 12:1624, 1625; 13:1752
  see also Legionnaire's disease
pneumonitis 6:853
pneumothorax 13:1751, 1752
podiatry 12:1626–1628
  see also feet
podophyllin 17:2397
poisoning 12:1629–1632
  carbon monoxide 1:59; 3:395; 12:1630, 1637–1638; 17:2320
  causing fits 5:583
  dementia and 4:459
  food see food poisoning
  headaches and 6:758
  lead 3:413; 4:573; 5:583; 8:1048–1050; 10:1394, 1395; 12:1630, 1638; 13:1746
    treatment 3:345; 8:1049
  methanol 10:1411
  toxic metals 2:230
    chelation therapy and 3:345, 346
  see also lead poisoning; mercury poisoning
  treatment 4:556; 12:1632
    use of emetics 4:562
  unconsciousness and 17:2321
  see also irritants; overdoses
  poison ivy, oak, or sumac 2:211
poliomyelitis (polio) 6:728; 12:1633–1635; 16:2285
  limping and 8:1077
  paralysis and 11:1492, 1493; 12:1635
  post-polio syndrome and 9:1259; 12:1635
  scoliosis and 14:1891
  treatment and outlook 12:1634–1635
  vaccination 7:911, 912; 12:1633, 1635; 13:1763; 16:2285; 17:2332
pollen 14:2003
pollution 12:1636–1641
  lead 8:1050; 12:1638
  light 12:1641
  noise 12:1641

radiation poisoning 12:1641
  soil 12:1640–1641
  visual 12:1641
  water 4:574; 12:1636, 1638, 1639–1640
  see also acid rain; air pollution; sick building syndrome
polyaromatic hydrocarbons (PAHs) 1:59
polyarthritis, symmetrical 13:1821
polychlorinated biphenyls (PCBs) 4:574
polydactyly (extra fingers) 2:257; 10:1305; 12:1613
polygenes 6:817, 818
polymerase chain reaction (PCR) 3:377–378
polymorphic light eruption 11:1564, 1565
polymorphs 2:225–227
polymyalgia rheumatica 9:1292
polyneuritis 6:728
polyps 6:727; 12:1642–1643
  cervical 3:339; 5:642; 6:733; 11:1488; 17:2327
  colon 3:386, 387; 12:1642, 1643
  in the intestines 12:1642
  nasal 10:1372, 1375; 12:1642, 1643
  in the rectum 13:1787
  in the uterus 5:642; 12:1642, 1643; 17:2327, 2329
polysaccharides 15:2120, 2121
polysomnographic (PSG) studies 7:958
polysplenia 6:805
porphyria 11:1565; 14:1958
"porter's neck" 1:122
Portuguese man-of-war stings 2:210, 211
port-wine stains 2:208, 209
positron emission tomography see PET scanning
postnasal drip 11:1557
postoperative care 12:1644–1647
postpartum depression and psychosis 4:465; 8:1062; 9:1247; 10:1322; 12:1648–1651
post-polio syndrome 9:1259; 12:1635
post-traumatic stress disorder (PTSD) 10:1358; 12:1652–1655; 15:2102
  complex 12:1653
postural drainage 3:295; 11:1580–1581
postural syncope 2:214, 215
posture 12:1656–1658; 14:1948
  Alexander technique and 1:65, 66
  during pregnancy 12:1656, 1677, 1678
  ligaments and 8:1069, 1072
  massage and 8:1144
  working with computers 13:1804, 1846
postviral fatigue syndrome see chronic fatigue syndrome
pot see marijuana
potassium 9:1234, 1235
  paralysis and 9:1292
  supplements 4:544, 545
  overdose 9:1234
potassium chloride 6:787
poultices
  bread and starch 15:2063
  see also compresses, hot
practolol 14:1956, 1957
prednisolone 7:914
prednisone 4:442
preeclampsia (preeclamptic toxemia; PET; proteinuric hypertension) 3:322; 7:931; 8:1106; 12:1659–1660; 17:2399
pregnancy 12:1661–1665
  alcohol taken during 5:633; 15:2080
  anemia 1:88

ankles, swollen 15:2146, *2147*
blood samples during 11:1511
"blossoming" during 12:1662
breasts 2:276; 12:1663, *1664*
  colostrum production 12:1663
  prevention of mastitis 9:1159
calcium during 3:310, 311; 12:1678
cancer during 13:1774
carpal tunnel syndrome and 3:322, 323
cervical incompetence 3:338
chicken pox and 3:350
constipation 3:404; 8:1045; 12:1662, 1675
cramp 4:437; 12:1662
cystitis 4:450
dangers of parasites during 11:1498
diabetes during 7:960
diagnostic techniques 12:1664–1665
  amniocentesis 1:84
  chorionic villus sampling 2:207; 3:367–368; 5:638; 7:877
  ultrasound 2:207, 285; 4:477, 479, *480*; 12:1664; 13:1869, 1870; 14:1893, *1894*; 17:2315, 2316–*2317*
  X rays 12:1664–1665, 1676; 17:*2431*
diet 2:206; 3:402; 4:491; 8:1127, 1128; 10:1379; 12:1662, 1665, *1675*, 1678
  to avoid listeriosis 8:1083
driving and 5:638
drugs (medicines) taken during 1:99; 3:401; 9:1170
  antibiotics 1:99
  painkillers 11:1478
  thalidomide 2:206; 3:402; 6:749; 9:1170; 11:1550; 16:2202–2204
ectopic 1:14; 4:541, 571; 6:733; 11:1521
  after hysterectomy 7:903
  after sterilization 15:2068, 2069, 2070; 16:2286
  the Pill and 10:1417
  salpingitis and 13:1860
edema 4:544; 12:1662–1663; 17:2399
estrogen levels 5:593
fainting in 5:611, 612; 12:1662
fatigue 5:618
fetal alcohol syndrome and 5:633
first signs of 12:1661
flatulence 5:645
fluoride taken during 5:651
food fads 1:113
frights during 3:401; 5:634
goiter 5:704
gonorrhea and 5:705
gum disease and 6:731
hair during 6:735
heartburn 5:592; 6:786, 787; 12:1661, 1662, 1675
hemorrhoids (piles) 5:637; 12:1662, 1675
hepatitis during 6:809, 810
high-risk 13:1839
increased urination 12:1662
intercourse during 5:634; 7:963; 12:1661, 1675
itches 7:988
lethargy in first few weeks 8:1056
lupus and 8:1105, 1106
malaria during 8:1122
manipulation of the fetus 8:1136
marijuana taken during 8:1137
mole changes during 9:1242
moods during 9:1246–1247
morning sickness 5:636, 645; 6:857; 9:1248–1249; 17:2391
multiple *see* multiple births
multiple births detected 12:1676
occupational hazards and 10:1394

older women and 1:84; 5:682; 6:749, 750
the pelvis and 11:1522, 1524
phantom 11:**1548–1549**
PKU sufferers and 11:*1558*, 1559
placenta previa 3:341; 9:1277; 12:1605
preeclampsia (preeclamptic toxemia; PET; proteinuric hypertension) 3:322; 7:931; 8:1106; 12:**1659–1660**; 17:2399
  rhesus (Rh) factor and 2:*234*–235; 12:1604; 13:1815–*1816*; 15:2081
  risk of birth defects 2:206; 4:506; 6:749, 750
slipped disks 14:1982
smoking during 5:638; 10:1361; 12:1604, 1665; 14:1995; 15:2080
snoring 14:2004
STDs and 12:1675; 14:1932, 1933, *1935*
stretch marks 9:1276; 12:1661, 1662, 1679; 15:2105, *2105*
swelling and puffiness 12:1659
sympathetic 1:13
tests for 12:1661; 15:2024
trimesters 5:634–639
trying to become pregnant 6:732
vaccinations during 2:206; 16:2284
vaginal discharge 12:1662
varicose veins 5:637; 12:1662, 1675–1676; 17:2344
weight after 10:1384
weight during 9:1248; 15:2105
while breast-feeding 8:1032
yeast infections 5:634
see also abortion; conception; fetus; labor; miscarriage; placenta; prenatal care; surrogacy
preimplantation genetic diagnosis (PGD) 5:677
premature babies 2:204, 279; 7:*933*; 10:1338; 11:1516, *1517*; 12:**1666–1669**
  giving oxygen to 11:1464, 1466
  see also neonatal intensive care unit
premedication 1:*91*, 93; 12:**1670**; 14:1902
premenstrual syndrome (PMS) 6:859; 8:1056; 9:1201, 1202; 12:**1671–1674**
  headaches 6:758
  treatment 12:*1674*
  light therapy 14:1898
prenatal care 12:1665, **1675–1679**, 1680
  to avoid preeclampsia 12:1660
  dangers of smoking 5:638; 10:1361; 12:1604, 1665
  dental care 12:1676
  diet 2:206; 3:402; 4:491; 8:1127, 1128; 10:1379; 12:1662, 1665, *1675*, 1678
    to avoid listeriosis 8:1083
  exercise 5:601, 634; 12:1665
  exercises(s) 11:1570; 12:1665, *1677*, 1678–*1679*
  nipples 12:1675
  obstetricians and 10:1389–1390
  posture 12:1656, *1677*, 1678
  prenatal clinics 6:769, 770
  routine checkups and tests 6:749; 12:*1659*, 1660, *1663*–1664, 1676
  vitamin or mineral supplements 5:638; 12:1675
    folic acid 2:206; 3:401; 5:638, 682; 10:1351; 15:2037, 2039; 17:2377
    iron 12:1675
  weight gain 12:1665
presbyacusis 4:455
presbyopia 5:608
prescribers 11:1551
prescriptions 11:1552, *1553*, 1554

preservatives, food 5:656
preventative medicine 12:1680–1684
priapism 12:1700; 14:1928; 16:2196
prickly heat 6:795; 11:1545; 12:**1685**; 15:2130
prick test, for allergies 14:1913
primal therapies 13:1735
primary (medical term) 4:474
prions 11:1509
proctalgia fugax 1:102
professional patient syndrome *see* Munchausen syndrome
progesterone 4:*566*
  breast development and 2:275
  the menstrual cycle and 9:1202; 11:1459
  in the Pill 17:2326
  pregnancy and 2:276
    morning sickness 6:857
  and the skin 8:1091; 14:1900
  to treat premenstrual syndrome 12:1674
prolactin 2:276; 4:*566*; 6:858, 859; 7:899; 8:1032; 12:1598, 1600
prolactin-inhibiting factor 7:899
prolactinomas 12:1598, 1600–1601
prolapse 11:1526; 12:**1686–1688**
  bladder (cystocele) 7:925; 12:1686, *1687*
  cord 12:1687–1688
  invertebral disk *see* slipped disk
  mitral valve 17:2341, 2342
  rectal 1:*103*; 12:1686, *1687*, 1688
  uterine (womb) 2:161; 6:733; 7:*904*, 905; 12:*1686*–1687, 1688; 17:2327, 2335
  vaginal wall 17:2335
promethazine 7:893
Propiobacterium acnes 1:31, 32, 34
prostaglandins 6:758; 7:948; 12:**1689**
  NSAIDs and 10:1369, *1370*
    aspirin 1:137; 12:1689
  used in abortions 1:14, 15, 16
  used to induce labor 7:933–934; 10:1322; 12:*1689*
prostate gland 5:590, 690; 12:**1690–1695**
  cancer 3:316; 5:690; 9:1187; 12:*1691*, 1694
    treatment and outlook 12:1694–1695; 13:1776
  enlargement 2:217, 218; 5:690; 12:*1690*, 1691–1692
  tests for 8:1020
prostatitis 5:690; 9:1284; 12:1690–1691
  rectal examination 12:*1694*
  surgery 10:1423; 12:*1695*
    removal 7:925; 10:1421; 12:1690, 1692, 1693–1694, *1695*
  uremia and 17:2322
prostatitis 5:690; 9:1284; 12:1690–1691
prostheses 12:**1696–1700**
  breast
    external 8:1145, 1146, *1148*; 12:*1698*, *1699*, 1700
    internal (implants) 8:*1145*; 10:1421; 12:1614, 1615, *1616*, 1698, 1700
  earbones 12:1696, *1699*, 1700
  joint replacement 7:**998–999**; 12:1698–1699
    hips 1:*122*; 2:*189*; 6:829, 830; 7:998, *999*, 1000; 10:*1438*; 12:1696, 1699
    knees 7:*998*, 999; 10:1430
  male genitalia 12:1700
  see also artificial limbs

protein 12:**1701–1702**
  dietary 4:488–489; 6:772, 773; 10:*1380*; 12:*1701*
  during pregnancy 12:1678
  genetically engineered 5:679
  genetics and 12:1702
  processed in the liver 8:1084–1086
  synthesis in the cell 5:683, *685*
protein C, activated 14:1915
Proteus spp.
  P. mirabilis 2:166
  P. vulgaris 2:166
Proteus syndrome 2:209
prothrombin 2:228; 17:2385
proton pump inhibitors 4:531; 6:787
protozoal infections 7:936; 11:1510; 12:**1703–1704**
Prozac 4:466; 13:1737, 1738; 16:2258
PRSP (penicillin-resistant *Streptococcus pneumoniae*) 1:98
pruritus
  of pregnancy 7:988
  pruritus ani 1:103
  pruritus vulvae 17:2393, 2394
  see also itches
pseudobulbar palsy 9:1258, 1259
pseudocyesis *see* phantom pregnancy
pseudohypoparathyroidism 11:1505
Pseudomonas aeruginosa 13:1758
psittacosis 12:*1624*, **1705**
psoriasis 4:469; 6:739; 7:989; 12:**1706–1708**
  tattooing and 16:2173
  types 12:*1706*, *1708*
psychiatry 12:**1709–1715**, 1716; 13:1734
psychic healing 5:614
psychoanalysts 12:1712
psychoanalytic therapies 13:1735
psychodrama 12:1715; 13:1735
psychogenic disorders 12:1712–1713
psychology 12:**1716–1718**; 13:1734
psychoneuroimmunology 15:2102
psycho-oncology 10:1399
psychoses 9:1207; 11:1540–1541; 12:1713, **1719–1722**
  antisclerotic 14:1911
  nervous breakdown and 10:1340
  paranoid 12:1720
    amphetamines and 1:87
  postpartum psychosis 12:1649, 1651
  senile 14:1911
  treatment 12:1722; 14:1905
  see also bipolar disorder; schizophrenia
psychosomatic problems 9:1206, 1209; 12:1714, **1723–1725**
  back pain 2:161
  self-healing and 5:614
  stress and 5:616
psychosurgery 12:1715
psychosynthesis 13:1735
psychotherapy 3:428; 9:1228; 11:1541; 12:1712, 1714; 13:**1733–1736**; 16:*2206*
  formal 12:1714
  Gestalt therapy 5:695–696; 13:1735
  insight-directed 12:1714
  the subconscious and 15:*2114*, 2115
  supportive-expressive 4:529
  to treat phobias 11:1563
  see also behavior therapy; hypnosis
psychoticism scale 11:1541
psychotropic drugs 13:**1737–1738**
psychoneuroimmunology 7:908
ptomaine poisoning 5:658
PTSD *see* post-traumatic stress disorder
ptyalin *see* amylase
ptyalism 13:1854

puberty 13:1739–1742
  acne and 1:31; 13:1739
  breastlike swellings in boys 2:275
  chubbiness 13:1739
  delayed, in boys 16:2195, 2196, 2250
  estrogen and 11:1459
  failure to menstruate 17:2335
  the larynx 13:1742; 17:2389
  stretch marks 15:2105
  testosterone and 13:1742; 16:2195–2196
  see also adolescence
public health 12:1680–1681; 13:1743–1746
Pudenz-Heyer shunt 7:880
puerperium 10:1390
pulled muscles 9:1292, 1294; 13:1747–1748; 15:2054
  treatment 13:1747, 1748
pulmonary disorders 13:1749–1752
  asbestosis 1:136; 12:1639; 13:1751
  bronchiectasis 6:741; 12:1623–1624; 13:1750, 1751
  cancer see cancer, lung
  chronic obstructive pulmonary disease (COPD) 3:370–371
    oxygen therapy for 11:1465, 1467
  edema 2:283; 3:348; 4:545; 17:2407, 2408
  fibrosing alveolitis 13:1751, 1752
  pneumoconiosis 2:282; 4:564; 12:1621; 13:1752
  pulmonary embolism 13:1751, 1752; 16:2215
  tuberculosis 16:2287–2289, 2290
  see also asthma; bronchitis; coughing; emphysema; lung and lung diseases; pleurisy; pneumonia
pulmonary function tests (PFTs) 3:371
pulse 3:373; 13:1753–1754
  rate
    fitness and 1:50; 11:1572, 1574
    irregular 6:781
    taking the 13:1753
    difficulty 17:2429
  see also heart, heartbeat
punch-drunk 2:266
punctures see wounds, puncture
purines, gout and 5:707
purple hearts 1:87; 15:2083
purpura 2:228; 3:318; 13:1755–1756
  Henoch-Schönlein 13:1755, 1756
  senile 13:1756
pus 2:225; 13:1757–1758
  in abscesses 1:21; 13:1757
  anchovy-sauce (chocolate-sauce) 13:1757
  in boils 2:255, 256
  in wounds 1:19
Putti-Platt operation 4:498
pyelograms, intravenous (IVPs) 4:475
pyelonephritis 17:2325
pyloroplasty 17:2314
pyorrhea and gingivitis 13:1759–1761
  gingivitis 6:731; 9:1263; 13:1759–1761
    acute ulcerative 6:731
    necrotizing ulcerative 13:1760
    halitosis and 6:740
  pyorrhea (peridontal disease) 4:461; 6:731, 759; 12:1610; 13:1759–1760, 1761
pyridostigmine 10:1313
pyrogen 5:641

Q

Q fever 13:1762
qigong (chi kung) 1:81; 3:358, 360–361
quadriplegia 3:336; 15:2043
quarantine 13:1763
  see also isolation
quinalbarbital 2:170
quinidine 13:1765
quinine 4:437; 8:1123; 13:1764–1765
  deafness and 4:455, 502
quinolones 1:100
quinsy 14:2012–2013; 16:2236–2237

R

rabies 13:1766–1769
  incubation period 7:927; 13:1766, 1767–1768
  vaccination 13:1766, 1769; 16:2270, 2280
race 2:252–253
radiation 8:1060; 11:1510
  a cause of cancer 8:1126; 13:1772
  a cause of leukemia 8:1061
  environmental 4:574; 12:1641
  mutations and 3:330
  UV 11:1469, 1470
  working with 10:1395
  see also Chernobyl disaster; radiation sickness
radiation therapy see radiotherapy
radiation sickness 13:1770–1771
radioisotope scans 2:268; 3:315; 10:1354, 1355
radionuclide scanning 4:477, 480
radiopharmaceuticals 2:190
radioiodine 13:1774; 16:2223
radiotherapy 3:314, 315–316; 10:1400; 13:1772–1776; 17:2435
  for lymphoma 8:1115
  in outpatients departments 11:1457
  as palliative treatment 13:1776
  postsurgery treatment using 13:1776
  radioactive implants 3:316; 10:1400; 12:1693; 13:1774
  side effects 13:1770–1771, 1776
radius 4:546, 547
radon 13:1839
Ramsay Hunt's syndrome 14:1939
ranitidine 6:786
rape 13:1777–1780; 14:1926, 1927
  post-traumatic stress disorder and 12:1652, 1653
rapid eye movement (REM) sleep 4:511, 512; 7:957; 13:1781; 14:1978–1980
rashes 13:1782–1784
  allergy 13:1782; 14:1969
    to tattoo pigments 16:2172, 2173
  chicken pox 2:223, 224; 3:349; 13:1782, 1783, 1784
  confluent 13:1783
  drug-induced 13:1784
  gold 13:1821
  herpes 6:825; 13:1784
  hives 6:831; 13:1783
  hookworm infection and 6:852–853
  lupus
    discoid lupus erythematosus 8:1105, 1106, 1107
    systemic lupus erythematosus 8:1105, 1107
  macular 13:1783
  maculopapular 13:1783
  measles 9:1163, 1164; 13:1782, 1783, 1784
  papular 13:1783

penicillin allergy 1:99, 100
photosensitive 11:1564, 1565; 15:2126
prickly heat 12:1685; 15:2130
purpuric 13:1755, 1756
pustular 13:1783
Rocky Mountain spotted fever 13:1845
rubella (German measles) 13:1784, 1849
scabies 13:1865, 1866
scarlet fever 13:1784; 14:1878, 1879
sex flush 5:590
shingles 14:1938, 1939
smallpox 14:1987, 1988
syphilis 13:1784; 14:1932, 1933; 15:2154, 2155
typhoid and paratyphoid 13:1784; 16:2297
typhus 16:2300
vesicular 13:1783
  see also dermatitis; diaper rash; eczema
Raynaud's syndrome 5:669; 6:747; 8:1105; 10:1378
  biofeedback and 2:183, 184
  scleroderma and 14:1888, 1889
RDAs (recommended daily amounts) 5:656
  vitamins 5:655, 656
reactive arthritis 13:1785–1786
  genitourinary (urogenital) 13:1786
rebirthing 13:1735
recovery position 1:134
recovery rooms 12:1644–1645
rectocele 12:1686
rectum 13:1787–1788
  cancer 13:1787, 1788
  fistula connecting to the vagina 5:644
  polyps 13:1787
  prolapse 1:103; 12:1686, 1687, 1688; 13:1787
Reed-Sternberg cells 6:833
reflexes 2:262; 3:364; 9:1264–1265, 1266; 10:1345; 13:1789–1792; 15:2040, 2041
  absence 13:1789, 1792
  behavioral 13:1792
  blinking 13:1789, 1792
  bodily function 13:1791
  breathing 13:1790, 1792
  conditioned 9:1253; 13:1789, 1792
  coordination and 3:414
  coughing 3:426
  knee-jerk 8:1025; 9:1266, 1267; 13:1791
  light 13:1410
  Moro 13:1791
  orientation reflexes 13:1791
  shivering 9:1264
  testing 4:475, 476; 11:1519
  vomiting 17:2391
reflexology 1:78, 80; 6:837; 8:1143; 13:1793–1794
reflux, gastroesophageal 6:786–787; 17:2313
  halitosis and 6:740
refracting heads 5:609
rehabilitation 13:1795–1799
Reich, Wilhelm 9:1230
reiki 1:81
Reiter's syndrome 13:1786; 17:2312
relaxation 9:1230, 1232; 13:1800–1802; 15:2103, 2104; 17:2405
  biofeedback and 2:182–183
  flotation therapy and 5:648, 649, 650

tai chi and 16:2166
  yoga and 13:1802; 17:2440, 2444
releasing factors (inhibitory factors) 7:899
renin 2:238, 239
renodialysis machines 8:1014–1015, 1016
repetitive strain injury (RSI) 10:1396; 11:1475; 13:1803–1804
repression 9:1192
research, medical 9:1170–1172
reserpine 2:198
respirators 13:1805–1806
respiratory distress syndrome 12:1667, 1668–1669
respiratory system
  health 2:283
  mucous membranes 9:1189, 1269
  phlegm and 11:1560
  see also breathing; lung and lung diseases
restricted environmental stimulation therapy (REST) 5:648
resuscitation 13:1807–1810
  after drowning 4:521, 522
  cardiopulmonary (CPR) 1:134, 135; 3:320, 321; 13:1807, 1808, 1809, 1810
  mouth-to-mouth see artificial respiration
retained products of conception (RPC) 17:2338
reticular formation 17:2318, 2319
retinal artery occlusion 2:222; 10:1411
retinal vein thrombosis 2:222
retina and retinal disorders 13:1811–1812
  disorders
    cotton wool spots 13:1812
    detached retina 2:220, 222; 5:608–609; 13:1811, 1812
    deterioration with Tay-Sachs disease 16:2174
    diabetic retinopathy 5:609; 13:1811, 1812
    hypertensive retinopathy 13:1812
    macular degeneration 2:220, 222; 8:1119; 13:1811, 1812
    retinal artery occlusion 2:222
    retinal vein thrombosis 2:222
    retinitis pigmentosa 2:222; 13:1811, 1812
  retina 5:606; 13:1811
    artificial sight and 2:191
    laser sugery on 2:221; 8:1041, 1042
    light-sensitive cells 10:1362, 1410; 13:1811
retinitis pigmentosa 2:222; 13:1811, 1812
retinoids 1:33
retinol 17:2373
retinopathy
  diabetic 5:609; 13:1811, 1812
  hypertensive 13:1812
retinoscopes 10:1413
retroviruses 5:680
Reye's syndrome 5:641; 10:1369; 11:1478, 1479; 13:1813–1814
rhesus (Rh) factor 2:233, 234–235; 12:1604; 13:1815–1816; 15:2081
rheumatic fever 6:788; 13:1817–1818, 1819; 15:2097
  heart valves and 13:1817; 15:2067; 16:2215, 2216; 17:2341
  symptoms 13:1818
  Saint Vitus' dance 13:1818, 1851
rheumatism 11:1581; 13:1819
rheumatoid arthritis 1:126; 3:323; 7:1002, 1003; 11:1581; 13:1820–1824
  in adults 1:122–123

in children 1:123
in the hands 6:746; 13:*1820*, 1821,
1823, *1824*
monitored using thermography
16:2207, 2208
stiffness and 8:1027; 15:2077
treatment 13:1823–1824;
15:2072–2073
rheumatoid factor 13:1821
rheumatoid nodules 13:1821
Rh factor *see* rhesus (Rh) factor
rhinitis 11:1560; 13:**1825–1826**; 14:2002,
2003
season allergic *see* hay fever
vasomotor 14:2003
rhinoplasty (changing shape of the
nose) 3:424, 425; 12:*1613*
rhinoviruses 17:2372
rhodopsin (visual purple) 10:1362;
13:*1812*; 17:2373
rhythm method 3:411; 13:**1827–1830**
rhytidectomy 3:424
rhytidectomy *see* face-lifts
ribosomes 3:331; 5:*685*; 9:1240
effect of tetracyclines on 16:2199
ribs 13:**1831–1834**
ankylosing spondylitis and 13:1834
cervical 13:1832
cracked 3:347; 13:*1834*
dislocated 13:1834
floating 13:1832
fractured 3:347; 13:1832–1834
joints 7:*1002*, 1003
osteoid bumps 13:1836
tumors in 13:1834
RICE (mnemonic) 1:50; 15:2051
ricin 2:186
rickets 2:260; 3:*311*; 11:1526;
13:**1835–1836**; 17:2381
rickettsia
Rocky Mountain spotted fever and
13:*1844*, 1845
typhus and 7:*937*, 938; 16:*2300*, *2301*
rickety rosary 13:1836
rifampin 1:99
rights, patient's bill of 7:873
rigor 14:1942
rigor mortis 4:458
rigors 5:640
ring pads 4:*519*
ringworm 7:938, *939*; 10:1315;
13:**1837–1838**; 14:1974
see also athlete's foot
risk analysis 13:**1839–1840**
risus sardonicus 16:2198
Ritalin 2:152; 13:1738
rituals 7:894
river blindness 11:*1500*, 1501; 16:*2282*,
2283, *2284*; 17:2419
RNA
messenger (mRNA) 5:683, *685*
transfer (tRNA) 5:*685*
road rage 13:**1841–1843**
robotics, and telesurgery 16:2180
Rocky Mountain spotted fever
13:**1844–1845**
Rogaine (minoxidil) 2:169; 14:1969
rolfing 8:1144; 13:**1846–1848**
Röntgen, Wilhelm Conrad 17:2431
Roosevelt, Theodore 15:*2059*
rosacea 1:34; 7:875
rosemary 10:1329
roseola infantum 5:588
roughage 1:102; 3:404; 4:490
roundworms (nematodes) 11:*1498*;
17:*2419–2420*
see also Ascaris
RSI *see* repetitive strain injury

rubella (German measles)
13:*1849–1850*
arthritis and 1:124
during pregnancy 13:1849, 1850
birth defects and 2:207; 3:326,
336, 402; 7:910; 13:1850
rash 13:1784, *1849*
subclinical infection 7:935
vaccination 2:206; 6:748; 7:910, 912;
13:1739, 1849, 1850
avoiding pregnancy after 13:1849
Rubin's test 7:945

S

sacrum 2:159; 11:1522
SAD *see* seasonal affective disorder
safety *see* accident prevention
Saint Vitus' dance 13:1818, **1851**
salazopyrin 3:383
salicylic acid 6:813; 17:2362–2363
saliva 1:67; 4:*494*; 5:702; 8:1149, 1261,
1269; 13:**1852–1854**
excess 13:1854
lack of 4:495; 8:1149; 13:1854
nervousness and 9:1262; 13:1852,
1854
salivary ducts 13:*1852*
stones in 9:1263; 13:*1854*
salivary glands 13:*1852*–1853
mumps and 9:*1283*–1284; 13:1854
tumors 13:1854
salmonella 2:166; 13:**1855–1857**
encephalitis and 11:*1513*
food poisoning and 5:657, 659;
7:928; 13:1855, *1856–1857*
paratyphoid and 13:1855, 1857;
16:2296
typhoid and 13:1855, 1857; 16:2295
Salmonella paratyphi 16:2296
Salmonella typhi 16:2295, 2296
salmon patches 2:208, 209
salpingitis 3:400; 6:733; 7:943;
13:**1858–1860**
salpingoophoritis 7:943
salt 9:1235; 13:**1861–1862**
dietary 5:653; 11:1484; 13:1861
edema and 4:544
loss 13:1862
cramp and 4:437; 11:1544
salt water as an emetic 4:562
salt gargle 16:2213
sarcoma 3:312; 16:2291
fibroids and 5:642; 17:2327
Kaposi's 1:56
osteogenic 2:260; 14:1966
SARS (severe acute respiratory
syndrome) 7:938, 962; 13:1763,
1863–1864
scabies 3:349; 11:1516; 13:**1865–1866**
scabs 2:*226*; 14:*1881*, 1972
scalded skin syndrome 15:2062
scalding 13:**1867–1868**
treatment 3:*304*; 13:1867, 1868
see also burns
scalp disorders *see* hair and scalp
disorders
scalpels 15:2137–2138
scans 13:**1869–1870**
see also CT scans; diagnostic
imaging; MRI; PET scanning;
ultrasound
scarlet fever (scarlatina) 14:**1878–1879**
rash 13:1784; 14:*1878*, 1879
scars 6:765; 14:**1880–1881**, 1971, 1972;
17:*2422*, *2423*, *2424*
acne 1:31; 14:1880

appendix-removal 1:109
discharge from 5:644
chicken pox 3:349; 13:*1782*,
1783
how to prevent 14:1881
keloid 7:*1005*; 14:1880, *1881*
numbness in and around 10:1376
plastic surgery and 12:1617
surgical, healing 15:2136
Schick test 4:497
Schilling test 11:1536
schistosomiasis (bilharzia) 11:*1499*,
1501; 16:2281, 2284; 17:*2420*, 2421
schizophrenia 9:1208, 1209, 1247, 1278;
12:1720; 14:**1882–1884**; 15:2150
cause 12:1722
hypochondria and 7:895
nervous breakdown and 10:1342
paranoid 10:1342
treatment 9:1209; 12:1710; 13:1737
sciatica 2:161–163; 8:1078, 1094, 1095;
10:*1349*; 14:**1885–1887**, 1983
diagnosis 10:1355
sclera 5:604
sclerodactyly 14:1888
scleroderma (systemic sclerosis)
14:**1888–1889**; 15:2148
sclerotherapy 3:424
scoliosis 8:1078; 11:1448; 14:**1890–1891**
scopolamine 12:1670
scotoma 10:1411
scrapie 4:438
scratches 1:19
scratch test 1:72, 73; 13:*1783*
screening 14:**1892–1895**
babies 14:1893
eye tests 10:1407
hearing tests 4:454
cancer 3:314–315; 14:1892
children 14:1893–1894
prenatal 14:1893
see also amniocentesis; chorionic
villus sampling; ultrasound,
during pregnancy
scrotum 11:1530
scurvy 2:260; 10:1379; 14:**1896–1897**;
17:2378
hemorrhaging and 6:804
sea sickness *see* motion sickness
seasonal affective disorder (SAD)
9:1186; 10:1353; 14:**1898–1899**;
17:2380
sebaceous glands 5:700; 14:*1900–1901*,
1971
acne and 1:32
cysts 4:446, 447; 6:726; 14:1900;
15:*2147*, *2148*
sties and 15:*2112*
seborrhea *see* dermatitis, seborrheic
seborrheic tendency 4:451
sebum 1:32; 6:735; 14:*1900*, 1901
secobarbital 7:893
secretin 6:857–859; 11:1487
secretion 5:598
sedatives 14:**1902–1905**
causing drowsiness 7:892
dangerous mixed with alcohol
7:892
premedication 1:*91*, 93; 12:*1670*;
14:1902
see also antidepressants;
antipsychotic drugs; sleeping
pills
seizures 2:215
epileptic *see* epilepsy, seizures
selective serotonin reuptake inhibitors
see SSRIs
selenium 5:655; 16:2250

self-healing 5:614
self-massage 9:1233
semen (seminal fluid) 3:399; 5:589,
590, 690; 14:**1906–1907**; 15:2035
see also sperm
semicircular canals 2:*167*; 17:2391
seminal fluid *see* semen
seminal vesicles 14:1906–1907, 1919;
15:2035
seminiferous tubules 5:689; 16:*2191*,
2194; 17:2347
senility 14:**1908–1911**
see also aging
senna 5:598; 8:1045–1046
sensate focusing 14:1925
sensitization 14:**1912–1913**
covert 2:177
sepsis 14:**1914–1915**
puerperal 17:2338–2339
septic shock 4:441; 14:1915, 1943
septicemia 2:236; 14:1914
serology 4:475
serotonin (5-HT) 2:198; 7:875; 9:1222;
16:2258
severe combined immune deficiency
(SCID) 5:677
sewage 4:574; 12:1636, 1639; 13:1744
sex 14:**1916–1925**
12 steps to sexual intimacy 2:246
frequency 14:1916
libido 8:1062–1063; 14:1920–1921,
1922
aging and 1:53
the Pill and 7:963; 10:1414;
14:1920–1921
pituitary gland and 12:1598
safe
while traveling 16:2273
see also contraception
sexual attraction 14:1917
sexual awareness 14:1917
sexual problems 14:1919–1925
dyspareunia (painful intercourse)
4:568; 7:965; 8:1034; 9:1269;
13:1860; 14:1924–1925, 1929
impotence 1:130; 5:590;
7:**919–920**; 11:1531; 14:1924
premature ejaculation 5:589,
590; 14:1924, 1928
sex therapy and 14:1925, *1929*
see also sexual dysfunction
what is "normal" 14:1922
see also intercourse; orgasm
sex changes 5:672, 673
sex education 1:45; 6:768, *769*
sex flush 5:590
sex hormones 12:1598
reduced 6:858
see also estrogen; progesterone;
testosterone
sex therapy 16:2206
sexual abuse 14:**1926–1927**
of children 3:353; 14:*1926–1927*
see also child abuse; incest
sexual dysfunction 14:**1928–1929**
female
failure to achieve orgasm
10:1424; 14:1929
lack of libido and sex difficulties
after childbirth 8:1062; 14:1921,
1928
male
impotence 1:130; 5:590;
7:**919–920**; 11:1531; 14:1924
Peyronie's disease 14:1929
premature ejaculation 5:589,
590; 14:1924, 1928
priapism 12:1700; 14:1928; 16:2196

sexual intercourse *see* intercourse
sexually transmitted diseases (STDs)
  1:22, 45; 7:943; 11:1530;
  14:1930–1935
  casual sex and 14:1931
  chlamydial infection 14:1931–1933,
    1935; 16:2192; 17:2338
  genital herpes 3:337, 341; 6:825;
    11:1531; 14:*1932*, 1933, 2009
  genital warts 11:1530; 14:1933, 1935;
    17:2393, 2395, 2396–2397
    treatment 17:2397
  kidney disease and 8:1018
  pregnancy and 12:1675; 14:1932,
    1933, *1935*
  prevention 14:1934–1935
  pubic lice 8:1066
  salpingitis and 13:1858
  thrush as 14:1934
  trichomoniasis as 16:2278–2279
  vaginal discharge and 14:1933–1934
  vulval inflammation and 17:2393
  where to go for help 14:1935
  see also AIDS; gonorrhea; syphilis
Seyle, Hans 15:2098–2099, 2101
shaking *see* tremor
shampoos
  dandruff and 4:451, 452; 6:739
  pH balanced 6:737
  to treat head lice 8:1065
shape, body 2:*253*–254
sheep
  cloning 3:377
  transgenic 5:681
shellfish
  allergy to 15:2145
  poisoning 8:1086
shell shock 10:1358; 12:1653; 15:2102
  see also post-traumatic stress
    disorder
shiatsu 1:80; 6:776; 8:*1144*; **14:1936–1937**
shift work 2:187
Shigella 2:166; 4:533, 573
shingles 2:224; 6:825; 10:1349;
  14:1938–1939
  back pain and 2:161, 163
  chicken pox and 3:349, 350; 6:825;
    14:1938
  lesions and rash 2:223; 7:*935*;
    10:*1349*; 14:*1938*, 1939
Shirodkar operation 3:338
shivering 9:1264; **14:1940–1942**;
  16:2183
shock 4:555; **14:1943–1947**
  after bites or stings 2:212
  anaphylactic 14:1945
  cardiogenic 14:1944, 1945, 1947
  causing loss of voice 10:1334
  coma and 3:395
  effects of 14:1946
  from bleeding 6:806
    internal 6:805; 14:1945
  from burns or scalds 3:304, 305;
    6:806; 13:1867, 1868; 14:*1943*, 1944
  hypovolemic 14:1944–1945
  neurogenic 14:1945
  outlook 14:1947
  psychological 14:1943, 1944
  septic (endotoxic) 4:441; 14:1915,
    1943, 1945, 1946
  surgical 4:540; 12:1646
  symptoms 14:1946
  treatment 14:1946–1947
  unconsciousness and 17:2320–2321
  wounds and 1:20
shock lung 14:1943, 1946
shoes 2:159; 3:299, *300*; 5:625, 628;
  7:885; 12:1628

aerobics 1:51–52
  children's 5:626
  sports 15:2052
short sight *see* myopia
shoulder **14:1948–1949**
  bandaging 4:*518*
  bursitis 3:*308*
  dislocated 4:*498*–499; 8:1069, *1135*;
    10:1433; 14:1948
  exercise 14:1949
  frozen 1:124; 6:799; 14:1949, 1968;
    15:2076
    hydrotherapy and 7:883
  impingement syndrome 3:308
  injury to, affecting the elbow 4:546
  ligaments 8:*1071*
  osteoarthritis 10:1437
  painful 11:*1475*
    treatment 6:764; 11:1580
  "rounded" 14:1948
  stiff 14:1949; 15:2076, 2078, *2079*
Siamese twins **14:1950–1951**
sibutramine 10:*1385*
sick building syndrome **14:1952–1953**
sickle-cell anemia 1:89, 90;
  14:1954–1955
  malaria and 16:*2201*
sickle-cell trait 14:1954
side effects 11:1554; **14:1956–1959**
  of antibiotics 1:100; 14:*1959*; 17:2364
sight *see* eyes and eyesight
sigmoidoscopy 4:501, 570; 14:1960
sign language 10:*1307*, *1308*
sildenafil (Viagara) 7:963; 14:*1928*
Silent Spring (Carson) 13:1839
silicon 16:2250
silicosis 10:1395; 14:1961
sinews *see* tendons
single-photon-emission computerized
  tomography (SPECT) 4:480
sinoatrial node (pacemaker) 6:*782*;
  9:1267; 11:1472
sinuses 5:644; 10:1372, 1373; 14:1962,
  1963
  radiation of pain from 15:2149
sinusitis 6:741; 9:1269; 10:1375; 13:1826;
  14:1962–1963
  headaches and 6:758, 759; 15:2150
sinusoids 17:2358
situs inversus 2:252
sixth disease 5:588
Sjogren's syndrome 8:1149
skeleton 9:1265; **14:1964–1968**
  backache and 2:258
  see also bones; cartilage; joints
Skene's glands 17:2394
skin, disorders, *see also* rashes
skin patch *see* transdermal patch
skin and skin diseases **14:1969–1975**
  dermatology 4:469–470
  disorders
    acne and pimples 1:31–34, 75;
      2:255; 7:*885*; 14:1880, 1970, 1974,
      1975
    Addison's disease 9:1181
    albinism 5:684, 686; 6:735; 7:*921*,
      922; 9:1181; 10:*1304*, *1305*
    allergic reactions 1:71, 73; 4:467,
      468, 487, 542, 543; 6:747, 795;
      14:*1974*; 16:2172, 2173
    athlete's foot 2:150; 7:886, *937*;
      13:1763, 1837; 14:1975; 17:2436
    birthmarks 2:208–209; 12:1613;
      14:1972, *1974*
    blackheads (comedones) 1:31, *32*;
      14:1901
    blisters 2:223–224; 3:300, 304,
      382; 7:*918*; 13:*1756*

boils 2:255–256; 13:1757
bruises (contusions) 3:298, 319;
  17:2422, 2423, 2424
calluses 3:417, 418; 12:1627;
  17:2362
cancer 2:192, 208; 3:316; 4:573,
  574; 6:726; 8:1125, *1126*;
  9:1182–1185; 11:1468, 1470;
  13:1776; 14:1975; 15:2024, 2127–2128
  in children 14:1972–1974
  corns 3:*417*–418; 12:1627; 17:2362
  cradle cap 14:1972–1973
  cysts 4:*446*–447
  dandruff 4:451–452; 15:2112
  dermatitis 1:71, 73; 4:467–468,
    481, 482; 7:946, *948*; 13:1782;
    14:*1974*, 2009
  eczema 2:224; 4:467–468,
    542–543; 14:1969, 1974–1975
  hives (urticaria) 6:831
  impetigo 2:223, 224; 7:918
  keloids 7:1005; 14:1880, *1881*
  melanoma 9:1182–1185, 1242,
    1243; 11:1470; 14:1975
  moles 2:209; 6:726; 9:1182, 1183,
    1184, 1242–1243; 11:1511; 14:1972,
    1974, 1975
  photosensitivity 11:*1564*–1565;
    15:2126, 2129
  psoriasis 4:*469*; 6:739; 7:989;
    12:1706–1708; 16:2173
  purpura 2:228; 3:318; 13:1755–1756
  ringworm 7:938, *939*; 10:1315;
    13:1837–1838; 14:1974
  rosacea 1:34; 7:875
  scleroderma (systemic sclerosis)
    14:1888–1889; 15:2148
  seborrhea (seborrheic
    dermatitis) 1:32; 4:468, 482, 483;
    7:988, 989; 13:*1783*
  stretch marks 9:1276; 12:1661,
    1662, 1679; 15:2105–2106
  sunburn 2:223; 3:303; 6:831;
    11:1470; 15:2126–2129; 16:2272
  swellings 15:2147–2148
  thrush 16:2220
  treatment 4:469–470
  verruca (plantar wart) 3:418;
    5:625; 7:886; 12:1627;
    17:2361–2363, 2395
  vitiligo 9:*1181*; 17:2388
  warts 6:726; 14:*1975*;
    17:2395–2397
  whitlow (paronychia) 6:747;
    10:1314; 17:2411, 2438
  see also rashes
skin
  aging 14:*1970*, 1975
  care 14:1975
  chemicals spilled onto 7:*981*
  cosmetics 3:*422*–423
  dry 14:*1901*
  excretion through 5:597–598
  glands *see* glands, apocrine; glands,
    sweat; sebaceous glands
  grafts 3:302, 304; 5:*709*, *710*–711;
    9:1221; 12:1612, 1615–1616
  greasy 14:1900, 1901
  hardening the 2:223
  pigmentation (color) 6:817; 9:1181,
    1183; 11:1468; 14:1971, *1972*
  specimens 15:2024
  structure 14:1969–1970,
    1971
  synthetic 2:190
  temperature 16:2208
  touch receptors 16:2239–2240
  wound healing 6:*765*; 14:1971–1972

wrinkles 14:*1970*; 15:2127;
  17:*2427*–2428
  see also hair; melanin; nails
skull 6:760
  bony lumps on 2:257
  fractured 5:*662*, 663; 6:760
  replacement surgery 10:1354–1356
  suture joints 7:1000
SLE *see* lupus
sleep and sleep problems
  14:1976–1980
  problems
    depression and 7:957, 958;
      8:1056–1057
    myoclonic jerks 16:2293, 2294
    narcolepsy 7:897, 899; 15:2083
    nightmares 4:511, 512; 14:1978
    PTSD and 12:1653
    sleeplessness *see* insomnia
    sleepwalking 14:1981
  sleep 5:620; 14:1976–1977
    amount necessary 14:1978
    in babies and children 1:85; 3:354;
      14:1976, *1977*, 1980
    brain activity 14:1977
    deprivation 14:1978
    dreaming 4:*511*–512; 5:620;
      9:1190, 1228; 13:1781;
      14:1978–1979; 15:2114
    "early birds" and "night owls"
      2:187, 188; 14:1976
    hallucinations when waking or
      falling asleep 12:1721
    induced by alcohol 6:752
    mind active during 9:1226
    rapid eye movement (REM) 4:511,
      512; 7:957; 13:1781; 14:1978–1980
    versus unconsciousness 17:*2319*
    wet dreams 5:589; 14:1906
    see also drowsiness
sleep apnea 16:2236
sleeping pills 5:620; 7:958, 959;
  14:1980
  dangerous mixed with alcohol
    7:892
  dangerous on long flights 7:993
  disadvantages 7:892, 957; 14:1978
  drowsiness and 4:523; 8:1057
  overdose, treatment 11:1462
  postoperative 3:412
  used for anxiety 1:104
sleeping sickness 12:1704;
  16:*2281*–2282
sleepwalking 14:1981
slings 4:516, *519*
slipped disk 2:160, 161–163; 3:325;
  14:1968, **1982–1985**
  fibrositis and 5:643
  paralysis and 11:1491–1493
  reoccurrence 2:163
  sciatica and 2:161–163; 10:*1349*;
    14:*1885*–1887, 1983
  scoliosis and 14:1890
  treatment 11:1446; 14:*1982*,
    1983–1985
  traction 16:2255
small intestine 1:68
  celiac disease and 3:*329*
  Crohn's disease 4:*442*–443
  digestion in 4:*494*–495
  duodenum 1:68; 4:494–495,
    530–531
  ileum 1:68
  jejunum 1:68
  typhoid in 16:*2295*, 2297
smallpox 9:*1217*; **14:1986–1988**
  a biological weapon 2:185, 186
  vaccination 7:910, 911, 912

smart drugs 14:1989
smears, cervical see Pap smear
smegma 11:1531
smell 14:1990–1994
    disorders 14:1993
        loss (anosmia) 14:1993; 16:2169,
            2170
    emotions and 2:262; 14:1993
    taste and 14:1992; 16:2169, 2170, 2171
smelling salts 5:611
smogs 1:59–60; 4:574; 12:1636, 1637
smoking 3:315; 6:768, 770–771; 8:1100;
        11:1510; 14:1995–1999
    addiction to 17:2416
    artery disease and 1:101, 118; 5:669;
        6:783
    cancer and 2:279, 283; 3:314; 8:1067,
        1104, 1126; 13:1749; 14:1996,
        1997–1998
    chest problems and 13:1750
    children starting 14:1997
    chronic bronchitis and 2:279; 3:294,
        426
    chronic obstructive pulmonary
        disease and 3:370
    the circulation and 1:120
    damage by free radicals and 1:101
    drugs
        cocaine 3:380
        marijuana 4:526; 8:1137
    during pregnancy 5:638; 10:1361;
        12:1604, 1665; 14:1995; 15:2080
    effect on the lungs 8:1103
    emphysema and 2:279; 3:294, 296;
        4:563–564
    filters on cigarettes 14:1996
    giving up 2:283; 14:1999
        acupuncture and 1:37
        the body recovering from
            10:1359; 14:1996
        constipation and 3:404
        flotation therapy and 5:649
        hypnosis and 7:890
        nicotine gum 14:1995
        nicotine patches 14:1995;
            16:2259, 2260
        weight and 10:1384
        withdrawal symptoms 10:1361;
            17:2417, 2418
    halitosis and 6:740, 741
    heart attacks and 6:783; 16:2214
    hoarseness and 6:832
    immediate effects 10:1359,
        1360–1361
    longevity and 1:53; 14:1998, 1999
    nicotine and 10:1359–1361;
        14:1995–1996
    nicotine staining 6:740
    phlegm and 11:1560
    public health and 13:1744, 1746
    reducing the effects of 14:1995,
        1996
    reflux esophagitis and 6:787
    secondary (passive) 10:1360;
        13:1840; 14:1999
    sense of smell and 14:1990
    sense of taste and 16:2169
    skin damage and 9:1185; 17:2428
    smoker's cough 3:371, 426; 5:603;
        8:1036
    teeth and 4:460; 14:1999
    the tongue and 16:2232
    vision and 3:388
    wheezing 17:2407
    why people smoke 14:1995–1997
    work-related diseases and 10:1392
snakebites 2:212; 14:2000–2001;
    16:2280

sneezing 10:1373; 11:1524; 14:2002–2003
    with hay fever 6:757
snoring 1:41; 14:2004–2005
snuff 9:1188
sodium 9:1234
    deficiency 8:1128
    pump 13:1861–1862
sodium bicarbonate 5:645
sodium cromoglycate 4:543; 6:757
soil, pollution 12:1640–1641
solvent abuse 4:526, 527;
    14:2006–2007
solvents, dangers of working with
    10:1393, 1395
somatoform disorders 10:1358
somatotropin see growth hormone
somatrophin 2:252
somnambulism see sleepwalking
sores 14:2008–2009
    canker (aphthous ulcers) 17:2311
    chrome 14:2009
    decubitus ulcers see bedsores
    genital 14:2009
    industrial 14:2009
    mouth, from solvent abuse 14:2007
    treatment 14:2008, 2009
    tropical 14:2009
    see also blisters; cold sores; ulcers;
        wounds
sore throat 11:1555, 1557; 14:2010–2013
    laryngitis 7:946; 8:1038, 1039;
        10:1335; 14:2011, 2013; 16:2212;
        17:2389
        acute 8:1036, 1037–1039
        chronic 8:1036, 1037, 1039
    peritonsillar abscesses (quinsies)
        14:2012–2013
    pharyngitis 11:1556, 1557; 14:2011
    streptococcal throat (strep throat)
        11:1555, 1556, 1557; 14:2010;
        15:2097; 16:2212
    treatment 14:2010, 2013; 16:2213
    see also tonsillitis
sound therapy 9:1231
spas 9:1272
spastic colon 15:2022–2023
spasticity 2:149; 3:335, 336
    speech difficulties and 10:1308
    see also cerebral palsy
special-care baby unit see neonatal
    intensive care unit
specimens 15:2024–2026
    blood tests 2:225; 4:475; 8:1029;
        15:2024–2025
    sputum tests 15:2025
    stool samples 15:2025
    urine tests 4:475; 5:596; 8:1029;
        12:1676; 15:2024, 2025, 2026
    for ketones 7:1006
    in pregnancy 15:2024
    for protein 8:1018, 1020
    see also biopsy; Pap smear
SPECT (single-photon-emission
    computerized tomography)
    4:480
speculum 6:734; 11:1488–1489; 15:2027
speech 10:1334; 15:2028–2031; 17:2389
    esophageal 8:1036; 17:2389
    the mouth and 9:1262–1263;
        16:2233
    problems 15:2030, 2031
        aphasia 1:107–108; 10:1308;
            15:2030
        in children 8:1081–1082; 15:2028,
            2030, 2032, 2033
        lisping 8:1081–1082; 11:1483;
            15:2060
        mutism 10:1307–1309

stammering and stuttering 1:107;
        15:2032, 2058–2061
    stroke and 1:107; 10:1307; 15:2030,
        2033, 2107, 2110
    signals 2:248
    see also voice
speech therapy 10:1309; 13:1798;
        15:2032–2033; 16:2206
    for aphasia 1:107, 108; 15:2110
speed (drug) 1:87
sperm 3:399–400; 5:589, 689; 14:1906;
        15:2034–2035; 16:2194
    analgesic abuse and 1:137
    chromosomes 5:683
    first produced 15:2034
    infertility and 1:129, 130; 7:943;
        14:1907; 16:2194
    life span 3:399; 6:732; 7:945;
        13:1827–1828
    low sperm count 1:131; 3:399; 5:689;
        7:943; 15:2034, 2035
    IVF and 7:974
    production 15:2034, 2035
    tested 9:1238
    for in vitro fertilization 7:971
    see also semen
spermatic cord 16:2192; 17:2347
spermicides 3:407–408, 409
sphincter(s)
    cardiac 1:67
    pyloric (pylorus) 1:68; 15:2088
sphygmomanometer 2:183; 4:475, 476;
        11:1569; 15:2036–2039
spina bifida 2:206, 207; 3:401, 402;
        4:574; 5:684; 10:1351;
        15:2037–2039, 2041–2043
    chance of having another child
        with 7:878; 15:2038
    detection 3:367; 17:2316
    hydrocephalus and 7:879
    inherited 5:682; 15:2037
    leg braces 10:1432
    prevention, folic acid supplements
        and 2:206; 3:401; 5:638, 682;
        10:1351; 15:2037, 2039; 17:2377
    treatment 3:402; 15:2039
        plastic surgery 12:1614
    types 15:2037–2039
        meningocele 10:1351; 15:2037,
            2039
        meningomyelocele 7:879;
            15:2039
    see also birth defects
spinal canal 6:761
spinal cord 6:761; 10:1344–1345;
        15:2040–2043
    analysis of touch and pain in
        16:2240–2241
    multiple sclerosis and 9:1280
    paralysis and 11:1492, 1493; 15:2043
    problems 15:2041–2043
        damage 11:1492, 1493; 15:2040,
            2043
        myelitis 15:2040, 2043
spinal fusion 7:1002
spinal tap 15:2042
spine (backbone)
    chiropractic and 3:362, 363
    curvature 11:1448; 14:1968
        lordosis (swayback) 13:1848
        osteoporosis and humpback
            11:1450, 1451
        scoliosis 8:1078; 11:1448;
            14:1890–1891
    injuries, rehabilitation 13:1795
    osteoarthritis 5:691; 10:1437
    osteopathy and 11:1448, 1449
    osteoporosis 11:1451

spinal anesthetics 8:1093
    see also epidural injections
spinal traction 16:2255
    see also back and backache; spinal
        cord; vertebrae
spiritual healing 5:614
spirochetes 2:165; 11:1510; 17:2402
spirometry and spirometers 3:371;
        13:1752
Spitz-Holter shunt 7:880
spleen 15:2044–2046
    enlarged 8:1109; 15:2045–2046
    feeling the 15:2045
    lacerations 8:1031
    multiple (polysplenia) 6:805;
        15:2044
    removal 8:1030, 1114; 15:2044, 2046
    ruptured 5:663; 8:1030; 15:2044,
        2046
splinters 15:2047
splints 15:2048–2049
    inflatable 15:2048
    joint, for rheumatoid arthritis 13:1822
spondylolisthesis 14:1968
sports injury 15:2050–2051, 2052–2055
    bursitis 3:308
    carpal tunnel syndrome 3:323
    cramp 4:437
    dislocations 15:2055
    first aid 1:50
    fractures 15:2050–2051, 2054
    hamstring injuries 6:743–744
    muscle stiffness 15:2054
    muscle strain 15:2054
    osteoarthritis and 10:1435
    prevention 8:1027
    pulled muscles 13:1747; 15:2054
    sprains 15:2055
    torn knee cartilage 3:325; 10:1434;
        15:2055
    torn muscles 9:1290, 1292
    to tendons 15:2054
    treatment 15:2051
        cold and hot 6:797, 799
    see also dislocation; fractures;
        pulled muscles; sprains; tennis
        elbow
sports medicine 15:2052–2055
    biofeedback 2:181
    spots before the eyes 2:219
    sprains 8:1072; 15:2056–2057
        ankles 6:764; 15:2057, 2145
        splints used for 15:2048
        sports injuries 15:2055
        treatment 15:2051, 2056, 2057
    springs, thermal 9:1272–1273
    sputum see phlegm
    squint 2:219; 4:505; 5:609
    SSRIs (selective serotonin reuptake
        inhibitors) 4:466; 13:1738
        see also Prozac
    staining, biopsy samples 2:193
    stammering and stuttering 1:107;
        15:2032, 2058–2061
    staphylococcus 2:164; 5:670; 11:1510;
        15:2062
        abscesses and 13:1758
        food poisoning and 5:657, 659;
            7:928; 15:2062
        name 15:2062
        pneumonia and 12:1623
        in skin lesions 2:255; 5:657; 7:918
        Staphylococcus aureus 1:34; 2:166;
            15:2062; 16:2247
            methicillin-resistant (MRSA)
                1:98; 11:1508; 15:2062
            toxic shock syndrome and 16:2247,
                2248

starch 15:2063–2064, 2121
broken down by amylase 11:1487;
15:2063
statin drugs 8:1119
steam cabinets 6:776
steatorrhea 5:624
Stelazine (trifluorperazine)
16:2256
stem cell 15:2065–2066
cloning and 3:378
embryonic 15:2065, 2066
stenosis 15:2067
aortic 15:2067; 17:2341
coronary artery 15:2067
laryngeal 15:2067
mitral 15:2067
pulmonary 15:2067
pyloric 1:67; 15:2067
spinal 8:1078
stercobilin 5:623
sterility see infertility
sterilization (microbial), for surgery
10:1404–1405; 15:2135–2136
sterilization (reproductive)
15:2068–2071; 16:2286
failure 16:2286
ectopic pregnancy and 15:2068,
2069, 2070; 16:2286
hysterectomy 7:905; 15:2069, 2071
involving the fallopian tubes
15:2069, 2070, 2071; 16:2286
involving the ovaries 15:2069, 2071;
16:2286
laparoscopic 8:1034; 15:2071
male see vasectomy
the menopause and 15:2070;
16:2286
reversal 15:2068; 16:2286
assessment 8:1034
sternum (breastbone) 12:1591
pigeon chest 3:347; 12:1590–1592
steroids 1:48; 15:2072–2073
for asthma 7:953, 954; 15:2072
for dermatitis 4:468
for eczema 4:543
immunosuppressive 7:914
produced in the body 6:859;
15:2072
side effects 14:1956–1957, 1959;
15:2073
structure 15:2073
stethoscope 4:474, 475; 15:2074–2075
stiffness 15:2076–2079
arthritis and 10:1436, 1437;
15:2077–2078
muscle 15:2054, 2076–2077
treatment 15:2076, 2078, 2079
Still, Andrew Taylor 3:362
stillbirth 15:2080–2082
Still's disease 1:123
stimulants 15:2083–2085
sports and 1:85
see also amphetamines
stings see bites and stings
stitch 1:49; 15:2086–2087
stitches see sutures
stomach 1:67–68; 15:2088–2090
cancer 6:741; 15:2090; 16:2292
cramps 5:599
gastritis 5:670, 671; 9:1269; 15:2088,
2089
mucous membrane 9:1188
removal 15:2088
"rumbling" 1:11
size 15:2088
stapling the walls of 10:1386
tumors 15:2090
ulcers (gastric ulcers) 1:11; 4:495;

5:581; 15:2088, 2089–2090;
17:2313, 2314
aspirin and 1:122; 11:1479
asymptomatic 17:2312
biopsy 2:192
bleeding from 6:803–804;
8:1042; 14:1945
body weight and 15:2090
causes 15:2089; 17:2313
gastritis and 5:671
gastroscopy and 4:570, 571;
8:1042
stomach or arm pain and
14:1948
treatment 2:157, 158; 5:581;
8:1042; 15:2090
stomach pump 4:562; 15:2091–2093
stomatitis 9:1263
aphthous (viral) 9:1263; 17:2311
stone therapy 6:798
stools see feces
stork marks 2:208, 209
strain 15:2098
see also tension
strains
eyestrain 9:1233
ligament 8:1072
pulled or strained muscles 6:799;
9:1292, 1294; 13:1747–1748; 15:2051,
2054
strangulation 15:2094–2096
strawberry marks 2:208, 209
strawberry tongue 14:1879
streptococcus 2:164; 5:670; 11:1510;
14:1914; 15:2097
glomerulonephritis and 8:1020
impetigo and 7:918
rheumatic fever and 13:1817, 1818
scarlet fever and 14:1878–1879
streptococcal throat (strep throat)
and 11:1557; 14:2010; 15:2097;
16:2212
Streptococcus fecalis 15:2097
Streptococcus mutans 15:2097
Streptococcus pneumoniae 15:2097
penicillin-resistant (PRSP) 1:98
Streptococcus pyogenes 2:166;
14:1878–1879; 15:2097
Streptococcus viridans 15:2097
streptomycin
balance and 9:1194
deafness and 4:455
stress 15:2098–2102, 2103
acne and 1:32
the blood-brain barrier and 2:230
blood pressure and 2:237
cancer and 3:314
family relationships and 5:616–617
the heart and 7:997
post-traumatic stress disorder
(PTSD) 10:1358; 12:1652–1655;
15:2102
psychosomatic symptoms and
5:616; 12:1723, 1724
ulcers and 4:530; 15:2102
see also anxiety; tension
stress management 15:2103–2104;
17:2405
biofeedback 2:181–183
meditation 1:75
rolfing and 13:1846
visualization 9:1231
see also relaxation
stress testing, cardiac 4:551; 11:1574
stretch marks 9:1276; 12:1661, 1662,
1679; 15:2105–2106
stroke 2:265, 267; 5:691–692; 6:803;
10:1347; 15:2107–2111; 16:2217–2218

assessment, MRI scans 2:269
associated with heart attacks
15:2108
brain scars after 14:1881
causes 2:267; 15:2107–2108; 16:2217
cerebral infarction (blood vessel
blockage) 1:121; 15:2107–2108,
2109; 16:2217
hemorrhage 15:2108, 2109
high blood pressure and 15:2107,
2108
fits and 5:583
limping and 8:1078
loss of second languages and 1:107
paralysis and 11:1490, 1493
affecting sense of touch 16:2239
patients at home 15:2110, 2111
prevention 15:2107, 2108, 2110–2111;
16:2261, 2262
risk 15:2108–2109
the sense of touch and 16:2239,
2242
sight and 2:222; 5:606–607; 10:1411
smart drugs 14:1989
speech and 1:107; 10:1307; 15:2030,
2033, 2107, 2110
transient ischemic attacks and
15:2109, 2111; 16:2261, 2262
treatment 1:108; 4:557; 5:692;
15:2109–2110
exercises 15:2111
hydrotherapy 7:881
occupational therapy 10:1397
physical therapy 11:1580; 15:2107,
2110
rehabilitation 13:1796, 1797
surgery 15:2107
strychnine 15:2084
stuttering see stammering and
stuttering
sty 2:256; 4:447; 6:799; 15:2112–2113
subconscious 9:1228; 15:2114–2115
sublingual glands 13:1261; 13:1853
submandibular glands 13:1853
sucrose 5:702; 15:2121
sudden infant death syndrome (SIDS)
15:2116–2117
suffocation 15:2118–2119
babies 1:135
first aid 15:2119
sugars 15:2120–2121
diabetes and 4:471, 473; 15:2121
dietary 5:702
teeth and 15:2120, 2121
white and brown 5:653
levels in the body 4:488; 7:960;
15:2121
see also glucose; sucrose
suicide 4:464; 15:2122–2125
assisted 15:2125
see also euthanasia
in the elderly 6:839
pacts 15:2124
teenage "suicidal gestures" 12:1630
sulfasalazine 4:443
sulfonamides 1:100
sulfur dioxide 1:28, 29, 60; 12:1638
summer flu see gastroenteritis
sunburn 3:303; 11:1470; 15:2126–2129
blisters 2:223; 15:2127, 2128
in children 15:2128, 2129
prevention 11:1470; 15:2128–2129
rash and itching from 6:831
treatment 15:2128; 16:2272
sunscreen 11:1470; 15:2128–2129;
17:2428
sunstroke (heatstroke) 6:796; 11:1545;
15:2130–2131

suntanning preparations 14:1970
superior vena cava 3:373
suppositories 15:2132–2133
suprachiasmic nucleus 2:187
surgeons 15:2139–2140
training 15:2134
surgery 15:2134–2140
brain see brain surgery
bypass 3:346, 420–421; 10:1402,
1403; 17:2357
for cancer 3:315
"clean" and "dirty" 15:2135
cosmetic 3:424–425; 12:1612, 1615
for moles 9:1243
dressings used after 4:515
effects of 12:1646–1647
hemorrhaging after 6:806
instruments used in 15:2136,
2137–2139
laparotomy 8:1035
LASIK 8:1043–1044
microsurgery 5:709; 9:1218–1221;
10:1434; 15:2139
minimally-invasive
(keyhole/laparoscopic) 6:764;
9:1236–1237; 15:2138, 2139
telesurgery and 16:2180
see also laparoscopy
open-heart 10:1401–1403
operating rooms and 10:1404–1406
operating tables 10:1406
plastic and reconstructive
12:1612–1617
postoperative care 12:1644–1647
respirators used during
13:1805–1806
risks 15:2136
side effects 13:1840
sterilization during 10:1404–1405
telesurgery 16:2180
tourniquets used in 16:2246
under hypothermic conditions
7:900
viewing rooms 10:1406
see also transplants
surrogacy 15:2141–2143
sutures (stitches) 8:1031; 12:1647;
15:2136–2137, 2138, 2144; 17:2425
abdominal, bursting 15:2138, 2144
absorbable (dissolving) 15:2144;
17:2422, 2425
internal 15:2144; 17:2422
nonabsorbable 17:2425
removal 15:2144
a stitched cut healing 6:765
swallowing 1:67; 5:592; 9:1261, 1262;
10:1334; 11:1484, 1556, 1557
difficulty in, pharyngeal web and
16:2211
swayback (lordosis) 13:1848
sweat see perspiration
sweep 7:932
swellings 15:2145–2148
see also edema; elephantiasis
swimmer's itch 11:1509
swimming 7:881; 8:1094, 1095; 11:1573
eczema and 4:542
otitis and 11:1452, 1453
Sydenham's chorea see Saint Vitus'
dance
symptoms 4:474–475; 15:2149–2152
see also diagnosis
synapses 2:157, 158; 10:1344
syncope see fainting
syndactyly 12:1613, 1614
synovectomy 1:126; 13:1824
synovial fluid 3:325; 4:547; 8:1025
synovitis 9:1189

syphilis 4:459; 6:803; 7:938; 11:1531; 14:1931; 15:2153–2155
congenital 14:1931
diagnosis 15:2153, 2154, 2155
latent 15:2154
neuralgia with 10:1349
pregnancy and 12:1675; 14:1931, 1932; 15:2154, 2155
primary sore or ulcer 15:2153–2154, 2155
rash 13:1784; 14:1932, 1933; 15:2154, 2155
spinal cord affected by 15:2042
tongue or lip ulcers and 17:2311
treatment 15:2155
ulcers or sores in the groin 15:2153–2154; 17:2314, 2334
warning 15:2155
syringing 4:454, 456, 537, 538; 15:2156–2157
systemic lupus erythematosus see lupus
systemic sclerosis see scleroderma

T

T3 (triiodothyronine) 16:2225
T4 see thyroxine
tachycardia 13:1754
tacrolimus 7:913, 914; 8:1024
Taenia saginata 17:2420–2421
Taenia solium 17:2421
tai chi 16:2165–2168
talipes equinovarus see clubfoot
tampons, retained
toxic shock syndrome and 16:2247, 2248
vaginal discharge and 17:2338
tantrums see temper tantrums
tapeworms 11:1498, 1500, 1501; 17:2419, 2420–2421
tarsal tunnel syndrome 3:322
tartar (calculus) 12:1609; 13:1761
taste 13:1853; 16:2169–2171, 2232–2233
appetite and 1:113
smell and 14:1992; 16:2169, 2170, 2171
taste buds 16:2169, 2171, 2232, 2233
tattooing 2:236; 6:809; 16:2172–2173
medical uses 16:2173
tattoo removal 8:1040, 1042; 12:1614; 16:2172, 2173
taurine 14:1989
Tay-Sachs disease 16:2174
detection 3:367; 16:2174
TB see tuberculosis
tea 14:1902, 1905; 16:2256
herbal 6:815; 11:1480
tear ducts 10:1373–1374
tears 4:444–445
teeth and teething 8:1149; 16:2175–2178
abscesses 1:21; 13:1758
absence of teeth 16:2178
bridges 4:463
broken teeth 16:2176
brushing 6:730, 731; 12:1608; 13:1761
canines 16:2175–2177
impacted 7:916
capped 4:462
color 16:2178
crowned 4:462, 463
decay (caries) 12:1609
halitosis and 6:740; 12:1608
deciduous (milk or baby) teeth 16:2175, 2176, 2178
filling 16:2176

delayed teeth 16:2178
dental care 4:460–461; 6:740
anesthetics 1:92–93; 8:1092; 10:1378
avoiding plaque 4:461; 12:1610
during pregnancy 12:1676
fluoride 4:461; 5:651–652; 12:1636; 16:2176
gums and gum diseases 4:461, 462; 6:730–731
heart murmurs and 9:1287
orthodontics 10:1425–1429; 16:2175, 2177
while wearing orthodontic appliances 10:1425, 1426
dentures 4:462–463; 8:1149
dietary sugar and 15:2120, 2121
impacted teeth 7:915–917; 14:2012; 16:2175
incisors 16:2175, 2176, 2178
loss 6:730, 731
molars 16:2176, 2178
mottling 5:651–652
overlapping or crooked 6:730; 13:1759
pain, radiation from sinuses 15:2149
permanent teeth 16:2176
premolars 16:2175, 2176
smoking and 4:460; 14:1999
stained by tetracyclines 16:2178, 2199
structure of a tooth 16:2178
teething 9:1262; 16:2176, 2177
transplants 10:1426
wired together 10:1384
wisdom 16:2177–2178
impacted 7:915, 916; 16:2175, 2177
infection and 15:2148
quinsy and 14:2012
X rays 17:2434
see also dental care; gums and gum diseases
Telehomecare 6:839
telemedicine 16:2179–2180
telephones, cellular 3:333–334
telomeres 1:55
temperature 16:2181–2184
basal metabolic rate and 17:2401
changes in a day 2:188
core 16:2181
exercise and 16:2181
fertility and 7:945
fevers 5:640–641; 6:759; 9:1214; 11:1545; 15:2150
shivering with 14:1940, 1942
treatment 5:641; 9:1177; 15:2150
heat loss and 6:762; 16:2183
normal 5:640; 6:795; 14:1940–1941; 16:2181
regulation 3:319; 6:847; 7:897, 898; 14:1940–1942; 15:2130; 16:2182–2183
biofeedback and 2:183
goose pimples 6:735; 14:1942
perspiration (sweat) 11:1543–1545; 15:2130–2131; 16:2183
shivering 14:1940, 1941, 1942; 16:2183
the rhythm method and 13:1828–1829, 1830
skin surface, and thermal imaging 16:2207, 2208
taking 16:2181, 2183–2184
temper tantrums 3:356, 413; 7:906
Tempra see acetaminophen
tendonitis 6:799
tendons 8:1069; 9:1265; 16:2185–2186
Achilles 5:626; 10:1433

cut through 16:2185
dislocated 16:2185
grafting 5:711
ruptured 10:1433
severed 1:20; 16:2185, 2186
sports injuries 15:2054
tenosynovitis 5:629; 8:1105; 16:2185, 2186; 17:2430
tenesmus, rectal 3:383; 13:1788
tennis elbow 1:124; 4:547; 6:799; 14:1968; 16:2187
tenosynovitis 5:629; 8:1105; 16:2185, 2186; 17:2430
tensilon 10:1312, 1313
tension 16:2188–2190
headaches and 6:758, 759; 9:1230
necessity of 13:1801–1802; 16:2188
treatment
massage 8:1142
mind-body therapy 9:1230
relaxation 13:1800–1801
see also stress
TENS (transcutaneous electrical nerve stimulation) 11:1482, 1579
testes (testicles) 5:689; 16:2191–2194; 17:2347
cysts 4:447; 16:2191, 2193–2194
hydrocele 16:2192, 2193–2194
descended 5:689
enlargement 16:2192
infection and inflammation
epididymitis 16:2193
orchitis 9:1284; 16:2193
infertility and 16:2194
one removed 16:2191
prosthetic 12:1700
removal 16:2192, 2193
temperature 15:2035
torsion or twisting 16:2191, 2192, 2193
tumors 16:2192, 2194
undescended 16:2192, 2195
varicocele 7:943–944; 16:2194
vasectomy and 16:2191
see also infertility
testosterone 1:48; 8:1062; 16:2191–2192, 2195–2196
deficiency 16:2196
excess
in men 16:2196
in women 16:2196
puberty and 13:1742; 16:2195–2196
sebaceous gland activity and 14:1901; 16:2196
transdermal patches 16:2260
tests
laboratory 8:1028–1029
laboratory see laboratory tests
tetanus 1:20; 2:236; 7:937, 938; 16:2197–2198, 2285; 17:2426
vaccinations 1:17; 2:206; 7:910, 911, 912; 8:1030; 16:2197, 2198, 2285; 17:2424, 2426
tetany 3:311; 11:1504
hyperventilation 6:745; 11:1504
tetracyclines 1:100; 4:468; 16:2199
side effects 11:1565; 14:1957; 16:2178, 2199, 2272
taken during pregnancy 1:99; 16:2178, 2199
tetrahydrobiopterin 11:1559
tetraiodothyronine see thyroxine
tetralogy of Fallot 2:243
texturizers 5:654
thalamus 2:263
epilepsy and 5:583
pain and 11:1475
the sense of taste and 16:2171

the sense of touch and 16:2241, 2242
thalassemia 1:88, 89, 90; 16:2200–2201
detection 3:367
thalidomide 8:1119; 16:2202–2204
taken during pregnancy 2:206; 3:402; 6:749; 9:1170; 11:1550; 16:2202–2204
victims using prostheses 12:1698
therapeutic communities (TCs) 4:528
therapy 16:2205–2206
complementary therapies 16:2206
see also alternative medicine
group therapy 5:713–714; 13:1736
mind-body therapy 9:1230–1233
see also physical therapy; psychotherapy; speech therapy
thermal imaging 16:2207–2208
thermistors 16:2184
thermometers 4:475; 16:2181, 2183–2184
theta-wave training 2:182
thiopental (pentothal) 2:170
thirst 16:2209–2210
symptom of diabetes 15:2152; 16:2209, 2210
threadworms (pinworms) 1:103; 7:988; 11:1498, 1501; 17:2419, 2420
throat 14:2011; 16:2211–2213
cancer 3:316
diphtheria and 4:497
infections, causing ear pain 16:2212
obstruction 11:1557; 16:2211, 2213
sore throat 11:1555, 1557; 14:2010–2013
laryngitis 7:946; 8:1036, 1037–1039; 10:1335; 14:2011, 2013; 16:2212; 17:2389
strep 11:1555, 1556, 1557; 15:2097; 16:2212
wartlike growths 17:2395
see also pharynx
thrombophlebitis 16:2214, 2215, 2218
thromboplastin 16:2214
thrombosis 1:119, 120; 16:2214–2218
arterial 16:2217
in the brain, and stroke 15:2107; 16:2217–2218
cerebral 16:2217–2218, 2262
coronary 3:419–420; 6:783–784; 16:2215–2216, 2217
see also heart attack
deep vein 2:223; 10:1417; 15:2146–2147; 16:2218; 17:2345
edema and 4:544
in the heart's atria or ventricles 16:2215–2216
obesity and 10:1385
the Pill and 10:1417; 16:2214
prevention, warfarin 16:2214, 2216
venous 16:2217
thrush (Candida; candidiasis) 7:987; 16:2219–2220; 17:2337, 2436
chronic mucocutaneous candidiasis 16:2220; 17:2437, 2438
genital 10:1368; 14:1934; 16:2220
in the mouth 9:1263; 16:2219, 2220; 17:2436, 2437
of the nails 16:2220; 17:2437, 2438
people at risk from 16:2219, 2220
diabetics 10:1368; 16:2219, 2220
on the skin 16:2220
diaper rash 4:481–482
feet 16:2220; 17:2436
systemic infections 17:2437, 2438
treatment 16:2220
vaginal discharge 6:733; 16:2220;

thrush (cont'd)
  17:2334, 2336
  see also yeast infections
thumb
  double 3:401
  great mobility 7:1002
  sucking 8:1081
thymomas 16:2222
thymus 5:700; 8:1113; 9:1187; 16:2221–2222
  tumors 16:2222
thyroid 10:1334–1335; 16:2223–2226
  cancer 5:704; 6:832; 13:1774;
    15:2096; 16:2225
    thermography and 16:2208
  effect of the pituitary on 4:567;
    6:847; 12:1599; 16:2224
  goiter 5:704; 10:1334; 16:2224, 2225,
    2226
  growth and 4:532
  metabolic rate and 16:2182; 17:2401
  overactive (thyrotoxicosis;
    hyperthyroidism) 5:704; 6:857;
    10:1332; 11:1450, 1503; 15:2150;
    16:2223–2224, 2226
    Graves' disease 16:2225–2226
    heat production and 16:2182
    treatment 13:1774; 15:2150;
      16:2223, 2224
    tremor and 16:2275
  radionuclide scans 4:477, 480
  removal 10:1332, 1421, 1422; 16:2225
  shivering and 14:1941
  thyroiditis 5:704; 16:2224, 2226
  tumors 4:567
  underactive (hypothyroidism;
    myxedema) 3:323; 5:699, 704;
    8:1055; 9:1214; 16:2223–2224,
    2226
    coma and 3:395
    congenital (cretinism) 16:2226
    growth and 4:532
    hair and 16:2224
    Hashimoto's disease and 5:704
    heat production and 16:2182
thyroidectomy 16:2225
thyroid hormone see thyroxine
thyroiditis 5:704; 16:2224, 2226
thyroid-stimulating hormone (TSH)
  4:567; 6:847; 7:899; 12:1599;
  16:2224
thyrotoxicosis (overactive thyroid;
  hyperthyroidism) 5:704; 6:857;
  10:1332; 11:1450, 1503; 15:2150;
  16:2223–2224, 2226
  Graves' disease 5:704; 16:2225–2226
  heat production and 16:2182
  treatment 13:1774; 15:2150; 16:2223,
    2224
  tremor and 16:2275
thyroxine (thyroid hormone; T4;
  tetraiodothyronine) 2:225, 226;
  4:566, 567; 6:847; 16:2224, 2250
  deficiency 4:532; 6:858; 10:1383
  goiter and 5:704
  causing postpartum depression
    12:1649
  too much 6:858
TIA see transient ischemic attack
ticks 2:211
  Lyme disease and 8:1108; 16:2199
  Q fever and 13:1762
  Rocky Mountain spotted fever and
    13:1844–1845
tics see twitches and tics
Tietze's disease 13:1831
tinea pedis see athlete's foot
tinnitus 10:1365; 16:2227–2228
  unilateral 2:227

tiredness 15:2150; 16:2229–2231
  chronic fatigue syndrome 3:369;
    10:1353
  old age and 5:620; 16:2229
  see also fatigue
tissue engineering 2:190
tissue expanders 16:2266
tissue fluid 3:319
tissues 2:254
tissue typing 16:2263, 2265
TNM classification 8:1098–1099, 1132
tobacco mosaic virus 17:2369, 2371
tocopherols 17:2382, 2384
toeing in see pigeon toes
toenails see nails
toes
  "ballet dancer's toe" 1:122
  fractured 5:627
  gangrenous 5:669
  gout 5:707
  reattached 9:1219
  stiffness 15:2079
togaviruses 17:2372
tomography
  computerized (axial) see CT scans
  positron emission see PET scanning
  single-photon-emission
    computerized (SPECT) 4:480
  X-ray 17:2434
tongue 16:2232–2234
  cancer 16:2234
  inflammation due to food allergy
    7:947
  injuries to 16:2234
  piercing 2:250, 251
  sense of taste 16:2169, 2232–2233
  strawberry tongue 14:1879
  structure 16:2169, 2170, 2232, 2233
  swallowing the 15:2118; 16:2232
  ulcers 16:2234; 17:2311
tonics 3:412; 15:2083, 2084; 16:2229,
  2231
toning lotions 3:423
tonsillectomy 8:1113; 14:2012–2013;
  16:2235, 2236, 2237
tonsillitis 2:281, 282; 8:1112; 14:2010,
  2011–2012; 16:2212, 2235,
  2236–2237
  swollen lymph nodes and 8:1109
tonsils 2:281; 11:1557; 16:2212, 2235–2237
  enlarged 16:2236
  peritonsillar abscess (quinsy)
    14:2012–2013; 16:2236–2237
  removal (tonsillectomy) 8:1113;
    14:2012–2013; 16:2235, 2236, 2237
  tonsillitis 2:281, 282; 8:1112; 14:2010,
    2011–2012; 16:2212, 2235,
    2236–2237
    swollen lymph nodes and 8:1109
  tumors 16:2237
  viral infections 16:2237
toothbrushes 6:731; 12:1608
toothpaste, fluoride 5:651, 652
tophi (chalk stones) 5:708
total allergy syndrome 16:2238
touch 16:2239–2242
  the brain and 2:264
touching 2:246
Tourette's syndrome 2:152;
  16:2243–2244, 2293, 2294
tourniquet 1:17; 16:2245–2246; 17:2422
toxemia 2:236
  preeclamptic (PET) 7:931
toxic confusional state 15:2150
toxicologists 11:1551
toxic shock syndrome 16:2247–2248
Toxocara canis 2:220
toxocariasis 11:1500

Toxoplasma gondi 2:220
trace elements 16:2249–2250
  harmful 16:2250
  see also minerals
tracheal tubes 13:1808
trachea (windpipe) 10:1333
tracheostomy 7:946; 8:1037; 13:1805;
  16:2251–2252; 17:2389
tracheotomy 10:1333; 16:2251
trachoma 2:220; 3:416; 16:2282
traction 16:2253–2255
  for fractures 10:1431–1432, 1433;
    16:2253, 2254, 2255
  intermittent 16:2253
tranexamic acid 17:2392
tranquilizers 1:104; 14:1903, 1904,
  1980; 16:2256–2258
  alternatives to 16:2256, 2257, 2258
  side effects 16:2272
  see also sedatives
transactional analysis 13:1735
transcutaneous electrical nerve
  stimulation (TENS) 11:1482, 1579
transdermal patch 16:2259–2260
Transderm Nitro 16:2260
transient ischemic attack (TIA)
  16:2261–2262
  strokes and 15:2109, 2111; 16:2261,
    2262
translocation 5:676–677
transpersonal therapy 13:1735
transplants 16:2263–2266
  artificial 16:2265
  brain 16:2263
  from animals 4:503
  heart 4:504; 6:791–794; 10:1422;
    16:2263, 2264, 2266
  kidney see kidney transplants
  liver 4:504; 8:1084; 16:2263, 2265,
    2266
  living donor 16:2264–2265
  lung 4:504; 13:1750
  marrow see marrow transplants
  pancreas 16:2264
  postoperative care 16:2266
  rejection 16:2265
  suppression of 6:794; 7:913, 914;
    8:1022, 1139; 15:2072, 2073; 16:2265
  umbilical cord blood 5:676, 677
  see also donors; grafting
transsexuals 5:672, 673; 16:2196
transurethral resection of the prostate
  (TURP) 12:1693
transvestites 5:673
trauma center 16:2267–2269
  see also emergency department
travel and health 16:2270–2273,
  2284–2285
  basic precautions 16:2282
  see also tropical diseases
travel sickness pills, overdose 4:562
tremor 16:2274–2275
  benign essential 16:2274, 2275
  intention 16:2275
  of Parkinson's disease 11:1506;
    16:2274
  physiological 16:2274, 2275
  red nucleus 16:2275
trench mouth 13:1760
Treponema pallidum 2:166; 14:1932;
  15:2155
TRH (TSH-releasing hormone) 16:2224
triage 4:560; 16:2268
triazolam 7:893
Trichinella 11:1499; 16:2276
trichinosis 16:2276–2277
trichlorethylene 10:1393
trichogram analysis 6:739

Trichomonas vaginalis 16:2278, 2279;
  17:2325, 2336, 2337–2338
trichomoniasis 12:1703; 14:1934;
  16:2278–2279; 17:2325, 2337–2338
  as a urinary tract infection 17:2325
tricyclic drugs 4:466
trifluorperazine (Stelazine) 16:2256
triglycerides 5:621
triiodothyronine (T3) 16:2225
trimeprazine 7:893
trochlea 4:546
trophoblastic disease 17:2327
tropical diseases 16:2280–2285
  see travel and health; under names of
    individual diseases
Trychophyton fungus 13:1837, 1838
trypanosomiasis 12:1704
  African see sleeping sickness
trypsin 4:494, 495; 11:1487
trypsinogen 11:1487
TSH see thyroid-stimulating hormone
tubal ligation 16:2286
tuberculosis (TB) 2:282; 7:927, 938,
  940; 13:1752; 16:2285, 2287–2290
  abdominal 16:2288, 2290
  arthritis following 1:124
  diagnosis 16:2289
  fatigue and 5:619
  meningitis following 9:1195
  miliary 16:2288
  open 16:2289
  pigeon chest and 12:1592
  pleurisy and 12:1619
  prevention 16:2290
    vaccination 7:912; 13:1763;
      16:2285, 2287, 2290; 17:2330
  silicosis and 14:1961
  of the spine 2:161
  treatment 2:282; 7:982; 9:1194;
    13:1750, 1752; 16:2288, 2290
  surgery 16:2287
tularemia, a biological weapon 2:185,
  186
tumors 16:2291–2292
  benign 3:312, 313; 8:1124, 1125; 16:2291
    see also fibroids; polyps
  malignant 8:1124–1126; 16:2291, 2292
    see also cancer
  mixed 9:1254
  pressing on the spinal cord 15:2043
  treatment 16:2292
tuning forks 4:454
tunnel vision 2:219; 13:1812
Turner's syndrome 10:1305
TURP (transurethral resection of the
  prostate) 12:1693
twelve-step facilitation (TSF)
  programs 4:529
twins 9:1274, 1276
  birth 2:204, 284
  can feel each other's pain 11:1476
  detected during pregnancy 12:1676
  identical 3:330, 400; 9:1274, 1275;
    11:1539, 1540; 12:1604
  nonidentical (fraternal) 3:400;
    9:1274, 1275, 1277; 11:1540;
    12:1604
    conception 13:1828
  the placenta and 12:1604, 1605
  Siamese 14:1950–1951
  tendency inherited 6:816
  see also multiple births
twitches and tics 16:2293–2294
  tics 9:1266; 16:2293, 2294
  Tourette's syndrome and 16:2243,
    2293, 2294
  twitches 16:2293–2294
Tylenol see acetaminophen

typhoid and paratyphoid
16:2295–2298
paratyphoid **13**:1855; **16**:2295, 2296, 2298
rash **13**:1784; **16**:2297
typhoid **4**:485, 533; **5**:623; **7**:937, 938; **13**:1855–1856; **16**:2285, 2295–2298
carriers **16**:2296, 2297
gallstones and **16**:2295
prevention **16**:2298
in the small intestine **16**:2295, 2297
treatment **16**:2297–2298
vaccination **7**:955; **16**:2285
typhus **4**:573; **7**:937, 938; **16**:2295, 2299–2301
epidemic **16**:2299, 2300, 2301
murine (endemic typhus) **16**:2299, 2300
scrub **16**:2300–2301
tyrosine **11**:1558–1559

U

ulcers **14**:2008; **17**:2310–2314
cancer/malignancy and **3**:312; **8**:1124
colon-wall **3**:387
decubitus see bedsores
diabetic foot, treatment **2**:190
duodenal (intestinal) **4**:495, 530, 531
bleeding from **6**:803–804; **8**:1042
body weight and **15**:2090
excess salivation and **13**:1854
kissing ulcers **17**:2313
pain **17**:2313
perforated **11**:1534, 1535; **17**:2313
treatment **2**:157, 158; **4**:531; **8**:1042; **15**:2138; **17**:2340
see ulcers, peptic
esophageal **17**:2313
in the groin **17**:2310, 2314, 2334
leg **1**:17; **17**:2310, 2312–2313, 2343
mouth **9**:1260, 1263; **14**:2008; **16**:2234; **17**:2310–2311
general disease and **17**:2311–2312
treatment **17**:2312
treatment in AIDS patients **16**:2204
peptic **7**:930; **17**:2313–2314
stress and **4**:530; **15**:2102
surgery for **17**:2312
see ulcers, duodenal; ulcers, stomach
skin
from chromium **10**:1392
rodent ulcers **14**:1975; **17**:2314
sepsis and **14**:1915
stomach (gastric) **1**:11; **4**:495; **5**:581; **15**:2088, 2089–2090; **17**:2313, 2314
aspirin and **1**:122; **11**:1479
asymptomatic **17**:2312
biopsy **2**:192
bleeding from **6**:803–804; **8**:1042; **14**:1945
body weight and **15**:2090
causes **15**:2089; **17**:2313
gastritis and **5**:671
gastroscopy and **4**:570, 571; **8**:1042
stomach or arm pain and **14**:1948
treatment **2**:157, 158; **5**:581; **8**:1042; **15**:2090
see ulcers, peptic
see sores
ulna **4**:546, 547

ultrasound **4**:478–479; **13**:1870; **14**:1893; **17**:2315–2317
breast scans using **8**:1132
for cataract removal **3**:326, 328
Doppler **4**:479
during pregnancy **2**:207, 285; **4**:477, 479, 480; **12**:1664, 1676; **13**:1869, 1870; **14**:1893, 1894; **15**:2143; **17**:2315, 2316–2317
taken with a full bladder **17**:2315
lithotripsy and **8**:1020
treatment (providing heat) **6**:797, 798; **11**:1579, 1580; **17**:2315
for hemophiliacs **6**:801
ultrasound-assisted lipoplasty (UAL) **8**:1080
umbilical cord **2**:203, 205
blood **5**:676, 677
prolapse **12**:1687–1688
unconsciousness **17**:2318–2321
after a blow to the head **17**:2318, 2320, 2321
coma and **3**:394–395; **17**:2321
common causes of **17**:2321
dealing with an emergency **4**:555–556
memory loss and **9**:1190
see also blackouts; fainting
undulant fever see brucellosis
Union Carbide disaster **4**:574
unipolar disorder **9**:1247
uremia **15**:2150; **17**:2322
ureters **2**:216; **17**:2324
urethra **2**:216–217; **5**:690; **8**:1017; **11**:1530; **17**:2323
birth defects **2**:207
ejaculation and **14**:1907
narrowing or obstruction **2**:217, 218
urethral syndrome **4**:449
urethral syndrome **4**:449
urethritis **11**:1531; **17**:2323, 2325
nonspecific **14**:1931–1933
uric acid, and gout **5**:707, 708; **10**:1306
urinary tract and disorders **17**:2324–2325
disorders
birth defects **2**:207; **17**:2325
cancer **17**:2325
cystitis **4**:449
infections **7**:925; **8**:1018; **17**:2324, 2325
urinary tract **2**:216–217, 252; **7**:926
see also bladder and bladder problems; kidneys and kidney diseases
urination
acute retention **12**:1692
bed-wetting **2**:217–218; **7**:925, 926
during cold weather **11**:1543
during the night **5**:598; **12**:1691
during pregnancy **12**:1662
incontinence **2**:218; **5**:693; **7**:925–926
spinal cord damage and **15**:2040
stress **7**:925; **12**:1687
prostate problems and **12**:1690, 1691, 1692
reflex **13**:1791
urine **5**:597
bacteria in **8**:1018
blood in **6**:803
color **2**:216, 217; **5**:598
biliary colic and **5**:668
jaundice and **5**:596; **7**:992
kidney failure and **8**:1020
protein in (proteinuria) **2**:239; **12**:1659
tests **4**:475; **5**:596; **8**:1029; **12**:1676; **15**:2024, 2025, 2026

for ketones **7**:1006
in pregnancy **15**:2024
for protein **8**:1018, 1020
urography, intravenous (IVU or IVP) **17**:2433
urticaria see hives
uterus (womb) **17**:2326–2329
conception and **3**:399, 400
dilatation and curettage (D & C) **4**:496; **5**:642; **9**:1202; **17**:2329
lining (endometrium) **4**:568; **9**:1203
position **17**:2326–2328
pregnancy and **17**:2326, 2328
problems **17**:2327
abnormal bleeding from **17**:2327
abnormal location of lining **6**:733; **17**:2327
absence **17**:2327
cancer **3**:316; **7**:905; **9**:1204; **14**:1934; **17**:2327, 2329
congenital malformation **17**:2327, 2328–2329
endometrial hyperplasia **17**:2327
endometritis **17**:2327
fibroids **5**:642; **6**:733; **17**:2327
polyps **5**:642; **12**:1642, 1643; **17**:2327, 2329
pregnancy outside the uterus **4**:541
prolapse **2**:161; **6**:733; **7**:904, 905; **12**:1686–1687, 1688; **17**:2327, 2335
removal see hysterectomy
trophoblastic disease **17**:2327
see also cervix and cervical smears
uveitis **17**:2311–2312
uvula **9**:1260; **11**:1483, 1485

V

vaccinations **2**:166; **7**:940; **9**:1216; **17**:2330–2332
attenuated vaccines **7**:911; **17**:2330
before traveling overseas **16**:2270, 2271–2272
during pregnancy **2**:206; **16**:2284
encephalitis and **4**:565
see immunization
vaccines, genetically engineered **5**:680–681
vaccinia see cowpox
Vacuflex **13**:1794
vagina **5**:690; **17**:2333–2335
absent **17**:2355
Bartholin glands **5**:690; **9**:1269
abscess **6**:733; **17**:2335
blocked **17**:2333, 2335
carcinoma **17**:2335
discharge **6**:733; **17**:2333, 2334, 2335, 2336–2339
bloodstained **3**:338; **5**:642; **17**:2339
during pregnancy **12**:1662
Pap tests and **11**:1489
of STDs **14**:1933–1934
thrush (Candida; candidiasis) **6**:733; **16**:2220; **17**:2334, 2336
trichomoniasis **14**:1934; **16**:2278, 2279; **17**:2336, 2337–2338
douching **5**:689
fistula **5**:644
lacerations **8**:1031; **17**:2333
menopause and **5**:593; **6**:856; **9**:1198, 1199; **17**:2334
prolapse into **2**:161; **6**:733; **7**:904, 905; **12**:1686–1687, 1688; **17**:2327, 2335
by intestines **12**:1686

unexplained bleeding from **3**:338; **4**:496; **5**:642; **6**:727; **9**:1202
vaginal wall prolapse **17**:2335
vaginismus **7**:919, 965; **14**:1924–1925; **17**:2334
vaginitis **17**:2336
atrophic **4**:496; **9**:1202; **17**:2334, 2335
of trichomoniasis **16**:2278, 2279; **17**:2336
yeast infection **7**:937; **17**:2436, 2437–2438
vaginal discharge **6**:733; **17**:2333, 2334, 2335, 2336–2339
after childbirth **17**:2338–2339
after miscarriage **17**:2338
bloodstained **3**:338; **5**:642; **17**:2339
caused by cancer **17**:2339
caused by chlamydia **17**:2338
caused by gonorrhoea **17**:2334, 2338
during pregnancy **12**:1662
from retained material **17**:2335, 2336, 2338
Gardnerella vaginalis infection **17**:2336, 2338
normal **17**:2334, 2336
during sexual arousal and intercourse **17**:2334
Pap tests and **11**:1489
of STDs **14**:1933–1934
thrush (Candida; candidiasis) **6**:733; **16**:2220; **17**:2334, 2336
trichomoniasis **14**:1934; **16**:2278, 2279; **17**:2336, 2337–2338
vaginal sponges **3**:410, 411
vaginismus **7**:919, 965; **14**:1924–1925; **17**:2334
vaginitis **17**:2336
atrophic **4**:496; **9**:1202; **17**:2334, 2335
of trichomoniasis **16**:2278, 2279; **17**:2336
vagotomy **2**:158; **17**:2314, 2340
Valium (diazepam) **7**:893; **14**:1903, 1904; **16**:2257
valves **6**:782; **17**:2341–2342
aortic **17**:2341, 2342
congenital abnormalities **17**:2342
grafting **5**:711
heart murmurs and **9**:1287–1289
heart valve disease **2**:215; **6**:788, 789; **9**:1287–1289; **16**:2215; **17**:2341–2342
mitral **17**:2341, 2342
prolapsing **17**:2341, 2342
pulmonary **17**:2341, 2342
replacement **6**:788; **10**:1401, 1402–1403; **12**:1698, 1699–1700; **17**:2341
rheumatic fever and **13**:1817; **15**:2067; **16**:2215, 2216
"Ross Switch" **15**:2136
tricuspid **17**:2341
vancomycin-resistant enterococci (VRE) **1**:98
varicella see chicken pox
varicocele **7**:943–944; **16**:2194
varicose veins **16**:2216, 2218; **17**:2343–2346
during pregnancy **5**:637; **12**:1662, 1675–1676; **17**:2344
edema and **4**:544
hemorrhoids and **6**:807
obesity and **17**:2344–2345
the Pill and **10**:1414
in the scrotum (varicocele) **7**:943–944; **16**:2194
swollen ankles and **15**:2146–2147
thrombophlebitis and **16**:2218

varicose veins *(cont'd)*
thrombosis and **16**:*2216*
treatment **17**:2343, *2345–2346*
ulcers and **17**:2312, 2343
varicose eczema **7**:987;
17:2345
venular flares and **17**:2344
variolation **7**:911
variola virus **14**:1986, *1987*, 1988
vasa deferentia **3**:400; **5**:689; **11**:1530;
14:1906, 1907; **16**:*2191*; **17**:2347
vascular disease, peripheral **1**:120
vasectomy **16**:2286; **17**:2347–2350
reversal **9**:1218, *1220*; **16**:2191; **17**:2347,
2348, 2349, 2350
VDRL test **15**:2154
vegans and veganism **17**:2351, 2352,
2353, 2354
illnesses associated with
17:2355
vegetarianism **4**:488, *489*; **10**:*1379*;
17:2351–2356
minerals and **9**:1234
see macrobiotics
veins **1**:119; **3**:373; **17**:2357–2358
bleeding from **6**:803
blood clots **15**:2146–2147; **16**:2218;
17:2357, 2358
grafts **5**:711
hepatic **17**:2358
intravenous infusions **7**:*970*
intravenous injections **7**:955–956
portal **16**:*2292*
thread veins or spider veins **3**:424;
4:553
valves **17**:2357, *2358*
varicose **16**:*2216*, 2218; **17**:2343–2346
during pregnancy **5**:637; **12**:1662,
1675–1676; **17**:2344
edema and **4**:544
hemorrhoids and **6**:807
obesity and **17**:2344–2345
the Pill and **10**:1414
in the scrotum (varicocele)
7:943–944; **16**:2194
swollen ankles and **15**:2146–2147
thrombophlebitis and **16**:2218
thrombosis and **16**:*2216*
treatment **17**:2343, *2345–2346*
ulcers and **17**:2312, 2343
varicose eczema **7**:987; **17**:2345
venular flares and **17**:2344
venlafaxine **4**:466
ventricular fibrillation **17**:2359–2360
ventricular septal defect **2**:242, *243*;
3:402
venular flares **17**:2344
venules **17**:2357
verruca (plantar wart) **3**:418; **5**:625;
7:886; **12**:1627; **17**:2361–2363, 2395
treatment **17**:2361, *2362–2363*
vertebrae **2**:159
cervical **6**:761; **10**:1332, *1335*
lumbar **14**:*1982*
strain on **14**:*1984*
osteopathic manipulation and
11:1448, 1449
osteoporosis **11**:*1451*
vertigo **4**:502; **17**:2364–2366
Ménière's disease and **9**:*1194*
positional **17**:2365, 2366
see dizziness
Viagara **7**:963; **14**:*1928*
vibration white finger **10**:1394, 1395,
1396
see also Raynaud's syndrome
vibrio **2**:164
Vibrio cholerae **3**:365

videoconferencing **16**:*2179*
villi **4**:*495*; **9**:*1189*
Vincent's organisms **13**:1760
viral hemorrhagic fevers **2**:186
virginity **17**:2367–2368, 2368
hymen and **7**:889; **17**:2367, 2368
internal examination and **7**:966
see abstinence
viruses **7**:935, 936; **11**:1510;
17:2369–2372
causing cancer **3**:314; **7**:935
causing fever **5**:641
coma and **3**:395
damaging effects **7**:939
encephalitis and **3**:395
infection by **7**:927
incubation period **7**:927, 928
lymphocytes and **8**:1113
prevention **17**:2372
reproduction **7**:*939*; **17**:2370
treatments **17**:2369, 2372
antibiotics ineffective **11**:1528;
17:2369
used in gene therapy **5**:679–680
vision **2**:220; **10**:*1411*, 1412–1413
double **4**:505
navigational **13**:1811
night **10**:1362
testing **10**:*1413*
tunnel **2**:219; **13**:1812
see eyes and eyesight
visualization **9**:1231
visual purple (rhodopsin) **10**:1362;
13:1812; **17**:2373
vitallographs **17**:2408
vitamin A **17**:2373–2374
an antioxidant **1**:*101*; **10**:1328, 1382
deficiency **5**:606; **8**:1118, 1128;
17:2373, 2374
during pregnancy **12**:1678
excess **17**:2373, 2374, 2387
genetically altered rice and **5**:675
night vision and **10**:1362
vitamin B **17**:2375–2377
B1 (thiamin) **17**:2377
daily requirements **17**:2376
deficiency **8**:1128; **12**:1722; **17**:2376
B2 (riboflavin) **17**:2376, 2377
daily requirements **17**:2376
deficiency **17**:2376
B3 (niacin; nicotinic acid) **17**:2377
daily requirements **17**:2376
deficiency **8**:1128
B6 (pyridoxine) **9**:1201, 1249; **12**:1674;
17:2375, 2376, 2377
deficiency **17**:2376
B12 (cyano-cobalamin) **17**:2376
deficiency **8**:1118; **11**:1536, *1537*;
15:2043; **17**:2355, 2376
excess **17**:2351
B13 (orotic acid) **17**:2377
B17 (laetrile) **17**:2377
biotin, deficiency **17**:2376
deficiency **5**:606; **7**:897; **8**:1118,
1128; **9**:1214; **11**:1536, *1537*; **17**:2375,
2376
during pregnancy **12**:1678
excess **17**:2375
folic acid (folacin) **17**:2376
supplements **2**:206; **3**:401; **5**:638,
682; **10**:1351; **15**:2037, 2039; **17**:2377
pantothenic acid **17**:2376
sources **17**:2377
supplements **17**:2377
toxicity **17**:2377
vitamin C **17**:2378–2379
an antioxidant **1**:*101*; **10**:1328, 1382;
17:2379

collagen formation and
14:1896–1897; **17**:2378
common cold and **3**:396
daily requirements **17**:2379
deficiency **2**:260; **3**:298; **5**:606;
6:804; **8**:1128; **10**:1379;
14:1896–1897; **17**:2378
people at risk from **17**:2379
during pregnancy **12**:1678
foods containing **14**:*1896*;
17:*2378–2379*
vitamin D **8**:1118; **17**:2380–2381
calcium absorption and **3**:*311*;
11:1504; **13**:1836
daily requirements **17**:2381
deficiency **2**:260; **3**:*311*; **5**:691; **8**:1128;
13:1835–1836; **17**:2381
veganism and **17**:2355
during pregnancy **12**:1678
excess **17**:2381, 2387
sunlight and **17**:*2380*
supplements **13**:1836
for babies **2**:272
types **17**:2380
vitamin E **4**:510; **17**:2382–2384
an antioxidant **1**:*101*; **10**:1328, 1382;
17:2384
daily requirements **17**:2384
deficiency **17**:2383
during pregnancy **12**:1678
iron supplements and absorption
of **17**:2382
overdosage **17**:2384
supplements **17**:*2383*
dangerous for babies **17**:2384
vitamin K **2**:228; **17**:2385–2386
during pregnancy **12**:1678
vitamins **4**:489–490; **10**:1381;
17:2387
RDA **5**:655, 656
supplements **8**:1127
during pregnancy **5**:638
for elderly people **5**:691
fatigue and **5**:619
fluorinated **5**:651
see under the names of each
vitamin eg: vitamin A
vitiligo **9**:*1181*; **17**:2388
vitreous humor **5**:606
vocal cords **8**:1036; **10**:1333–1334;
16:2212; **17**:2389
artificial **17**:2389
hoarseness and **6**:832; **8**:1039
nodes or polyps on **6**:832; **8**:*1037*,
1039; **10**:1335
see larynx and laryngitis
vocal nodes **6**:832; **8**:*1037*
voice **8**:1037
loss **10**:1308
through shock **10**:1334
puberty and **17**:2389
see speech
voice box *see* larynx
voice synthesizers **3**:*335*
volatile organic compounds (VOCs)
1:59
volvulus neonatorum **15**:2094
vomiting **10**:1330; **15**:2088–2089;
17:2390–2391
in babies **1**:69
projectile **1**:67, 69
blood **4**:495; **17**:2391
bulimia and **1**:*95*, 96; **10**:1384;
17:2391
in children **1**:69
"coffee grounds" material **4**:495;
17:2391
emetics and **4**:562

food poisoning and **4**:531;
5:657–658
with a hangover **6**:752
induction, not recommended when
corrosives are swallowed **7**:981
with morning sickness **9**:1248, 1249;
17:2391
motion sickness **9**:1253–1254; **10**:1330,
1331; **17**:2390, 2391
psychogenic **10**:1331
treatment **7**:1004; **17**:2390, 2391
unpleasant foods and **11**:1484
see also nausea
von Economo's disease **8**:1057
Von Recklinghausen's disease *see*
neurofibromatosis
von Willebrand factor (vWF) **17**:2392
von Willebrand's disease **17**:2392
vulva **5**:690; **17**:2393–2394
problems **6**:733
cancer **17**:2393
inflammation **17**:2393, 2394
pruritis vulvae **17**:2393
warts **17**:2393
vulvitis **17**:*2394*
vulvovaginitis **5**:705; **17**:2437

W

walking, and the feet **5**:625–626
warfare, biological and chemical *see*
biological and chemical warfare
warfarin **16**:2214
interaction with aspirin
14:*1957–1958*
warts **6**:726; **14**:*1975*; **17**:2395–2397
adult **17**:*2396*, 2397
filiform **17**:2396
genital **11**:1530; **14**:1933, 1935;
17:2393, 2395, 2396–2397
treatment **17**:2397
plantar *see* verruca
seborrhoeic **14**:*1975*
tattooing and **16**:2173
treatment **17**:2397
wartlike growths in the throat
17:2395
washing **7**:885
hands **5**:657; **7**:884, *887*
compulsive **3**:397, *398*
wasp stings **2**:210, 212
water
acid rain and **1**:29
balance, hypothalamus and
7:898–899
daily requirement **8**:1017
drinking water **4**:573
fluoridation of **5**:651, 652; **13**:1744
lead in **8**:1048–1049
mineral water **9**:1234
pollution **4**:574; **12**:1636, *1638*,
1639–*1640*
public health and **13**:1744
water brash **7**:930
water pills **4**:544
wax *see* earwax
wax treatments **6**:799; **11**:1579
waxy flexibility **14**:1882
weakness **15**:2150
weapons, biological and chemical *see*
biological and chemical warfare
weight **17**:2398–2401
charts **10**:*1383*
chubbiness in adolescents **13**:1739
gain
during the menstrual cycle **1**:112
stretch marks and **15**:*2105*, 2106

loss 17:2398, 2403
  cancer and 6:727
  eating disorders and 1:*94–95*, 96
  exercise and 1:49; 5:600
  flotation therapy and 5:649
  in health spas 6:774
  liposuction not recommended
    for 8:1079
  as a symptom of a disorder
    17:2399–2400
  visualization techniques 9:1232
  metabolic rate and 9:1214; 17:2401
  overweight
    children 10:1383
    cholesterol and 3:366
    the circulation and 3:372
    the hips and 6:828
    runs in families 6:816; 10:1383
    snoring and 14:2005
    the Pill and 10:1416;
      17:2398–2399
    unexplained loss of 15:2152
    see also obesity
weight training 9:1294
Weil's disease 17:2402
wellness 17:2403–2405
well-woman clinics 14:1895
welts 13:1783
Wernicke's encephalopathy 12:1722
West Nile virus 17:2406
wet lung (shock lung) 14:1943, 1946
wet nurses 8:1032
wheat, food value 6:773
wheelchairs 11:1495, *1497*
wheezing 17:2407–2408
whiff test 17:2338
whiplash injury 10:1334, *1335*;
  13:*1747–1748*; 17:2409–2410
whipworms 17:*2420*
whiteheads 1:31
whitlow (paronychia) 6:747; 10:1314;
  17:**2411**, 2438
whooping cough 3:426; 17:**2412–2415**
  treatment 17:2413–2414
  vaccination 7:911, 912; 11:1516;
    17:2412, *2413*, 2414–2415
willow bark 6:813
Wilm's tumor 17:2325
Wilson's disease 9:1235; 16:2249, 2250
windpipe (trachea) 10:1333
withdrawal symptoms 17:**2416–2418**
  fits 5:583
  from alcohol abuse 1:61; 6:742;
    17:2417, *2418*
  heroin or morphine 6:823; 17:2416,
    2417–2418
womb see uterus
workstations 11:*1493*
World Health Organization (WHO)
  13:1746
worms 17:**2419–2421**
  appendicitis and 1:110
  in the feces 5:623
  tests for 15:2025
  filarial 17:2419
    elephantiasis and 4:554; 8:1112;
      16:2283
  flukes
    liver fluke 8:**1088–1089**; 11:*1500*,
      1501; 17:2420, *2421*
    see schistosomiasis
  from undercooked or raw food
    17:2419, *2421*
  hookworms 2:241; 6:**852–853**;
    11:1499, *1500*, 1501; 17:2419–2420
  malnutrition and 16:2282
  roundworms 11:*1498*; 17:2419–2420
    see also Ascaris

tapeworms 11:1498, 1500, 1501;
  17:2419, *2420–2421*
threadworms (pinworms) 1:103;
  7:988; 11:1498, 1501; 17:2419, 2420
trichinosis and 16:*2276–2277*
whipworms 17:*2420*
wounds 17:**2422–2426**
  foreign bodies in 17:2426
  gunshot 17:2422
    treatment 17:2425
  healing 6:*765*; 14:*1971–1972*;
    17:2423
    zinc and 16:2250
    see also scars
  infections 17:2425–2426
    tetanus and 16:2197; 17:2424,
      2426
  needing medical attention 1:19
  puncture 1:*19*, 20; 17:2423, 2425
  splinters 15:**2047**
  treatment 17:2424–2425
    cleaning 1:*18*
    dressings 1:*17, 18*; 4:*513–515*
  see also abrasions and cuts; bruises;
    lacerations
wrist 17:**2429–2430**
  carpal tunnel syndrome 1:124;
    3:**322–323**; 6:747; 10:1344, 1396;
    13:*1804*
  dislocation 17:2430
  fractures 3:323; 5:660;
    17:2429–2430
  rheumatoid arthritis 13:*1823,
    1824*
  stiffness 15:2078
  tenosynovitis 5:629; 17:2430
  weak 17:2429
Wucheria bancrofti 4:554; 17:*2420*

X

xanthelasma 3:366
xenobiotics 14:1953
xenografts (animal tissue grafts)
  5:709, 710
X rays 4:*478*; 13:*1772–1773*; 17:**2431–2435**
  angiography and 4:478; 10:1355
    carotid angiograms 17:*2357*, 2431,
      2434
  arthrograms 17:2432
  barium liquids and 2:*171–172*; 4:*443*,
    478; 17:2433
  contrast 4:478
  dental 17:*2434*
  digital radiography 17:2433–2434
  during pregnancy 12:*1664–1665*,
    1676; 17:*2431*
  endoscopy and 4:570
  intravenous urography 17:2433
  mammography 2:192; 3:*312*;
    8:**1129–1132**; 16:*2292*; 17:2432
  risks from 11:1510; 17:2435
    "10 day rule" 5:*682*; 17:2435
    cancer 3:312
    during pregnancy 2:206, 285;
      4:478; 5:682; 17:2431
    leukemia 8:1059
    mutations 10:1306
    negligible for radiation sickness
      13:1770
  teleradiology and 16:2180
  therapy, heat treatment unwise
    after 6:798
  used in radiotherapy 13:*1772–1774*;
    17:2432
  see arteriograms; CT scans;
    myelography

Y

yeast, baker's 9:*1216*
yeast infections 7:938; 17:**2436–2438**
  causes 17:2436–2437
    see also thrush
  dandruff and 4:451
  diaper rash and 4:*481–482*
  oral 9:1263; 11:1484; 17:*2436*, 2438
  treatment 17:2438
  vaginal 7:*937*; 17:2436, 2438
    during pregnancy 5:634
  yellow fever 2:186; 16:2285; 17:**2439**
    vaccination 16:2272, 2285; 17:2439
Yersinia pestis 12:1607
yin and yang 1:37; 3:358; 5:650; 8:1116
  shiatsu and 14:1937
  tai chi and 16:2165
yoga 1:80; 5:602; 11:1477; 17:**2440–2445**
  during pregnancy 12:*1679*; 17:2444
  relaxation and 13:*1802*; 17:2440,
    2444
yttrium 5:698
"yuppie syndrome" 3:369

Z

Zantac 6:*786*
zest 17:**2446**
Ziehl-Neelsen stain 16:2289
zinc 9:1235; 16:2249, 2250
zinc pyrithione 6:739
zolpidem 7:893
Zovirax (acyclovir) 3:382; 14:1939